Neurologic Catastrophes in the Emergency Department

Neurologic Catastrophes in the Emergency Department

Eelco F. M. Wijdicks, M.D.
Professor of Neurology, Mayo Medical School,
Consultant, Department of Neurology, and
Medical Director, Neurological/Neurosurgical Intensive Care Unit,
Saint Mary's Hospital and Mayo Medical Center, Rochester, Minnesota

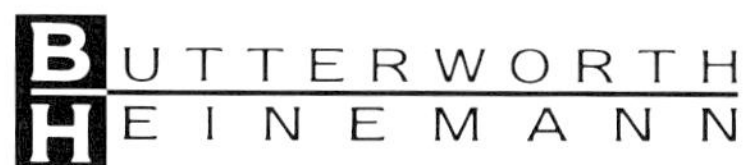

Boston Oxford Auckland Johannesburg Melbourne New Delhi

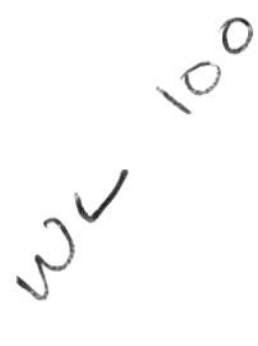

Butterworth–Heinemann

A member of the Reed Elsevier group

Nothing in this publication implies that Mayo Foundation endorses any of the products mentioned in this book. Care has been taken to confirm the accuracy of the information presented and to describe generally accepted practices. However, the authors, editors, and publisher are not responsible for errors or omissions or for any consequences from application of the information in this book and make no warranty, express or implied, with respect to the contents of the publication.

The authors, editors, and publisher have exerted every effort to ensure that drug selection and dosage set forth in this text are in accordance with current recommendations and practice at the time of publication. However, in view of ongoing research, changes in government regulations, and the constant flow of information relating to drug therapy and drug reactions, the reader is urged to check the package insert for each drug for any change in indications and dosage and for added warnings and precautions. This is particularly important when the recommended agent is a new or infrequently employed drug.

Some drugs and medical devices presented in this publication have Food and Drug Administration (FDA) clearance for limited use in restricted research settings. It is the responsibility of health care providers to ascertain the FDA status of each drug or device planned for use in their clinical practice.

Recognizing the importance of preserving what has been written, Butterworth–Heinemann prints its books on acid-free paper whenever possible.

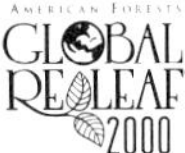

Butterworth–Heinemann supports the efforts of American Forests and the Global ReLeaf program in its campaign for the betterment of trees, forests, and our environment.

Library of Congress Cataloging-in-Publication Data

Wijdicks, Eelco F. M., 1954-
Neurologic catastrophes in the emergency department / Eelco F. M. Wijdicks.
p. cm.
Includes bibliographical references and index.
ISBN 0-7506-7055-X
1. Neurological emergencies. I. Title.
[DNLM: 1. Nervous System Diseases. 2. Critical Care.
3. Emergencies. WL 140 W662n 2000]
RC350.7.W55 2000
616.8'0425--dc21
DNLM/DLC
for Library of Congress 99-32437
CIP

British Library Cataloguing-in-Publication Data

A catalogue record for this book is available from the British Library.

The publisher offers special discounts on bulk orders of this book.
For information, please contact:

Manager of Special Sales
Butterworth–Heinemann
225 Wildwood Avenue
Woburn, MA 01801-2041
Tel: 781-904-2500
Fax: 781-904-2620

For information on all Butterworth–Heinemann publications available, contact our World Wide Web home page at: http://www.bh.com

10 9 8 7 6 5 4 3 2 1

Printed in the United States of America

*To my beloved wife, Barbara-Jane, and children,
Coen and Marilou, who are requisite to my happiness*

Contents

Preface

The first 60 minutes ("golden hour") in acute neurologic emergencies remain critical, and failure to intervene immediately may result in poor outcome.

Currently available books on neurologic emergencies in the emergency department do not reach beyond the basics of neurologic examination and interpretation of the findings. This book tries to fill the need for a resource for neurologists, emergency room physicians, and neurosurgeons who evaluate, treat, and transfer patients with catastrophic neurologic disorders. Critical care neurology is often interdependent with other clinical disciplines, and the book should also be useful for any physician in the emergency department who interacts with neurologists. The material is written from a neurologist's perspective, but the approach by emergency department physicians is reflected as well.

This monograph completes my three-part book project on critical care neurology. The third book not only offers a practical approach to major neurologic disorders but also links early management in the emergency department with more prolonged care in the intensive care unit. It focuses on rapid but accurate neurologic assessment, on the most useful bedside tests, and particularly on interpretation of neuroradiologic images. The organization of the book is standardized, with a major focus on priorities of initial stabilization. I have placed great emphasis on the predictive value of diagnostic tests when they are available. The chapters are interspersed with flow diagrams to facilitate decision making and boxed capsules covering major topics in the subject under discussion. The text is brief to facilitate reading. It is aimed to quickly explain, not to fully discuss, complex topics. It is intended to reflect the train of thought and action in the emergency department.

This book draws on new material on evaluation and management of major neurologic disorders, but at the risk of presumption I feel compelled to state that it is also the result of years of contemplation of these problems and all that I could find to read on the subject. However, in a discipline in its formative years, the "whats" are plentiful and the "whys" fewer. I hope this book is an informative guide to the recognition and management of acute neurologic catastrophes at their early stage of presentation and finds its way to neurologists, neurosurgeons, neuroradiologists, emergency physicians, residents, and fellows in these specialties.

E.F.M.W.

Acknowledgments

I owe a debt of gratitude to Secretarial Services, the Section of Publications, Medical Illustration, Computer Graphics, and the Plummer Library for their support. I would like to thank Julienne M. Montgomery, Kristy K. Hockens, Roberta J. Schwartz, John L. Prickman, Sharon L. Wadleigh, David A. Factor, Paul W. Honermann, Sandra Borgschatz, and my secretary, Stacy R. Schultz. They kept me going when all seemed Sisyphean. I am fortunate for the ways that Susan F. Pioli and Leslie Kramer from Butterworth–Heinemann Publishers managed this monograph.

E.F.M.W.

Part I

Evaluation and Management of Evolving Catastrophes in the Neuraxis

Chapter 1
Altered Arousal and Coma

Catastrophic brain injury has widespread effects, among them coma. Coma permeates the practice of all physicians. Elucidating the cause of coma cannot be compartmentalized into a simple algorithm, and novices become petrified when a hastily ordered computed tomography (CT) scan and initial laboratory results are normal. The priorities in evaluation of comatose patients have changed considerably with the arrival of magnetic resonance imaging (MRI). It may have encouraged a misconception that the cause of coma is easily established with CT scans or MRI. Relying solely on neuroimaging tests can be counterproductive and potentially dangerous. Albeit less common, failure to recognize diabetic coma, thyroid storm, acute hypopituitarism, fulminant hepatic necrosis, nonconvulsive status epilepticus, or any type of poisoning while wasting time performing neuroimaging tests and waiting for cerebrospinal fluid results may potentially lead to a rapidly developing neurologic fiasco.

The circumstances under which comatose patients are discovered can also be misleading. For example, a patient found next to an empty bottle of analgesic medication may have fulminant meningitis, traumatic head injury with skin lacerations may be a consequence of a fall from acute hemiplegia or brief loss of consciousness, and patients with massive intracerebral hematomas may be intoxicated. Another dramatic situation occurs when a patient with diabetes consumes a little alcohol but fails to have dinner and is brought in comatose and smelling of alcohol but profoundly hypoglycemic.

The causes of coma are many. Structural injury to the brain results in coma if it closely follows or directly affects the relay nuclei and connecting fibers that make up the ascending reticular activating system (ARAS) (Capsule 1.1). Evaluation of comatose patients requires a systematic approach exploring five major categories: (1) unilateral hemispheric mass lesions that compress or displace the diencephalon and brain stem, (2) bilateral hemispheric lesions that damage or compress the reticular formation in the thalamus, interrupting the projecting fibers of the thalamus-cortex circuitry, (3) lesions in the posterior fossa below the tentorium that damage or compress the reticular formation, (4) diffuse brain lesions affecting the physiologic processes of the brain, and (5), less commonly, psychiatric unresponsiveness, mimicking a comatose state (Table 1.1). Poisoning and drug abuse are common in the emergency room and thus receive proportionally more attention in this chapter.

Three major issues in the clinical approach to comatose patients are discussed. First, this chapter merges a thorough physical examination with a neurologic examination. Second, it emphasizes stabilization. Many stabilizing measures are simple, require virtually no specific skills, are easily mastered, and should be applied by physicians without delay. Third, it consolidates the priorities of diagnostic tests and provides recommendations for

Capsule 1.1. Ascending Reticular Activating System (ARAS)

The role of the ARAS is to arouse and maintain alertness. Despite identifiable structures, its definition remains conceptual. Coma is understood as a dysfunction of this anatomic neural network, which spans a large part of the rostral upper pons, mesencephalon, and thalamus and projects to the cerebral cortex of both hemispheres. Populations of neurons situated in the tegmentum of the pons and mesencephalon, intralaminar nuclei of the thalamus, and posterior hypothalamus are linked to the basal forebrain and associated cortex (Figure 1.1). These networks communicate through neurotransmitters, such as acetylcholine, norepinephrine, serotonin, and dopamine, and through activation of the forebrain produce wakefulness.

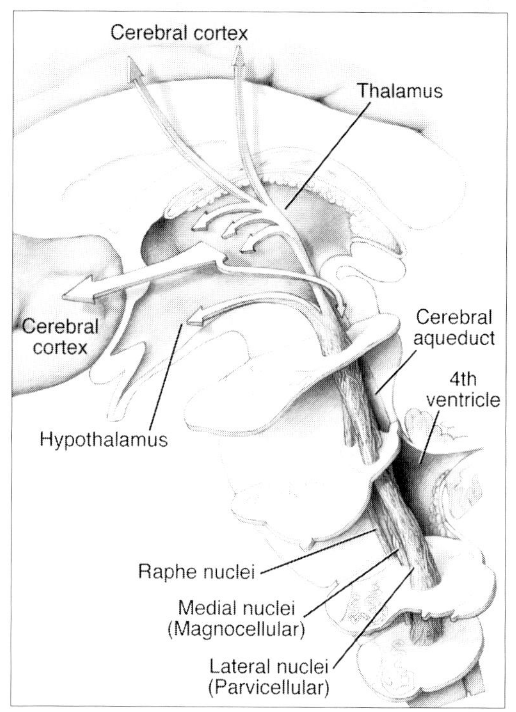

Figure 1.1.

definitive management and triage in each of the major categories.

Examination of the Comatose Patient

An examination that sorts out representative localizing neurologic findings remains of great importance in assessing the nature of coma, but equally important are a reliable history and a general physical examination.

The onset of coma may provide a clue. Acute onset in a previously healthy person points to aneurysmal subarachnoid hemorrhage, a generalized tonic-clonic seizure, traumatic brain injury, or self-induced drug poisoning. Relatives, bystanders, and police may all provide important data when patients are suddenly found comatose. Gradual worsening of coma most often indicates an evolving intracranial mass, a diffuse infiltrative neoplasm, or a degenerative or inflammatory neurologic disorder.

General Clinical Features

The general appearance of the patient may be deceptive, but extremely poor hygiene or anorexia may indicate alcohol or drug abuse. A foul breath in most instances means poor dental and periodontal hygiene or alcohol consumption. The classic types of foul breath should be recognized. These are "dirty restroom" (uremia), "fruity sweat" (ketoacidosis), "musty, fishy" (acute hepatic failure), "onion" (paraldehyde), and "garlic" (organophosphates, insecticides, thallium).

Fever and particularly hyperthermia (more than 40°C) in comatose patients may indicate an inflammatory cause, such as acute bacterial meningitis or encephalitis, but can occur in massive pontine hemorrhage, aneurysmal subarachnoid hemorrhage, and traumatic head injury. It may originate from direct compression, ischemia, or contusion of the hypothalamus. Hypothermia (less than 35°C) indicates exposure to a cold environmental temperature, a systemic illness, or intoxication. In patients with a devastating traumatic brain injury, it may be a systemic sign of brain death or acute spinal cord transection.

Examination of the skin may provide important additional findings leading to the cause of coma. Bullae or excoriated blisters at compression points are nonspecific in most comatose patients but may indicate barbiturate overdose[1] (Color Plate 1). Petechiae in the axilla strongly indicate fat emboli in acute unresponsiveness in a patient with a long bone fracture and rapidly developing pulmonary edema (Color Plate 2). The skin should be carefully inspected for needle marks in multiple sites outside the cubital fossa. (Scars in the cubital fossa alone may indicate that the patient is a blood donor or receives regular blood transfusions.) Significant periorbital ecchymosis ("raccoon eyes") and retroauricular ecchymosis (Battle's sign) indicate midface or skull base fractures; they should be carefully looked for but often become apparent after the patient has been transferred from the emergency department. The skin should be touched at different areas to assess its texture; both dry skin and skin drenched in sweat may point to certain intoxications (Table 1.2). Dry skin in a comatose patient (particularly the feet and axilla) points to overdose of a tricyclic antidepressant and characteristically is associated with tachycardia, fever, and cardiac arrhythmias. (As discussed in a later section, because electrocardiographic abnormalities can be entirely absent in tricyclic antidepressant overdose, its recognition may be extremely difficult.) Profuse sweating should always point to organophosphate pesticide poisoning or severe hypoglycemia.

Hypertension is a common clinical feature in coma associated with acute structural lesions and therefore has little predictive value. Hypertension usually subsides after the sympathetic outburst associated with the initial insult wanes, but unexplained surges of hypertension indicate poisoning from certain drugs, such as amphetamines, cocaine, phenylpropanolamine, hallucinogens, and sympathomimetic agents. Conversely, hypertension should be considered a cause of diffuse encephalopathy only in patients with profound hypertension (diastolic values ≥140 mm Hg), documented seizures, and papilledema, key signs that are often preceded by visual hallucinations.

Table 1.1. Classification and Major Causes of Coma

Structural brain injury
- Hemisphere
  - Unilateral (with displacement)
    - Intraparenchymal hematoma
    - MCA occlusion with swelling
    - Hemorrhagic contusion
    - Cerebral abscess
    - Brain tumor
  - Bilateral
    - Penetrating traumatic brain injury
    - Multiple traumatic brain contusions
    - Multiple cerebral cortical infarcts (vasculitis, coagulopathy, cardiac thrombus)
    - Bilateral thalamic infarcts
    - Lymphoma
    - Encephalitis (viral, paraneoplastic)
    - Gliomatosis
    - Acute disseminated encephalomyelitis
    - Anoxic-ischemic encephalopathy
    - Cerebral edema
    - Multiple brain metastasis
    - Acute hydrocephalus
    - Leukoencephalopathy (chemotherapy or radiation)
- Brain stem
  - Pontine hemorrhage
  - Basilar artery occlusion
  - Central pontine myelinolysis
  - Brain stem hemorrhagic contusion
- Cerebellum (with displacement)
  - Cerebellar infarct
  - Cerebellar hematoma
  - Cerebellar abscess
  - Cerebellar glioma

Acute metabolic-endocrine derangement
- Hypoglycemia
- Hyperglycemia (nonketotic hyperosmolar)
- Hyponatremia
- Hypernatremia
- Addison's disease
- Hypercalcemia
- Acute hypothyroidism
- Acute panhypopituitarism
- Acute uremia
- Hyperbilirubinemia
- Hypercapnia

Diffuse physiologic brain dysfunction
- Generalized tonic-clonic seizures
- Poisoning, illicit drug use
- Hypothermia
- Gas inhalation
- Basilar migraine
- Idiopathic recurrent stupor

Psychogenic unresponsiveness
- Acute (lethal) catatonia, malignant neuroleptic syndrome
- Hysterical coma
- Malingering

(MCA = middle cerebral artery.)

Table 1.2. Important Skin Abnormalities That May Have Discriminatory Value in Assessment of Coma

Sign or symptom	Meaning
Acne	Long-term anticonvulsant use
Bullae	Barbiturates, sedative-hypnotic drugs
Butterfly eruption on face	Systemic lupus erythematosus
Cold, malar flush, yellow tinge, puffy face	Myxedema
Dark pigmentation	Addison's disease
Dryness	Barbiturate poisoning, anticholinergic agents
Edema	Acute renal failure
Purpura	Meningococcal meningitis, thrombocytopenic purpura (bloody diarrhea!), vasculitis, disseminated intravascular coagulation, aspirin intoxication
Rash	*Streptococcus pneumoniae* (maculopapular) or *Staphylococcus aureus* (limited petechial) meningitis
Wetness	Cholinergic poisoning, hypoglycemia, sympathomimetics, malignant catatonia or sympathetic storms, thyroid storm

Combinations of change in vital signs may suggest certain poisonings. They are summarized in Table 1.3 and may be helpful in narrowing down the endless list of possible intoxications.

Neurologic Features

It should reflect the astuteness of a clinical neurologist to first evaluate whether the patient truly is comatose, in a locked-in syndrome, or malingering. In a locked-in syndrome, an acute structural lesion in the pons causes a nearly uncommunicative state, which spares pathways to oculomotor nuclei of the mesencephalon and reticular formation. Before pain stimuli are applied, the patient should be asked to blink and look up and down. This immediately suggests a locked-in syndrome despite the frequent finding of pupil abnormalities and primitive motor responses. Grim accounts have been published of failure to appreciate this entity.[2]

The depth of coma should be documented because it indicates prognosis in certain causes. Many coma scales have been devised, but only the Glasgow coma scale (a combination of the best possible eye, motor, and verbal responses, as summa-

Table 1.3. Common Changes in Vital Signs in Coma From Poisoning

Toxin	Blood pressure	Pulse	Respiration	Temperature	Additional signs
Amphetamines	↑	↑	↑	↑	Mydriasis
Arsenic	↓	↑	~	~	Marked dehydration
Barbiturates	↓	~	↓	↓	Bullae, hypoglycemia
Beta-adrenergic antagonists	↓	↓	~	~	Seizures
Carbon monoxide	~	~	~	~	Seizures
Cocaine	↑	↑	~	↑	Mydriasis, seizures
Cyclic antidepressants	↓	↑	~	↑	Mydriasis
Ethylene glycol	~	↑	↑	~	Anion gap and osmol gap, metabolic acidosis
Lithium	↓	~	~	~	Seizures, myoclonus
Methanol	↓	~	↑	~	Anion gap and osmol gap, acidosis
Opioids	↓	↓	↓	↓	Miosis
Organophosphates	↓	↓/↑	↑/↓	~	Fasciculations, bronchospasm, hypersalivation, sweating, miosis
Phencyclidine	↑	↑	~	↑	Miosis, myoclonus
Phenothiazines	↓	↑	~	↓/↑	Dystonia
Salicylates	~	~	↑	↑	Anion gap, metabolic acidosis, respiratory alkalosis
Sedative-hypnotics	↓	~	↓	↓	Bullae

(↑ = increase; ↓ = decrease; ~ = no change.)

Table 1.4. Glasgow Coma Scale

Eye opening	4	Spontaneous
	3	To speech
	2	To pain
	1	None
Best motor response (arm)	6	Obeying
	5	Localizing pain
	4	Withdrawal
	3	Abnormal flexing
	2	Extensor response
	1	None
Best verbal response	5	Oriented
	4	Confused conversation
	3	Inappropriate words
	2	Incomprehensible sounds
	1	None

rized in Table 1.4) has been tested for its reliability in daily clinical practice.[3,4] The need for the scale arose when researchers in Glasgow realized that a standard language had to be used rather than vague statements such as "He seems a bit brighter today."[5] The individual components have been graded, at times summed to a score between 3 and 15, but grading coma by sum scores of the Glasgow coma scale alone is misleading, because the sum scores represent different levels of decreased consciousness. A noxious stimulus, if needed, must be standardized: compression of the nailbed with the handle of the reflex hammer, compression of the supraorbital nerve, or compression of the temporomandibular joint (Figure 1.2).[6]

The components of the Glasgow coma scale (Figure 1.3) are as follows:

1. *Eye opening*. By definition, patients in coma have their eyes closed. Spontaneous eye opening, however, does not portend awareness. Patients in a persistent vegetative state usually have open eyes and frequent spontaneous blinking. Eye opening can be produced by aural stimulus, such as a loud voice, or noxious stimulus. Obviously, one should take care not to use both a loud voice and a noxious stimulus at the same time, and eye opening is difficult to assess in patients with facial trauma or periorbital edema.

2. *Motor response*. The motor response is one of the most important elements in the neurologic examination of the comatose patient. Motor response is graded from "following commands or obeying" to "no response after a noxious stimulus." It is important to note whether the legs are crossed, because this indicates relaxation and is never seen in patients in acute distress. It additionally is useful to ask the patient to follow simple commands rather than to squeeze a hand alone, because reflex grasping may be misinterpreted as obedience. An example of a simple command is to ask the patient to show a thumbs-up, fist, or victory sign.[7] For localization of a pain response, the arms should either cross the midline toward a contralateral nail bed compression or reach above shoulder level toward a stimulus

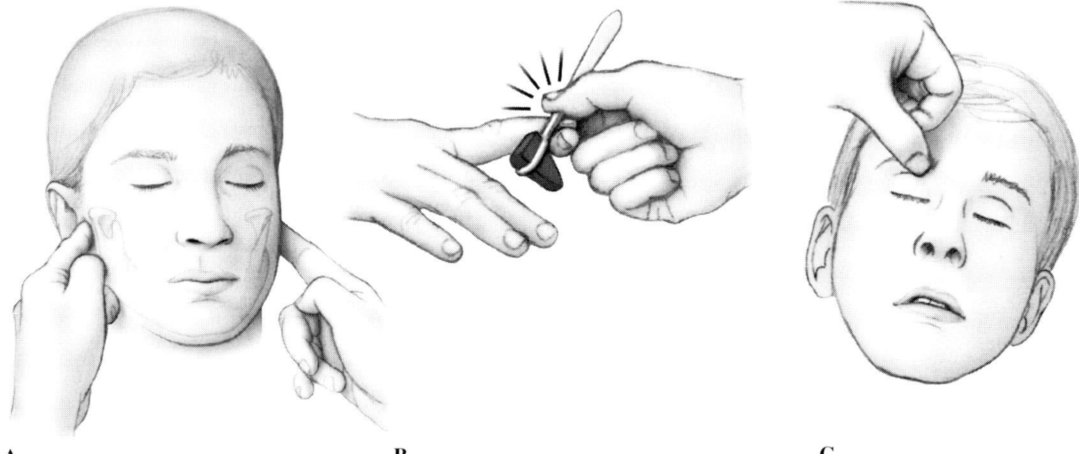

Figure 1.2. Methods of noxious pain stimuli. **A.** Compression of temporomandibular joints. **B.** Compression of nailbed with handle of reflex hammer. **C.** Supraorbital nerve compression.

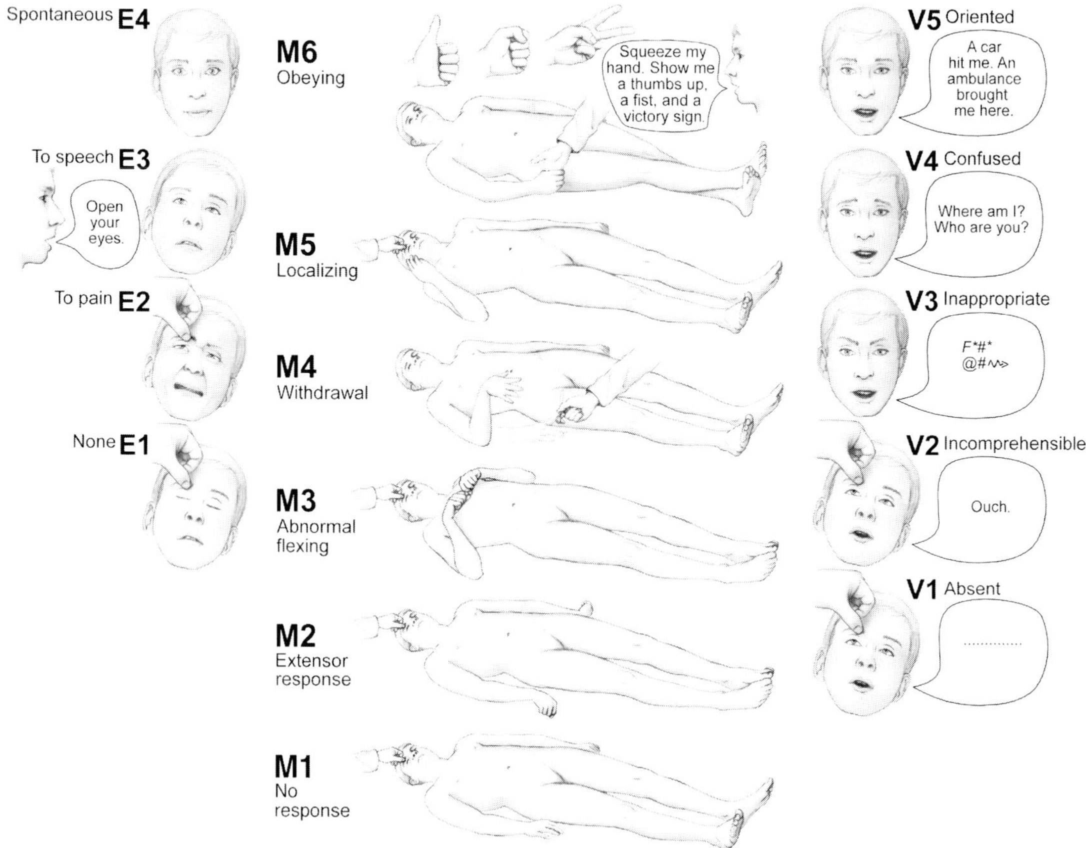

Figure 1.3. Glasgow coma score (see Table 1.4 and text for explanation).

applied to the face. Withdrawal to pain is quick, usually involving only flexion and not arm or wrist flexion and adduction (snap back response). Motor responses may include the so-called primitive responses. Both abnormal flexor responses (decorticate rigidity) and abnormal extensor responses (decerebrate rigidity) are nonlocalizing, indicating bilateral hemisphere diencephalic or brain stem lesions. Abnormal extensor responses imply more severe dysfunction but not necessarily a worse prognosis. These responses are not typically seen in coma from poisoning. An abnormal flexion response in the arms is indicated by stereotyped, slow flexion of the arm, wrist, and fingers, with adduction in the arms and extension, internal rotation, and plantar flexion of the legs. An abnormal extension response in the arms consists of adduction and internal rotation of the shoulder and pronation of the hand. By convention, the "best" motor response is scored when the difference between left and right is noted.

3. *Verbal response*. A normal verbal response is speech that implies awareness of self, environment, and circumstances. The patient knows who he is, where he is, and why he is there. Confused conversation is conversational speech with disorientation in content. Inappropriate speech is intelligible but consists of isolated words only and may include profanity and yelling. The term "incomprehensible speech" refers to the production of fragments of words or moaning or groans alone. Lack of speech (mutism) is rare.

Meningeal irritation should be assessed but becomes less apparent in patients with deeper stages of coma (e.g., no eye opening to pain, primitive motor responses, and moaning only). Muscle tone

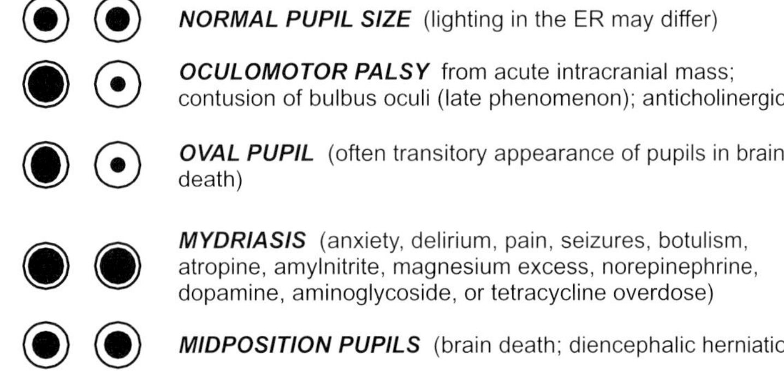

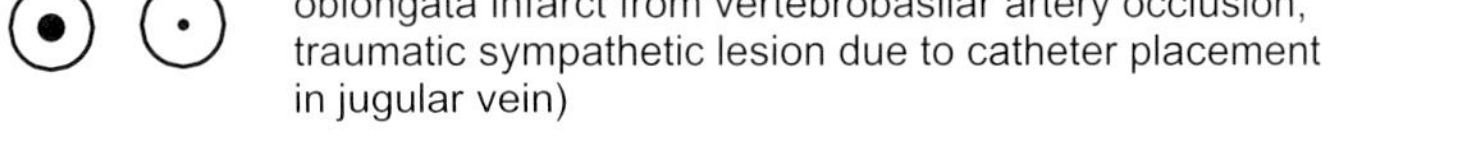

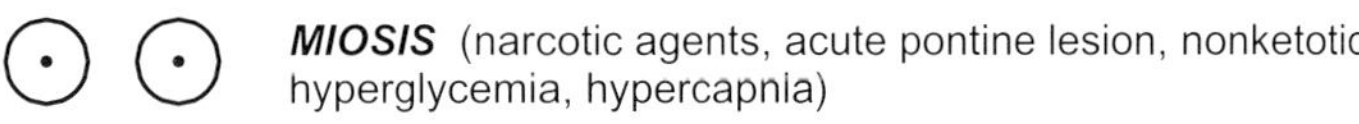

Figure 1.4. Pupil abnormalities in coma.

can be flaccid (normal in coma but may indicate intoxication with benzodiazepine or tricyclic antidepressant poisoning) or rigid (e.g., neuroleptic agents, etomidate, strychnine, malignant catatonia, or malignant hyperthermia). Abnormal movements such as twitching in the eyelids (may indicate seizures), tremors, myoclonus (anoxic encephalopathy, lithium intoxication, penicillin intoxication, pesticides), asterixis (acute renal, liver, or pulmonary failure), and shivering (sepsis, hypothermia) should be noted and integrated into the examination.

Examination proceeds with the cranial nerves. The size of the pupils and whether they are equal, round, oval, or irregular should be noted. It is important to understand the meaning of a unilateral dilated, fixed pupil (frequently designates uncal herniation); bilateral fixed, midposition pupils (frequently designate diencephalic herniation, brain death, or intoxication with scopolamine, atropine, glutethimide, or methyl alcohol); and pinpoint pupils (frequently designate narcotic overdose, acute pontine lesion, or syphilis [Argyll Robertson pupils]). The pupillary reactions to an intense beam from a flashlight are studied for both eyes. A magnifying glass may be needed to evaluate questionable pupillary responses, particularly in patients with small pupils. Pupillary abnormalities and their significance are shown in Figure 1.4.

Subhyaloid hemorrhage (Color Plate 3) is seldom seen in coma but when present implies aneurysmal subarachnoid hemorrhage. Papilledema (Color Plate 4) indicates acutely increased intracranial pressure but also is present in some patients with acute asphyxia.

Absence of spontaneous eye movement should be documented, along with lateral deviation to either side or disconjugate gaze at rest. Spontaneous eye movements—opsoclonus, ocular bobbing, and refractory nystagmus—may be seen in coma. Spontaneous nystagmus has no localization value and may occur in diffuse brain injury. The oculocephalic responses are evaluated in conjunction with passive, brisk horizontal head turning, and, if appropriate, the response to vertical head movements can be tested as well. (In patients with any head or spine injury, the oculocephalic responses should not be tested, because movement may luxate the cervical spine if fractured and immediately cause spinal cord trauma.) Oculovestibular responses are tested by irrigating each external auditory canal with 50 mL of ice water with the head 30° above the horizontal plane. Comatose patients exhibit tonic responses with conjugate deviation toward the ear irrigated with cold water. Bilateral testing can be done by rapidly squirting 50 mL of ice water in each ear, resulting in a forced downward eye movement. Forced gaze deviation indicates a large hemispheric lesion at the site looked at. Abduction of the eye only on the side being irrigated implies a brain stem lesion (internuclear ophthalmoplegia) as a cause of coma (Figure 1.5).

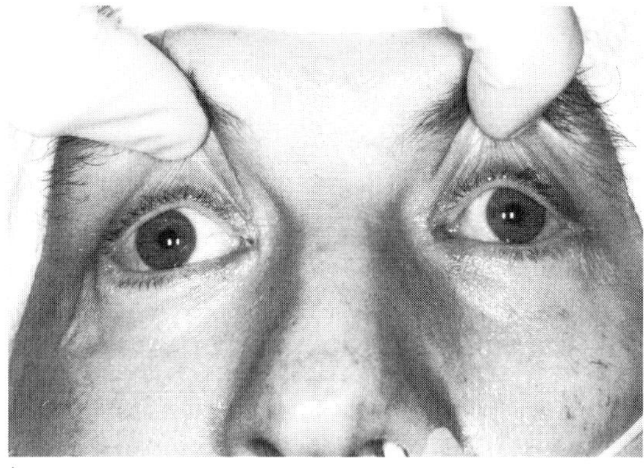

A

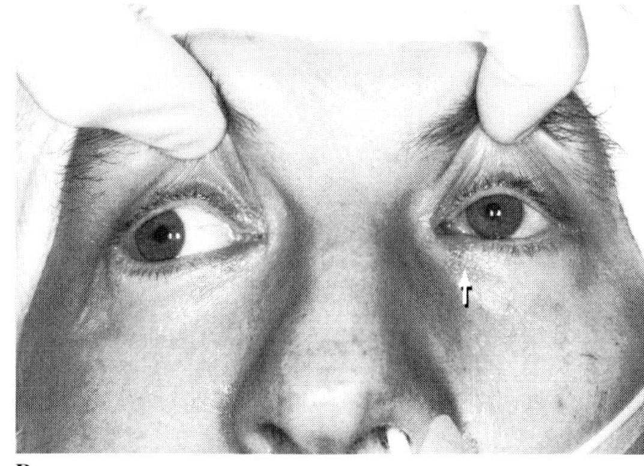

B

C

Figure 1.5. Internuclear ophthalmoplegia associated with acute pontine lesion. Adduction paralysis (*arrow*) can be elicited by cold water irrigation of the right ear (**B**) or the left ear (**C**).

Finally, corneal responses are tested by drawing a cotton wisp fully across the cornea. Spontaneous coughing or coughing after tracheal suctioning is recorded (to-and-fro movement of the endotracheal tube is not an adequate stimulus). Absence of coughing may indicate either that the neurologic catastrophe has evolved into brain death or that sedative drugs and neuromuscular blocking agents for emergency intubation have markedly muted these responses.

Brain Death

The clinical diagnosis of brain death is strongly suspected when all brain stem reflexes are absent in a comatose patient, but the cause of the catastrophic event should be known and demonstrated to be irreversible, which may include antidotes.[8,9] Brain death can be diagnosed in the emergency department but remains a presumptive diagnosis, and organ donation should not proceed directly from this location. Any physician assessing a patient with brain death should be very sensitive to the possibility that confounding causes may be present, particularly in patients admitted directly to the emergency department. Even when a catastrophic brain lesion is demonstrated on neuroimaging, the circumstances should be considered ambiguous until the history is complete and, if appropriate, a toxicologic study has ruled out drug ingestion.

The accepted clinical criteria for brain death are shown in Figure 1.6. The technical procedure for the apnea test is shown in Table 1.5.

Assessment of Patients with Structural Causes of Coma

These lesions are often acute (hemorrhage, infarct, abscess) or may be a critical extension of an infiltrating tumor or giant mass impinging on these structures. The boundary in the vertical axis is the lower pons. Destructive lesions below this level may lead to

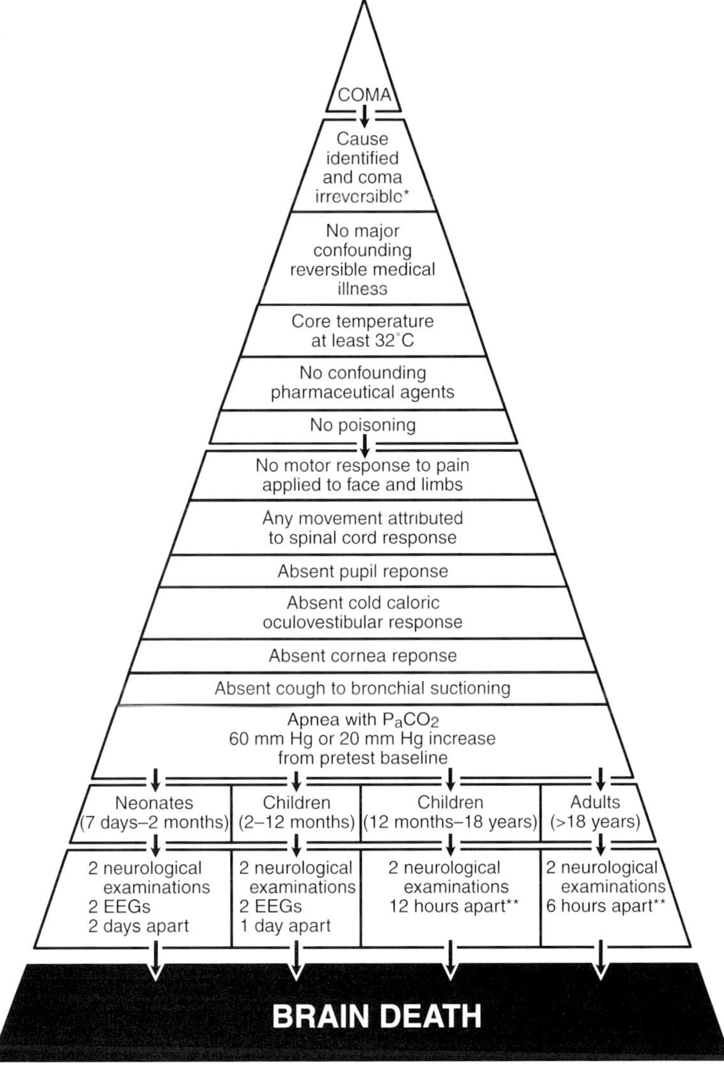

Figure 1.6. Brain death diagnosis and guidelines for confirmatory testing. (*Evidence preferably based on CT scan or CSF. **Confirmatory test such as cerebral angiography, nuclear scan, or transcranial Doppler ultrasonography may obviate observation over time.)

acute dysfunction of autonomic nuclei, resulting in failure to drive respiration or vascular tone. Coma or impaired consciousness in medulla oblongata lesions therefore is only an indirect consequence of hypercapnia or hypotension-induced global hemispheric injury. These lesions do not involve the ARAS structures and thus do not produce coma or hypersomnia.[10] These medullary structural lesions may involve hemorrhages (often arteriovenous malformation or cavernous hemangioma), metastasis, lateral or medially located medullary infarct, or an inflammatory lesion such as a bacterial or fungal abscess.

Tegmental pontine lesions interrupt the ARAS midway but result in impaired consciousness only with bilateral injury. The base of the pons does not participate in arousal; therefore, large lesions such as infarcts or central pontine myelinolysis do not impair consciousness but may interrupt all motor output except vertical eye movement and blinking initiated by centers in the mesencephalon. As alluded to earlier, this "locked-in syndrome" is often mistaken for coma until blinking and repeated up and down eye movements seem to coincide with questions posed to the patient. Communication is difficult, but cognition is intact, and patients may express their wishes for future care through code systems. It is a medical travesty if this disorder is not recognized, because the suffering of the patient, who

Table 1.5. The Apnea Test

Prerequisites:
- (1) core temperature ≥36.5°C (4.5°C higher than the required 32°C for clinical diagnosis of brain death)
- (2) systolic blood pressure ≥90 mm Hg
- (3) euvolemia
- (4) eucapnia
- (5) normoxemia

Connect a pulse oximeter to the patient.

Disconnect the ventilator.

Deliver 100% O_2, 6 L/minute (place a cannula close to the level of the carina).

Look closely for respiratory movements. Respiration is defined as abdominal or chest excursions that produce adequate tidal volumes.

Measure arterial PO_2, PCO_2, and pH after approximately 8 minutes and reconnect the ventilator.

If respiratory movements are absent and arterial PCO_2 is ≥60 mm Hg or there is an increase of 20 mm Hg in the PCO_2 over a baseline normal value, the apnea test result is positive (supports the clinical diagnosis of brain death).

If respiratory movements are observed, the apnea test result is negative (does not support the clinical diagnosis of brain death), and the test should be repeated.

Table 1.6. Diagnostic Considerations in Patients with Single Intracranial Mass

Immunosuppressed	Not immunosuppressed
Toxoplasma	Astrocytoma
Lymphoma	Oligodendroglioma
Progressive multifocal leukoencephalopathy	Glioblastoma multiforme
	Solitary metastasis
Aspergillus	Bacterial abscess
Mucormycosis	Sarcoidosis
Nocardia lymphoma	Aneurysm (giant)
Cysticercosis	Histoplasmosis
Echinococcus	Coccidioidomycosis
Schistosomiasis	Blastomycosis
Amebiasis	Multiple sclerosis
Mycobacteria	Meningioma
	Radiation necrosis

is unable to express the ability to communicate, is immeasurable.

Mesencephalic damage usually is seldom seen in isolation and more commonly occurs from extension of a lesion in the thalamus (e.g., destructive intracranial hematoma) or as a result of occlusion of the tip of the basilar artery, producing similar infarcts in both thalami and in the mesencephalic tegmentum.

Bilateral thalamic damage resulting in coma most often involves the paramedian nuclei, but damage to interlaminar, ventral lateral, or lateral posterior nuclei may impair consciousness by interrupting the thalamic cortex and thalamocortical projections. Infarcts in the distribution of the penetrating thalamogeniculate or anterior thalamic perforating arteries are the most common causes of bilateral thalamic damage, but an infiltrating thalamic tumor or infiltrative intraventricular masses in the third ventricle can produce sudden coma. Ganglionic hemorrhages may extend into the thalamus and compress the opposite thalamus.[11] Bithalamic hematoma is more commonly seen as an extension of pontine hematoma (see Chapter 7). Combined thalamic and mesencephalic damage may result in so-called slow syndrome, characterized by immobility, voicelessness, flat emotions, and somnolence most of the day.[10]

Bihemispheric structural damage may involve the white matter or cortex, or both, and a diversity of disorders may produce damage severe enough to reduce arousal. The most notable disorders are anoxic encephalopathy destroying most of the cortical lamina, multiple brain metastatic lesions, multifocal cerebral ischemia from vasculitis, multiple emboli from a cardiac source, markedly reduced global cerebral blood flow from acute subarachnoid hemorrhage, cerebral edema, hydrocephalus, blunt head trauma causing extensive scattered lesions in white and gray matter structures, and encephalitis (see Table 1.1).

Assessment of Patients with Acute Unilateral Hemispheric or Cerebellar Mass

Two major clinical manifestations may be observed in patients with an acute hemispheric mass: first, direct destruction of brain tissue leading to clinical features related to the involved lobe, and, second, remote effects from herniation and buckling of essentially normal tissue.

The differential diagnosis in unilateral brain masses is extensive (Table 1.6). Masses in the frontal lobe that are located on the right (in right-handed persons) may enlarge to impressive tumors that may not be detected by even the most meticulous neuro-

Capsule 1.2. Mechanisms of Herniation

Acute unilateral hemispheric masses may produce herniation syndromes from their volume or from surrounding edema. Whether displacement horizontally or vertically correlates with changes in consciousness and evolution of clinical signs remains a matter of some controversy. An alternative provocative but meritorious view is that horizontal shift measured by CT or MRI correlates better with early changes in consciousness in acute unilateral masses.[12,13] The diencephalic structures are compressed and dislocated toward the opposite site of the mass lesion. Bilateral masses "pinch" the upper brain stem rather than push it down. In addition, direct destructive damage of the thalamus with compression of the opposite dorsal thalamus may produce in the process bilateral involvement of the ascending reticular activating system and may cause coma despite an impressive shift in all directions[13] (e.g., large, destructive putamen hematomas). The significance of vertical displacement thus may be vastly overrated, and early thalamus damage may be key. However, advances in neuroimaging studies have allowed us to identify the development of mesencephalon ischemia from progressive vertical shift or disappearance of the fourth ventricle from brain stem impaction, suggesting that rostrocaudal deterioration is key in the development of progressive stages of herniation.[14] However, it is not certain whether these changes on MRI are the defining moment of irreversibility.

logic examination. A left frontal lobe mass, particularly if the lesion extends posteriorly, is manifested by Broca's aphasia. Its characteristics are distinct; the patient is constantly unable to repeat an exact sentence, speaks in short phrases and with revisions, and makes major grammatical errors together with loss of melody in lengthier narratives. Frontal lobe syndrome has been well recognized and appears in many guises, such as loss of vitality and prominent slow thinking. It may be manifested by weird behavior, sexual harassment, cynically inappropriate remarks in an attempt to be humorous, or intense irritability. Any executive function requiring planning ahead or some type of organization and planning is disturbed but may be covered up by euphoria, platitudes in speech, or "robotic-like" behavior, with preservation of social graces.

Masses in the temporal lobe may also generate changes in behavior and therefore may remain unnoticed or be delayed in recognition. Left-sided masses may change a normal personality into one of depression and apathy. More posterior localization in the temporal lobe may produce Wernicke's aphasia. This classic type of aphasia is recognized by continuously "empty" speech, often with syllables, words, or phrases at the end of sentences and characteristically with incomprehensible content (e.g., one of our patients, asked to define "island," responded, "place where petos . . . no trees . . . united presip thing," and to define "motor," "thing that makes the drive thing"). Involvement of the nondominant temporal lobe may be manifested by an upper quadrant hemianopia and nonverbal auditory agnosia (inability to recognize daily familiar sounds, such as loud clap, sound of a pager, and tearing of paper).

Parietal lobe masses also produce effects that depend on localization. Right parietal lesions usually cause neglect of the paralyzed right limb up to entire unawareness but also cause marked inertia and aloofness. Dominant (left in right-handed persons) parietal lobe impairs normal arithmetical skills, ability to copy three-dimensional constructions (such as making interlocking rings with index finger and thumb), recognition of fingers, and right-left orientation. A nonfluent aphasia may occur as well. Occipital lobe masses produce hemianopia. When only the inferior occipital cortex is involved, achromatopsia (loss of color vision in a hemianoptic field) or color naming (only in a right-sided hemianoptic field from a left occipital lesion) may result. Extension into the subcortical area from edema might produce alexia without agraphia in a left occipital lesion.

The quintessential patterns of brain herniation are (1) cingulate herniation, (2) central syndrome of rostrocaudal deterioration (herniation of the diencephalon structures, such as the thalamus), (3) uncal herniation, and (4) upward or downward herniation of brain tissue of the posterior fossa (Capsule 1.2).

Cingulate herniation is often asymptomatic and typically a diagnosis made by CT scanning or MRI.

It most frequently is a prelude to central or uncal herniation, when masses shift brain tissue even more. The cingulate gyrus is squeezed under the falx, but unless the anterior cerebral artery occludes (producing infarction and edema with frontal release signs and abulia), no major neurologic manifestation can be expected.

Central or diencephalic herniation occurs when a mass located medially forces the thalamus-midbrain through the tentorial opening. During this downward shift, the brain stem caves in and becomes distorted, and the shearing off of penetrating vessel from the basilar artery fixed to the circle of Willis results in irreversible brain stem damage.

Signs of central herniation have been recognized by the evolution of midposition or small bilateral pupils with sluggish light responses. At the same time, respiration becomes rapid, often with intermittent Cheyne-Stokes breathing. Patients barely localize pain stimuli and may fidget with bed linen or show a withdrawal response. Further progression results in extensor posturing and development of midposition pupils (diameter, 5 to 6 mm) unresponsive to light, disappearance of oculocephalic reflexes, and irregular gasping. Central herniation may progress to a midbrain stage in a matter of hours but then halts or very slowly progresses further (Figure 1.7). Central herniation may progress rapidly, but it is possible that the earlier signs of drowsiness, increased respiratory drive, and development of worsening motor responses are not appreciated by the physician or wrongly attributed to a new insult to the opposite hemisphere (e.g., in patients with a recent ischemic stroke).

Uncal herniation denotes displacement of the uncal gyrus, which is part of the temporal lobe, into the incisura tentorii. Uncal herniation has a more apparent presentation, with sudden appearance of a wide pupil with loss of light response. Ptosis, adduction paralysis, and diminished elevation are seen. Level of consciousness is reduced further when the uncus forces itself through the tentorium, flattening the midbrain and shifting it to the opposite direction. Contralateral hemiparesis occurs when the brain stem truly is squeezed against the opposite tentorial edge, damaging the pyramidal long tracts (classically named after Kernohan, the Kernohan notch). The midbrain displaces horizontally and may rotate if the compression is off center. The process can progress only more vertically, or the brain stem buckles and is squashed (Figure 1.8). Compression of the brain stem causes smaller pupils (often misinterpreted by novices as "improvement of fixed pupil" after administration of mannitol). Damage to the pons may lead to a transient locked-in syndrome.[15] Many of these features can be recognized on neuroimaging (see Figure 1.8).

Acute cerebellar masses (e.g., hematoma) are manifested by acute inability to walk, gaze palsy, and excruciating headache. Vomiting is common, and many patients can only crawl to the bathroom. Approximately 60% of the patients have a noticeable ataxia and nystagmus on examination before level of consciousness deteriorates from upward or tonsilar herniation.

Upward herniation occurs when the brain stem is lifted upward or when cerebellar tissue, particularly the vermis, is squeezed through the tentorial notch into the supracerebellar cisterns. The effects of brain stem compression and upward herniation are impossible to distinguish clinically but consist of progressive paralysis of upward gaze and further lapse into a deeper coma. Pupils become asymmetrical and finally contract to pinpoint size when pontine compression advances. MRI can document these anatomical changes with accuracy[16] (Figure 1.9).

Assessment of Patients with Poisoning or Drug Abuse Causing Coma

Intentional poisoning and drug abuse are common causes of coma in patients admitted to emergency departments (Capsule 1.3). The distribution of causes clearly depends on the geographic location of the hospital. The most common substances used for self-inflicted death by poisoning are tricyclic antidepressants, salicylates (particularly children), and street drugs. In the elderly, suicide attempts and unintentional intoxication through misjudgment of dose remain leading circumstances.

This section reviews the most commonly encountered poisonings causing coma. It is hardly possible to discuss all drugs that may cause coma; in fact, many do when ingested in enormous quantities. Polydrug abuse or intentional intoxication

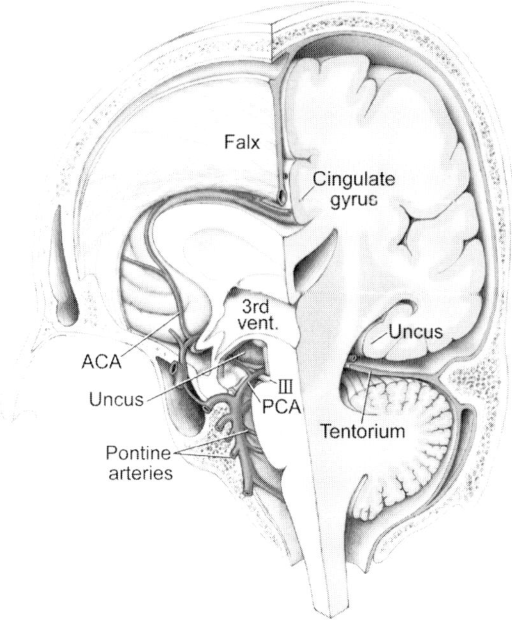

A

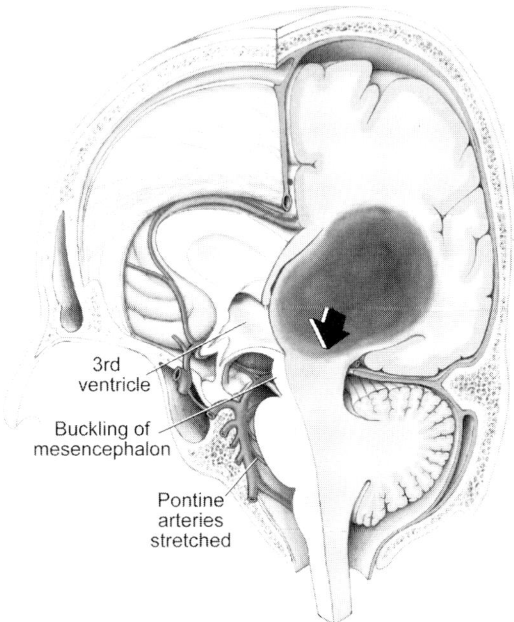

B

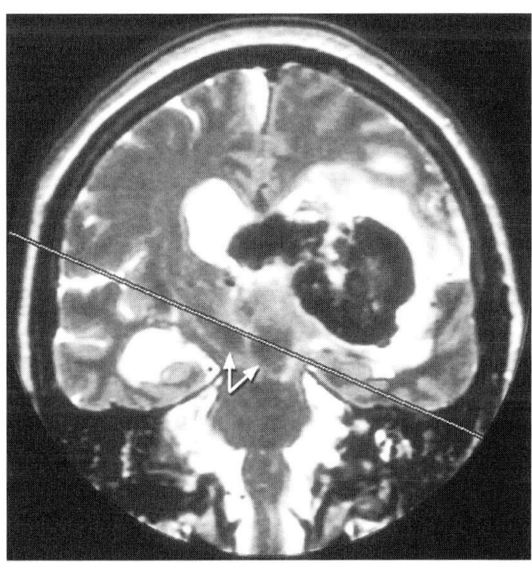

C

Figure 1.7. Normal anatomy (**A**), sketch of central or diencephalic herniation (**B**), and corresponding magnetic resonance image (**C**). Note downward movement of the brain stem. The red nuclei, usually horizontally aligned, have tilted (*arrows*). Ischemic brain stem lesions are the result of tearing of the penetrating arteries. (ACA = anterior cerebral artery; PCA = posterior cerebral artery; vent. = ventricle; III = third cranial nerve.)

often results in widely different clinical presentations. Many of the drug overdose cases are so complicated and difficult to diagnose that physicians are left with a dizzying array of possibilities. There is a potential flaw of presenting these intoxications in a simplistic fashion, but some clinical patterns are truly exemplary and should be recognized at first appearance.[17]

Central Nervous System Depressants

Central nervous system depressants first impair vestibular and cerebellar function. Therefore, nystagmus, ataxia, and dysarthria accompany or even precede the first signs of impaired consciousness.

Diagnosing an overdose of central nervous system depressant agents remains difficult, and one

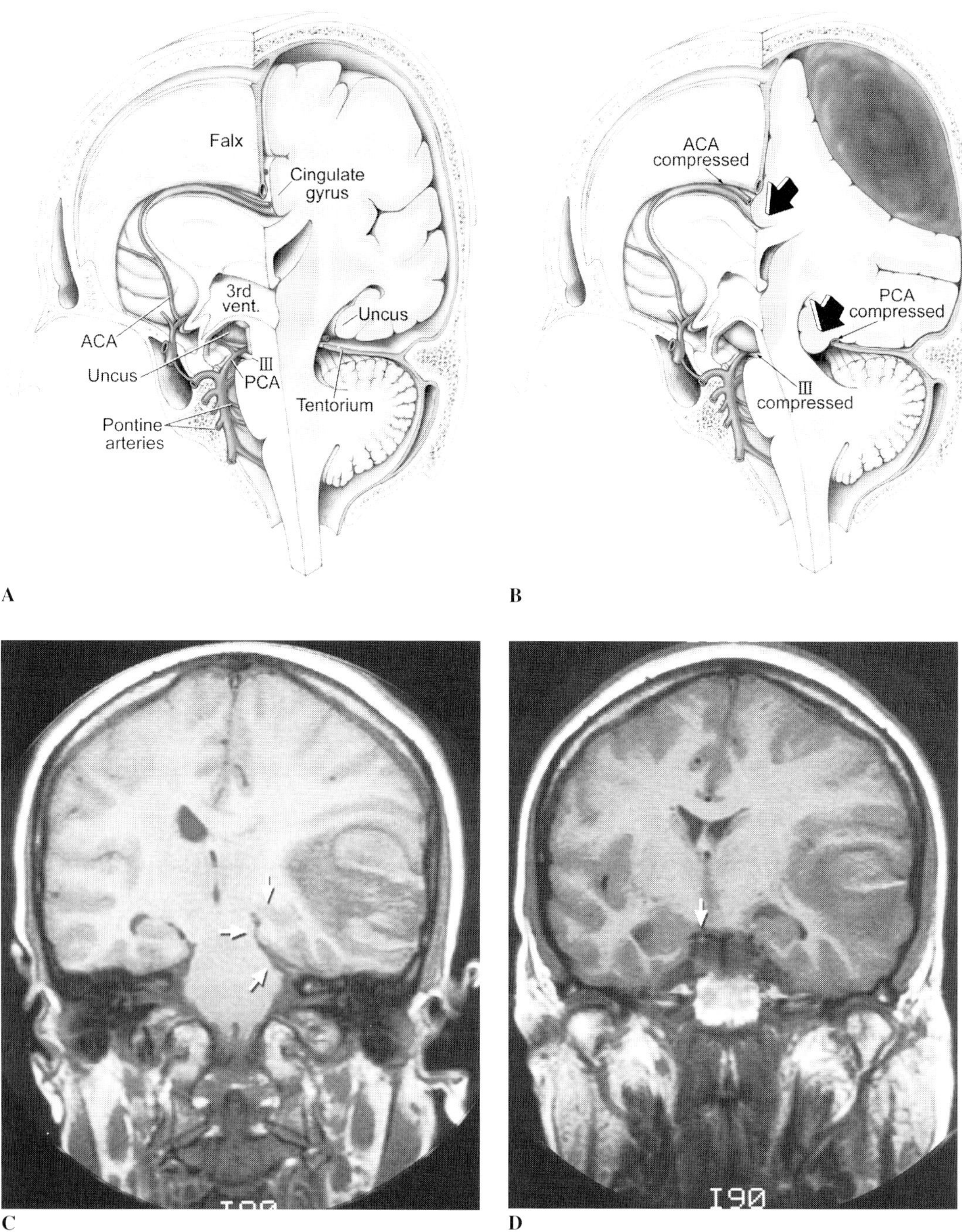

Figure 1.8. Normal anatomy **(A)**, sketch of uncal herniation **(B)**, and corresponding magnetic resonance image **(C–D)**. Note uncal herniation **(C)** (*arrows*) and disappearance of the oculomotor nerve due to compression **(D)** (*arrow* points to opposite oculomotor nerve). (ACA = anterior cerebral artery; PCA = posterior cerebral artery; vent. = ventricle; III = third cranial nerve.)

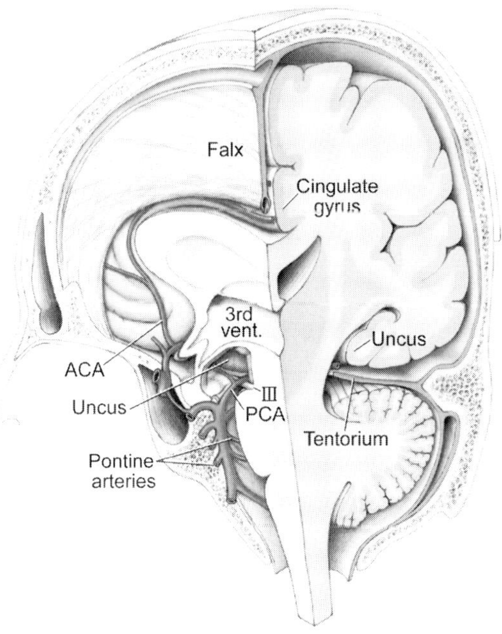

A

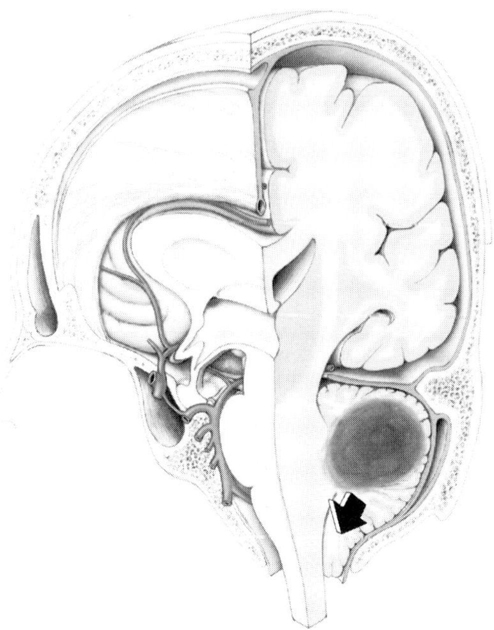

B

Figure 1.9. Normal anatomy **(A)**, sketch of tonsillar herniation **(B)**, and magnetic resonance images **(C)** (*arrows* point at orien tation lines). The iter of the aqueduct, usually located on the horizontal line drawn from the anterior tuberculum sellae to the confluence of the straight sinus and great vein of Galen, is upwardly displaced. The cerebellar tonsils are herniated below the line of the foramen magnum. (ACA = anterior cerebral artery; PCA = posterior cerebral artery; vent. = ventricle; III = third cranial nerve.)

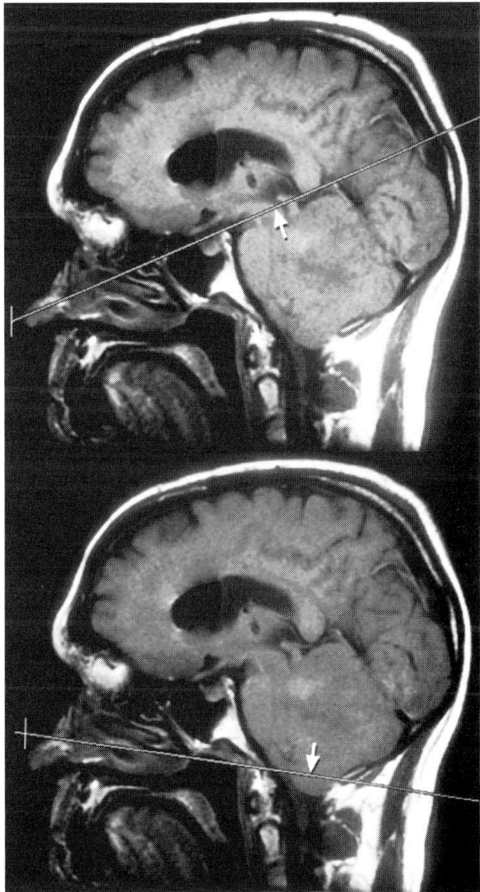

C

Capsule 1.3. Mechanisms of Toxin-Induced Coma

Coma induced by poisoning may result from at least five mechanisms. First, a chief factor may be hypoglycemia. Because many toxins cause profound hypoglycemia, early intravenous administration of glucose in any comatose patient has been advocated. Common examples are salicylates, β-adrenergic blockers, and ethanol.

Second, in other toxins, hypoxia is the main mechanism underlying coma and is produced by interference of oxygen transport, tissue utilization of oxygen, or simply displacement of oxygen by another gas, such as an industrial gas. Hypoxia can also be produced by acute pulmonary edema (e.g., cocaine) or aspiration pneumonitis (e.g., after seizures).

Third, a major mechanism of coma is depression of neuronal function involving the γ-aminobutyric acid (GABA)-benzodiazepine chloride iodophor receptor complex. The mechanism of action through GABA, one of the major central nervous system neurotransmitters, is increased output of GABA, which also leads to reduction of the turnover of acetylcholine, dopamine, and serotonin, culminating in a marked hypnotic-depressant effect. Opioids, however, exert their depressant effects on the central nervous system through a different set of receptors.

Fourth, toxins may cause seizures, usually as a terminal manifestation, which may be followed by a postictal decreased level of consciousness or nonconvulsive status epilepticus.

Fifth, structural central nervous system lesions may be caused by the toxin itself or may have resulted from traumatic head injury. Coma in poisoning or drug abuse may be due to spontaneous intracranial hematoma (e.g., amphetamine or cocaine overdose) or hemorrhagic brain contusions associated with a fall.

may fail to appreciate the dangerous potential of some agents (e.g., tricyclic antidepressants).

Ethanol

Alcohol intoxication is a frequent cause of reduced arousal. Alcohol ingestion can be fatal, but for death to occur, extreme quantities of ethanol should have been consumed, and more often an alcoholic binge is combined with consumption of other depressant drugs, leading to respiratory arrest or respiratory airway obstruction from vomiting.[18,19]

The development of acute alcohol intoxication depends not only on the blood alcohol concentration but also on the rapidity of the increase in blood and on tolerance, which is significantly increased in sots (typically, they are able to "drink someone under the table"). The clinical features of alcohol intoxication in relation to blood alcohol level are thus unreliable and apply only to naive drinkers. The clinical presentation of alcohol intoxication is well known and involves ataxia, dysarthria, loss of rapid reaction to sudden danger, and a feeling of high self-esteem that can lead to a series of misjudgments, including driving despite warnings from passengers. Aggression to well-intended restraint may lead to fistfights in susceptible persons and significant head injury.

Seizures are uncommon as a direct result of alcohol consumption but may be associated with severe hyponatremia (e.g., after consumption of large quantities at "beer fests"). Alcohol intoxication may mimic or coincide with many neurologic disorders, including hepatic encephalopathy, hypoglycemia, subdural hematoma, fulminant bacterial meningitis, and central pontine myelinolysis. Progressive confusion and combativeness in a previously alcoholic person, particularly if associated with tremors, marked (often initially unexplained) hypertension, and tachycardia, may indicate alcohol withdrawal and delirium. Recognition of profound alcohol withdrawal may become difficult, particularly if patients have passed well into a stage of agitation and decreased alertness.

The diagnosis of acute drunkenness seems straightforward, but laboratory confirmation and exclusion of confounding metabolic derangements are needed. Crucial laboratory tests should include measurement of serum alcohol level, arterial blood gases (to exclude hypoventilation), electrolytes, blood glucose, calcium and magnesium, and serum osmolality. Routine drug screens should be performed at all times to rule out other ingested drugs of abuse. A large osmolar gap is compatible with alcohol intoxication (see section on laboratory tests). When truly measured, the legal limit in many states is 1,000 μg/mL, and toxic levels are usually more than 2,000 μg/mL.

Management of patients in stupor or coma from alcohol intoxication consists of endotracheal intubation to protect the airway, thiamine intravenously, rewarming, liberal intravenous fluids, treatment of recurrent seizures, if any, and frequent assessment and management of potential hypoglycemia.

Barbiturates

Barbiturates are hypnotic-sedative agents that should be considered a cause of coma in drug addicts rushed into emergency departments. It is not surprising to find that barbiturates have been taken with other street drugs, and they may considerably deepen the level of coma.

Barbiturates significantly differ in duration of action (Table 1.7). They are very powerful stimulants of the inhibitory neurotransmitter γ-aminobutyric acid (GABA), resulting in early depression of respiratory drive. In the event of overdose, these differences often determine the time on the mechanical ventilator.

Depending on the degree of central nervous system depression, barbiturate overdose produces flaccid coma with initially small reactive pupils advancing to light-fixed, dilated pupils in near-fatal doses, often with associated profound hypotension from direct myocardial depression, a clammy skin, and hypothermia. Bullous skin lesions ("coma blisters") can be seen at pressure points and are very uncommon at other sites, suggesting skin necrosis from ischemia rather than a specific cutaneous toxicity.

The depth of coma can be estimated by measurement of barbiturate levels and by an electroencephalogram, which in severe cases may show isoelectric tracing, mimicking brain death, but more commonly displays a burst suppression pattern.

Management of barbiturate coma is supportive, with full mechanical ventilation until cough reflexes return. Vasopressors, such as dopamine, are needed to support blood pressure. When long-acting barbiturates have been ingested, hemodialysis may be indicated to reduce the time spent in coma.

Table 1.7. Classification of Barbiturates

Ultra-short-acting (DA, 0.3 hour)	Thiopental Thiamylal Methohexital
Short-acting (DA, 3 hours)	Hexobarbital Pentobarbital* Secobarbital†
Intermediate-acting (DA, 3–6 hours)	Amobarbital‡ Aprobarbital Butabarbital
Long-actıng (DA, 6–12 hours)	Barbital Mephobarbital Phenobarbital§ Primidone

(DA = duration of action.)
*Also known as "yellow jackets."
†Also known as "red devils."
‡Also known as "blue heavens."
§Also known as "purple hearts," "goofballs," and "downs."

With the improvement in intensive care support and hemodialysis, outcome is difficult to predict on the basis of depth of coma. An earlier landmark study by Reed et al.[20] found that mortality was high in patients with respiratory failure, hypotension, and coma for more than 36 hours, but these data may not apply in modern times.

Tricyclic Antidepressants

The prescription of antidepressant drugs for patients with severe depression may lead to use by the patient for a suicide attempt. This is possibly also related to the observation that it takes 2 to 3 weeks to achieve the antidepressant effect, and thus patients with suicide tendencies may take all the medication at once. Tricyclic overdose is one of the principal causes of death in intensive care unit series of drug overdosing.[21] By virtue of the profound cardiac toxicity of the drugs, death can be imminent in some patients on arrival in the emergency room.

Coma from tricyclic antidepressant toxicity may progress to a loss of all brain stem reflexes and apnea, mimicking brain death. However, coma with no response to painful stimuli occurred in only 13% of 225 patients with tricyclic overdose.[22] Tricyclic overdose may be manifested by delirium from cholinergic blockade, and some patients have other manifestations, such as dry skin, hyperthermia, and dilated pupils.[23] Seizures are common within hours of ingestion, often emerge at peak serum concentration, but seldom evolve into status epilepticus.[24]

A widened QRS interval on the electrocardiogram is a common manifestation, and at least initially cardiac arrhythmias may be absent. In a significant overdose, the management of cardiac arrhythmia determines care and can involve a temporary pacemaker. Sodium bicarbonate (50 mEq of $NaHCO_3$, 1 mEq/mL) should be administered to produce alkalosis, which inhibits sodium channel blockade by tricyclic antidepressants, a mechanism thought to be responsible for cardiac arrhythmia. Seizures can be managed with intravenous administration of phenytoin, but because of its own risk of producing cardiac arrhythmias, this agent probably is indicated only if seizures reoccur.

Lithium

Toxic manifestations of lithium are most often a result of incorrect dosage. Anticholinergic manifestations are common, including flushing of the face, dilated pupils, fever, and dry skin.[25]

With increasing blood levels, a rather slowly progressive clinical picture seems to emerge, characterized by myoclonus, hand tremor, and slurring of speech. This may further progress to delirium, acute mania, dystonic movements, oculogyric crises, facial grimacing, and, finally, stupor. Serum lithium levels are reasonably correlated with the severity of toxicity, which is serious when these levels reach or exceed 2.5 mEq/L.[25]

Restoration of sodium and water balance, which is disturbed by a lithium-induced nephrogenic diabetes insipidus, is key in its management. Hemodialysis or peritoneal dialysis should be instituted immediately in most cases.

Benzodiazepines

Patients with a benzodiazepine overdose seldom are in need of a long hospital stay unless coingestions have occurred. Massive exposure to benzodiazepines results in coma, but with appropriate support, neurologic morbidity is rare. Coma can be profound, but most patients awaken within 2 days; recovery times are longer with increasing age.[26]

The clinical presentation of benzodiazepine poisoning is nonspecific, and coma with extreme flaccidity is common.[27] Respiratory depression may not be evident, and hypoxic respiratory drive often becomes clear only when a pulse oximeter is connected to the patient on arrival in the emergency department.

The use of flumazenil is controversial, because seizures from acute withdrawal have been reported. A more recent study in 110 patients contradicted these risks and demonstrated that flumazenil is safe.[28]

Abuse of Illicit Drugs

It is not possible to gather all illicit drugs under one umbrella and discuss them in a few paragraphs. This section discusses some of the most commonly encountered examples of drug overdose. For complex problems, readers should refer to major toxicology textbooks,[29,30] available in most emergency departments, or a recent neurology text.[31] Not infrequently, these unfortunate, poorly nourished patients are found hypothermic or next to an empty syringe, bottle of liquor, or unlabeled pillbox.

Phencyclidine

Phencyclidine (slang: "angel dust") is rising in popularity among illicit drug users and users in college, and thus the prevalence of phencyclidine overdose is increasing in emergency rooms. Phencyclidine is usually packed in tablets and sold as powder or mixed with marijuana (slang: "wacky weed").[30]

Phencyclidine is a potent anesthetic agent, acting on both γ-aminobutyric acid and dopamine systems. Its clinical manifestations are highly unusual, with deep anesthesia and coma but a facial appearance of being fully awake.[32] Typically, a strong pain stimulus is not registered by the patient, and this sign should immediately point to phencyclidine as a toxin. Commonly, phencyclidine produces hypertension, tachycardia, salivation, sweating, and bidirectional nystagmus. Many patients act violently, demonstrate bizarre behavior, and speak endlessly.[33] Distortion of body image and vivid visual hallucinations may occur, and some patients are catatonic, which additionally may lead to rhabdomyolysis. When the patient's condition progresses to coma, cholinergic signs are obvious, with significant frothing, flushing, sweating (often with typical strings of large sweat droplets on the forehead), and miosis.[32,33]

Many patients recover fully with adequate ventilator support, but some may continue to manifest a schizophrenia-like picture of withdrawal, negativism, and delusions, which suggests chronic use of phencyclidine.

Cocaine

Cocaine blocks the presynaptic uptake of norepinephrine and dopamine and causes excitation.[34] Its recreational use is widespread, either by intranasal snorting or by smoking after dissolution in water and the addition of a strong base (so-called crack).

The clinical presentation after inhalation, smoking, or intravenous injection is characteristic. Patients have hypertension, widely dilated pupils, and tachypnea. Seizures often occur after the initial "rush."[35] In severely intoxicated patients, progression to generalized tonic-clonic epilepticus is not unusual.[36,37]

Coma from cocaine overdose may have other origins. These are cardiac arrest producing a profound anoxic-ischemic encephalopathy, intracerebral or subarachnoid hemorrhage from brief malignant hypertension (with only up to 50% of patients truly harboring a vascular malformation or aneurysm suggesting a direct relationship with the cocaine), and, finally, bilateral cerebral infarcts as a result of diffuse vasoconstriction[38–40] or long-standing occlusive disease of major cerebral arteries.[41]

General measures for cocaine overdose often include management of hyperthermia with cooling blankets or fans, β-adrenergic blockade or lidocaine to treat ventricular tachycardia, and careful monitoring for the possible development of acute myocardial infarction and recognition of status epilepticus.

Opiates

Acute opiate overdose may be produced by heroin (diacetylmorphine) or deliberate use of massive doses of narcotic drugs used for pain control. Fentanyl dermal patches, particularly, have become popular for pain control, and the absorption of this very potent opioid is so erratic that rapidly progressive stupor may occur.[42]

The clinical manifestations of opiate overdose include miosis, hypoventilation, and flaccidity. Brain stem reflexes may become lost, and the preserved light reflex in patients with extremely small pupils may be impossible to discern. Severe hypoxia from hypoventilation or florid pulmonary edema may be a major contributory factor to coma. Seizures appear more commonly with meperidine and propoxyphene.

Management of opioid poisoning has been facilitated by the use of naloxone or naltrexone. These opiate antagonists are without major adverse side effects, and dramatic reversal of coma is seen.

Arterial blood gas values are supportive in opioid overdose, demonstrating marked hypoxia and hypercapnia from hypoventilation. A point that cannot be emphasized strongly enough is that because serum drug screens do not identify opioids, urine samples are needed for detection. For other examples, see Appendix 1.1.

Naloxone is administered in doses of 0.4 to 2.0 mg repeated at 1- to 2-minute intervals. The effect is brief. An intravenous drip of naloxone is justified only in patients with a profound overdose resulting in hypotension and ventricular tachyarrhythmias.

Environmental and Industrial Toxins

Exposure to these toxins, whether intentional or accidental, frequently alters consciousness and produces prolonged coma long after the toxin has been eliminated, washed out, or neutralized. Important clues, if any, to environmental poisoning are dead pets and distinctive odors (from often-added sulfur-containing compounds) detected by neighbors.

The effect of these toxins on the central nervous system can be catastrophic, with a high probability of adverse neurologic outcomes.

Carbon Monoxide Poisoning

Carbon monoxide remains one of the leading causes of death by poisoning. Exposure to this odorless gas is possible at the time of a fire, from poorly vented fireplaces, from furnaces, and in any closed space where internal combustion engines have been used without ventilation. In most instances, suicide can be implicated, but one-third of admitted patients are victims of accidental circumstances.

Carbon monoxide readily binds to hemoglobin, with a 200 times greater attraction than oxygen. The cerebral injury due to carbon monoxide poisoning, however, is a cumulation of factors. Early animal studies by Ginsberg[43] clearly showed that the pathognomonic lesions can be produced only by carbon monoxide and hypotension and not by inhalation of carbon monoxide alone.

Carbon monoxide poisoning causes a shift of the hemoglobin dissociation curve to the left, which reduces oxygen unloading (Haldane effect). Through binding with myoglobin, carbon monoxide may trigger cardiac arrhythmias, hypotension, and hypoxemia from pulmonary edema, adding to the injury.[44]

The neuropathologic changes (selected from the most severe cases at autopsy) are predominant in the white matter, with demyelination and edema, and in the hippocampus, cerebellum, and globus pallidus. These lesions may be detected on CT scans;[45] they predict a severely disabled state as the best possible outcome.[46,47] MRI may more clearly delineate these abnormalities, which emerge even within hours of exposure, but only in patients with levels high enough to lead to coma (virtually always more than 50% carboxyhemoglobin levels).[48]

The symptoms preceding coma from carbon monoxide poisoning are nonspecific and vague, including headache, dizziness, and shortness of breath, all suggesting a developing viral illness. A cherry red appearance of the skin is very uncommon; it signals a near-fatal exposure.[43] Other clinical findings are retinal hemorrhages, dark color of retinal arteries and veins, and pulmonary edema. Rhabdomyolysis may be related to pressure necrosis in patients immobilized for an unknown length of time.

The most important laboratory test is the determination of a carbon monoxide hemoglobin level, which may be "falsely low" if oxygen has been administered in the emergency room or if the time between exposure and blood testing is more than 6 hours, which is approximately the half-life of carboxyhemoglobin (a 5% level of hemoglobin carbon monoxide can be attributed to smoking). Other laboratory test results that are more or less supportive are metabolic acidosis, increased creatine kinase, and cardiac ischemia on electrocardiography.

Management of carbon monoxide poisoning is treatment with 100% oxygen with a sealed face mask. Hyperbaric oxygen increases the amount of dissolved oxygen 10 times and may significantly shorten the duration of coma.[49] Hyperbaric oxygen is not routinely available, but there are no hard data to prove better outcome with this therapy. This observation strengthens the concept that additional factors, such as hypotension, are equally important in carbon monoxide's damaging effect. Hyperbaric oxygen therapy may, however, be the preferred approach in comatose patients and patients with significant cardiac ischemia despite initial breathing of 100% oxygen.

Cyanide

Cyanide poisoning should be entertained in any coma of undetermined cause, particularly in laboratory or industrial workers. A well-recognized intentional cause is the ingestion of nail polish removers.[50] Prevalence of cyanide poisoning is low, but its effects can be reversed with antidotes.

Cyanide has an unusual mechanism of action. By interacting with cytochrome oxidase (an essential enzyme in the mitochondrial electron transport chain), it greatly reduces production of adenosine triphosphate. Consequently, significant lactate acidosis results from a shift in anaerobic metabolism. Additionally, cyanide, like carbon monoxide, shifts the hemoglobin dissociation curve to the left and directly binds with the iron of hemoglobin, reducing the delivery of oxygen to the brain and other vital organs.[51]

Coma from cyanide poisoning is often accompanied by hypoventilation from central inhibition of the respiratory centers, severe lactate acidosis, bradycardia, hypotension, and rapidly developing pulmonary edema. A bitter almond or musty smell has been linked to cyanide poisoning, but recognition of its odor is impossible for many physicians.[51]

The supportive laboratory finding is lactate metabolic acidosis, which may be combined with respiratory alkalosis from hyperventilation to overcome hypoxia or respiratory acidosis from hypoventilation. Plasma cyanide can be measured, but correlation with the degree of coma is poor, and testing is thus impractical.

Cyanide poisoning has a good outcome when treated with the Lilly cyanide antidote kit. This contains amyl nitrite (by crushing of pellets and inhalation by patients), sodium nitrite, and sodium thiosulfate (intravenous, 50 mL of a 25% solution). The effect is based on conversion of hemoglobin into methemoglobin, which combines with cyanide but easily breaks down into free cyanide, which then combines with sodium thiosulfate and is eventually eliminated in the urine.

Reliable neurologic data on outcome are not available. Parkinsonism and dystonia have been reported, with associated lesions in the basal ganglia detected by CT scanning and with improvement in some instances.[52,53]

Toxic Alcohols

Methanol, ethylene glycol, and isopropyl alcohol are used in many commercial products, including antifreeze (ethylene glycol) and solvents (methanol). Isopropyl alcohol is best known as rubbing alcohol. The alcohols produce virtually similar laboratory effects, the most noticeable of which is a high anion gap metabolic acidosis.[54]

Methanol infrequently causes coma, but a fatal outcome is likely if it occurs. Methanol more commonly produces delirium and blurred vision. Careful examination reveals hyperemia of the optic disk, and blindness may follow as a result of the toxic effect of formaldehyde on retinal ganglion cells. Bilateral necrosis of the putamen is highly characteristic, frequently becoming apparent on neuroimaging studies in comatose patients only after several weeks.[55] However, the brains of patients dying of methanol poisoning may be normal or variably show congestion, edema, petechiae, and necrosis of the cerebellar cortex.

Several features of methanol poisoning are of interest. First, a latent period (up to 12 hours) is typical, making it very difficult for bystanders to understand the sudden occurrence of a lapse into coma, and thus more often a recent catastrophe is suggested. Second, prominent restlessness with vomiting and curling up from abdominal cramps may be followed by seizures before a lapse into unresponsiveness. Treatment is focused on correction of the acidosis with bicarbonate, but in comatose patients extracorporeal hemodialysis is imperative. Although the outcome can be very satisfactory, permanent neurologic disability may occur.[56]

Ethylene glycol is most commonly known as a major component of antifreeze and many detergents.[57] Suicide is the most common reason for ingestion, and then mortality is high. The metabolites produce toxicity, and the clinical features preceding coma are dramatic. Marked gait ataxia, nystagmus, paralysis of the extraocular muscles, and ocular bobbing are followed by generalized tonic-clonic seizures or profound myoclonus and, because of severe hypocalcemia, tetanic contractions. Lactic acidosis and an osmolar gap are characteristic laboratory features, but diagnosis is confirmed with the demonstration of calcium oxalate crystals in the urine.[57] Ethylene glycol poisoning is often treated with hemodialysis and high doses of ethanol up to intoxication of the patient (plasma ethanol target is 1,000 μg/mL). In a recent study, an inhibitor of alcohol dehydrogenase (fomepizole) was successful in preventing renal damage by inhibiting toxic metabolites such as oxalate. Fomepizole is an expensive alternative to ethanol but is without toxic effects. Intravenous loading of 15 mg/kg is followed by 10 mg/kg every 12 hours for 2 days, with a further increase to 15 mg/kg every 12 hours until the plasma ethylene glycol concentration is less than 20 mg/dL.[58]

Finally, isopropyl alcohol is rather potent, producing rapidly developing coma, always with severe hypotension from cardiomyopathy. The typical acetone breath should point to this toxin. The characteristic oxalate crystals in ethylene glycol are not found in isopropyl poisoning. Management involves gastric lavage; because the onset of coma is rapid, recovery from the stomach can still be substantial.

Miscellaneous Intoxications

In this section, poisonings that are of great clinical importance and are proportionally frequent or that produce striking clinical features are discussed.

Salicylates

As a result of safety packaging, the incidence of salicylate poisoning has substantially decreased, but it is still prevalent in children.

Salicylates may take some time to dissolve in the acidic stomach milieu but then are rapidly absorbed, and blood levels are maximal within 1 hour. After exposure to a massive dose, the pharmacokinetics are different, and through a complex mechanism the half-life of salicylates increases to 15 to 20 hours from a baseline level of 2 to 4 hours in therapeutic doses.[59]

Salicylates equilibrate rapidly with cerebrospinal fluid, and the levels of salicylates in cerebrospinal fluid appear to correlate better with outcome than do serum levels.[60] Determination of salicylate levels in cerebrospinal fluid, however, is cumbersome, because salicylates significantly interfere with platelet function and prolong prothrombin time.

The mechanism of action of salicylates is not entirely clear. It may involve (1) uncoupling of the oxidative phosphorylation and blocking of glycolysis, producing a metabolic acidosis; (2) direct stimulation of the brain stem respiratory centers leading to respiratory alkalosis, independent of an already compensatory response to the induced acidosis; and (3) increased metabolic demand from increased glycolysis to compensate for the uncoupling in (1), which may result in profound hypoglycemia.[59]

Salicylate poisoning should always be considered in restless, hyperventilating patients. Hyperthermia and purpura due to platelet dysfunction in the eyelids and neck may occur, simulating fulminant acute meningococcal meningitis. Pulmonary edema may occur and may become rapidly life-threatening. Severe acidemia caused by increased lipid solubility of salicylates in an acidic environment facilitates the entry of salicylates into the brain.

The laboratory features of increased anion gap, metabolic acidosis, and respiratory alkalosis are well appreciated and should lead to measurement of serum salicylate levels or, more practically, ferric chloride testing of the urine. Purple discoloration of the urine is diagnostic, and the test has good predictive value. A plasma salicylate level of 6 mg/dL usually is correlated with seizures and coma.

Management of salicylate poisoning involves gastric lavage, activated charcoal, and forced alkaline diuresis. Alkalization is performed with sodium bicarbonate or, in less severe cases, acetazolamide.

Acetaminophen

Acetaminophen is a substance in many nonprescription drugs, and as a result, poisoning is common. Usually, however, extremely large doses (plasma level >800 μg/mL) are required to directly depress consciousness; more likely, the development of acute hepatic necrosis or hepatorenal syndrome causes coma.[61]

Overdose of acetaminophen proceeds in phases, but liver damage can occur within 24 hours after ingestion. The biochemical basis for acute liver necrosis has been elucidated and is the rationale for therapy with *N*-acetylcysteine. In normal situations, acetaminophen is metabolized in the liver through either sulfation or glucuronidation and only a small fraction through the P-450 oxidase system, which produces an active metabolite that has the potential for liver necrosis. Overloading of the glucuronidation system by large ingestion of acetaminophen increases the formation of toxic metabolites. Decreased glutathione stores, as in patients with long-term antiepileptic drug use or chronic alcoholism, may increase the probability of liver necrosis after acetaminophen intoxication.[62,63]

Clinical features of acetaminophen overdose are nausea, vomiting, diaphoresis, and abdominal pain in the right upper quadrant but no depression in consciousness unless hepatic failure develops. Hepatic encephalopathy, with its characteristic asterixis and myoclonus, develops approximately 4 days after ingestion. Brain edema may become a feature in fulminant hepatic failure when patients lapse into stupor.

Together with *N*-acetylcysteine loading, management is largely supportive. *N*-acetylcysteine is metabolized to cysteine, which functions as a precursor for glutathione and serves to restore the glutathione scavenging.

Liver transplantation may be needed, and its consideration leads to an ethical quagmire in patients who used acetaminophen for a suicide attempt.

Antiepileptic Drugs

Overdose with antiepileptic drugs is most often intentional, but every now and then a prescription blunder or drug interaction that reduces metabolism can be implicated. Coma from antiepileptic drug overdose is not common, and most often nonspecific signs, such as dizziness, tremor, nystagmus, and profound ataxia, occur. Paradoxically, antiepileptic drug overdose may produce seizures, and the risk, at least in carbamazepine overdose, is increased in patients with a seizure disorder.[64]

Acute overdose of phenytoin (estimated serum levels >50 μg/mL) is characterized by rapid ataxia, dysarthria with combative behavior, and hallucinations, very seldom followed by generalized tonic-clonic seizures and progression to flaccid coma.

Management is supportive, with mechanical ventilation, charcoal to minimize further absorption, and benzodiazepines (e.g., lorazepam) or barbiturates (e.g., phenobarbital) in the rare event that seizures occur.

Carbamazepine is widely used in neurologic disorders. Its side effects are reminiscent of those of tricyclic antidepressants because of structural similarities, and neurologists, who are usually the primary health care providers, should appreciate this potential threat to life.[65–67] Respiratory depression is common in carbamazepine overdose, and prospective studies have found a median duration of 18 hours. Coma occurs in 20% to 50% of the reported series of carbamazepine overdose.[65,66] Fatal outcome may reach 15% of patients, most often affecting those in coma, with seizures, and with resuscitation for cardiac arrest; ingestion often exceeds 100 tablets.[65,68] Other manifestations of carbamazepine overdose are hypothermia, hypotension, tachycardia, and a diverse range of cardiac arrhythmias from its anticholinergic properties.[65,68]

Management is focused on cardiac manifestations, and problems similar to those in tricyclic antidepressant overdose should be anticipated. Recovery from carbamazepine overdose can be protracted, with fluctuating level of consciousness for many days.

Valproate toxicity is notable for its association with acute liver failure, but this devastating side effect has occurred only in young children and with concomitant use of other antiepileptic agents.[69] Massive ingestions (>200 mg/kg) produce coma with pinpoint pupils and hypertonia. As in acetaminophen poisoning, fulminant hepatic failure may produce many of the earlier manifestations of asterixis, myoclonus, and nystagmus.

Assessment of Acute Metabolic or Endocrine Causes of Coma

Acute metabolic derangements may produce reduced arousal and, when unrecognized, coma. Typical examples are hypoglycemia, hyponatremia, acute uremia, and acute liver failure. Overt hemiparesis, pupil abnormalities, and gaze preference are conspicuously absent on neurologic examination, but asterixis, tremor, and myoclonus predominate when deep coma sets in. Hyperglycemic nonketotic hyperosmolar coma is a notable exception, probably because of previous strokes in these patients with severe cerebrovascular risk factors. The mechanisms of these conditions causing hypometabolism in the brain are poorly understood, but many of these disorders cause diffuse cerebral edema (see Chapter 2); seizures intervene or cardiorespiratory resuscitation results in diffuse anoxic-ischemic damage (see Chapter 3). Endocrine crises, such as rarely encountered Hashimoto's thyroiditis (thyroid coma), Addison's disease, and panhypopituitarism, may be responsible for coma, and hormones of the hypothalamic pituitary axis should be measured in unexplained coma. The laboratory values compatible with marked impairment of consciousness are shown in Table 1.8. Coma should be attributed to other causes if the biochemical derangement is less severe.

Table 1.8. Laboratory Values Compatible with Coma* in Patients with Acute Metabolic and Endocrine Derangements

Derangement	Serum
Hyponatremia	≤110 mmol/L
Hypernatremia	>160 mmol/L
Hypercalcemia	≥3.4 mmol/L
Hypermagnesemia	≥5 μg/L
Hypercapnia	≥70 mm Hg
Hypoglycemia	≤40 mg/dL
Hyperglycemia	≥800 mmol/L

*Sudden decline in value is obligatory.

Neuroimaging and Laboratory Tests

CT scanning of the brain is particularly useful when the neurologic examination reveals localizing symptoms. Acute lesions in the brain stem and cerebellum may not be visualized on CT. Patients with acute basilar artery occlusion or evolving cerebellar infarction often have normal CT findings on admission, and MRI is needed to resolve the cause of the coma (Figure 1.10A). It may also demonstrate sparing of the ARAS in locked-in syndrome (Figure 1.10B).

CT findings in patients with altered consciousness, hemiparesis, or gaze preference are often abnormal. One should particularly evaluate whether basal cisterns are present on CT scans, because they

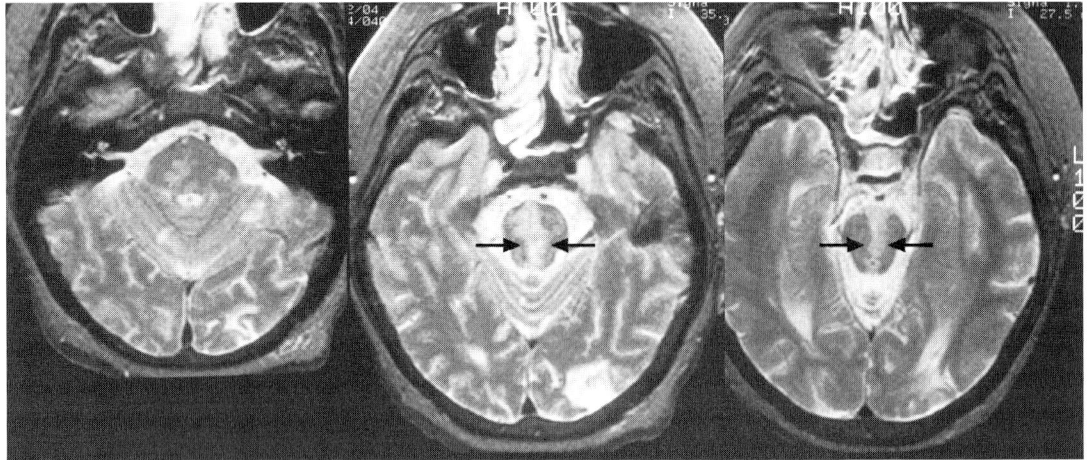

A

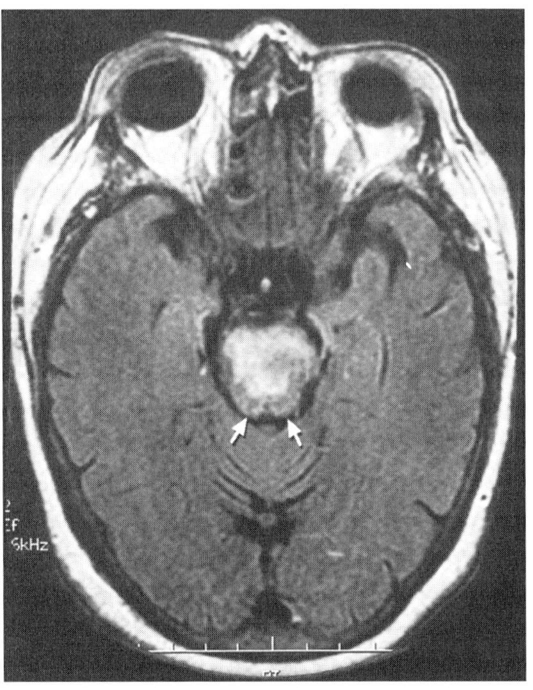

B

Figure 1.10. A. Linear hyperintensity (*arrows*) on magnetic resonance imaging (T2-weighted) in a patient with basilar artery occlusion. **B.** Locked-in syndrome. Note sparing of tegmentum (*arrows*).

may be filled in early uncal herniation.[70] Contralateral hydrocephalus may be present, usually caused by compression at the level of the foramen of Monro.[70] The ambient cistern is usually effaced, and an enlargement of the temporal horn is seen (Figure 1.11).

CT of the brain defines the existence of a mass, its remote effect, and edema and may hint at a cause. However, because of multiplanar views, MRI is more sensitive in recording the extension of the mass but also may reveal necrosis, pigments (deoxyhemoglobin, melanin), or fat, which may suggest the underlying pathologic condition. MRI clearly identifies giant aneurysms that may mimic tumors on CT.

In the emergency department, the CT scan appearance of a mass is most often characteristic enough to determine an early plan of action. Soli-

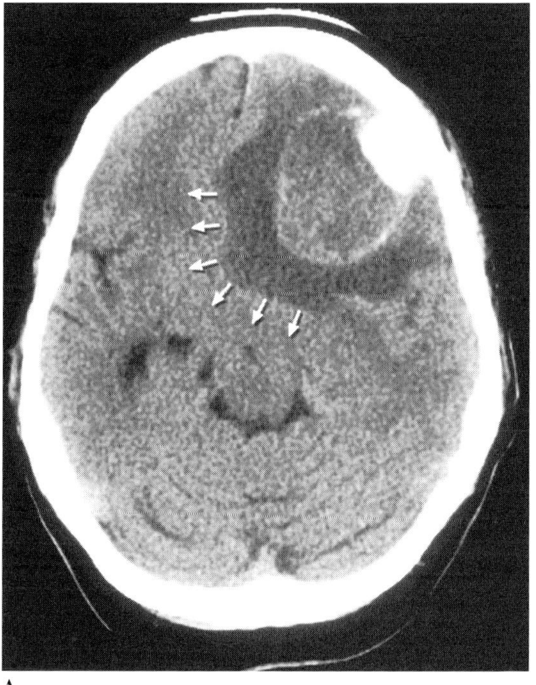

A

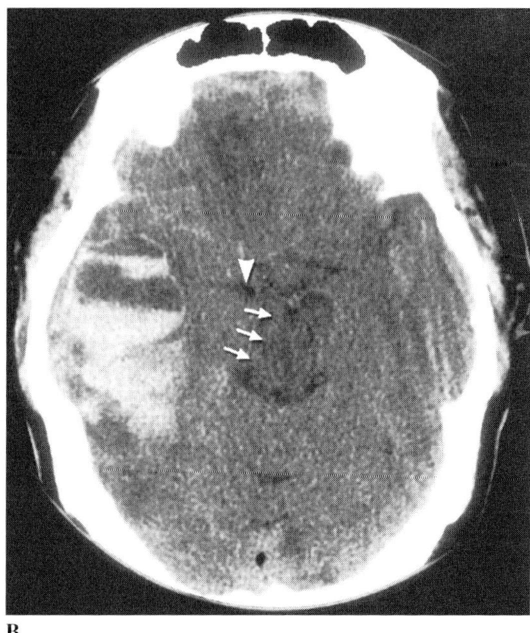

B

Figure 1.11. Patterns of herniation on computed tomography scans. **A.** Meningioma with massive edema causing distortion of the diencephalon (*arrows*) and cingulate herniation (*arrows*). **B.** Large intracranial hematoma in the temporal lobe causing shift of the temporal lobe (see tip of temporal horn [*arrowhead*]) and brain stem distortion (*arrows*) typical of uncal herniation.

tary lesions in nonimmunosuppressed patients most commonly represent intra-axial brain tumors or abscess. On unenhanced images, low density may represent tumor with edema. The degree of edema may reflect the degree of malignancy; rapidly growing tumors, such as glioblastoma, produce much more surrounding edema. Edema is also comparatively common in metastasis.

Most intracranial masses are hypodense, but hyperdense masses may point to a meningioma or lymphoma or hemorrhage into a tumor. Speckled calcification inside a mass, an important CT scan finding, is present in more than 50% of patients with an oligodendroglioma but may point to an inflammatory cause, particularly parasite infestation, such as cysticercosis, and less common disorders, such as paragonimiasis and echinococcosis.[71,72] They are often seen in areas other than the cystic mass, indicating calcium deposits in necrotic brain tissue.

Intracranial mass of inflammatory origin has become a much more common presentation in the emergency department from the increase in transplantation surgery and the AIDS epidemic.

Brain abscesses, usually from toxoplasmosis, are very commonly associated with AIDS infection. Toxoplasmosis seldom appears as a single mass, although one large mass may predominate. Basal ganglia localization is typical, and hemorrhage may occur. Tuberculoma or aspergillosis should be considered as well.[46,52] MRI can be helpful, because a dark (hypointense) T2 signal inside the mass is often found. The most common CT and MRI findings in comatose patients are summarized in Table 1.9.

Normal findings on neuroimaging, with no clinical evidence of an acute cerebellar infarction or acute basilar artery occlusion, should prompt immediate examination of the cerebrospinal fluid to search for possible central nervous system infection. Failure to exclude a potentially treatable central nervous system infection may have devastating consequences. The evaluation of cerebrospinal fluid findings in meningitis and encephalitis is further discussed in Chapters 10 and 11.

Neuroimaging is an obligatory study in patients with possible brain death. The results of neu-

Table 1.9. Frequent Abnormalities on Neuroimaging Studies in Coma

	Findings	Suggested disorders
Computed tomography scan	Mass lesion (brain shift, herniation)	Hematoma, hemorrhagic contusion, MCA territory infarct (see also Table 1.4)
	Hemorrhage in basal cisterns	Aneurysmal SAH, cocaine abuse
	Intraventricular hemorrhage	Arteriovenous malformation
	Multiple hemorrhagic infarcts	Cerebral venous thrombosis
	Multiple cerebral infarcts	Endocarditis, coagulopathy, CNS vasculitis
	Diffuse cerebral edema	Cardiac arrest, fulminant meningitis, acute hepatic necrosis, Reye's syndrome, encephalitis
	Acute hydrocephalus	Aqueduct obstruction, colloid cyst, pineal region tumor
	Pontine or cerebellum hemorrhage	Hypertension, arteriovenous malformation, cavernous malformation
	Shear lesions in the white matter	Head injury
Magnetic resonance imaging	Bilateral caudate and putaminal lesions	Carbon monoxide poisoning
	Hyperdense signal along sagittal, straight, and transverse sinuses	Cerebral venous thrombosis
	Lesions in corpus callosum, white matter	Severe head injury
	Diffuse confluent hyperintense lesions in white matter, basal ganglia	Acute disseminated encephalomyelitis, immunosuppressive agent or chemotherapeutic agent toxicity, metabolic leukodystrophies
	Pontine trident-shaped lesion	Central pontine myelinolysis
	Thalamus, occipital, pontine lesions	Acute basilar artery occlusion
	Temporal, frontal lobe hyperintensities	Herpes simplex encephalitis

(CNS = central nervous system; MCA = middle cerebral artery; SAH = subarachnoid hemorrhage.)

roimaging studies or cerebrospinal fluid examination should be generally compatible with the diagnosis of brain death. Thus, one should expect a large mass lesion producing brain tissue shift with herniation or an intracranial hemorrhage with enlarged ventricles. Other validating CT scan findings are multiple, large acute cerebral infarcts, massive cerebral edema, multiple hemorrhagic contusions, and cerebellar-pontine lesions compressing or destroying the brain stem.

Normal brain images in brain death can be seen immediately after cardiac arrest, carbon monoxide poisoning, asphyxia, acute encephalitis, and cyanide or other fatal poisoning.

Abdominal radiographs can be helpful in establishing whether the patient has ingested any tablets or foreign objects. Examples of radiopaque pills are chloral hydrate, trifluoperazine, amitriptyline, and enteric-coated tablets; however, many tablets may have dissolved before the patient is admitted to the emergency department.

Electrocardiography can be useful, and results are nearly always abnormal if intoxication is due to phenothiazines, quinidine, procainamide, or tricyclic antidepressants. Tricyclic antidepressant overdose characteristically produces widening of the QRS complex and QT prolongation. Widening of the QRS complex considerably increases the risk of seizures associated with tricyclic antidepressant overdose.[24] Electrocardiographic findings are also important in confirming hypothermia as a cause of coma (typically, the QRS complex widens and ST elevation occurs, suggesting a "camel's hump").

When poisoning is strongly considered as a cause of coma, simple bedside tests are essential to rule out toxins before time-consuming toxicologic screening is performed. However, most poisons and illicit drugs do not cause significant laboratory derangements. In fact, if abnormalities are found in a comatose patient, they may be more representative of poor nutrition, dehydration, or a rapidly developing febrile illness.

Acid-base abnormalities, however, may point to certain toxins.[17] A high anion gap acidosis is most common. The most prevalent toxins are shown in Table 1.10. Often, a high anion gap acidosis indicates ethylene glycol or methanol ingestion. Increased lactate, particularly when venous lactate can entirely account for a decrease in serum bicarbonate, may point to previous, often undetected, seizures, shock, and early sepsis.

The anion gap is calculated from the serum electrolytes. Normally, more cations (sodium and potassium) than anions (chloride and bicarbonate) are present, causing an anion gap of 11 to 13 mEq/L. Generally, potassium is deleted from the equation because its extracellular contribution in the anion gap is minimal; therefore, the equation becomes as follows: anion gap = $(Na^+ - [Cl + HCO_3^-])$. Increases in the anion gap result from the additional presence of an anion. Most of the time, it is lactate that increases in serum and creates an anion gap, often originating from poor tissue perfusion. However, additional urine testing is needed to further differentiate the cause of an increased anion gap. Ethylene glycol is another common contender when an increased anion gap is found. Urine microscopy can help demonstrate the additional presence of calcium oxalate crystals.

Salicylates usually produce a combined acid-base abnormality, and respiratory acidosis is often present.[59] The PCO_2 decrease in metabolic acidosis can be calculated ($PCO_2 = [1.5 \times (HCO_3)] + 8 \pm 2$), and a lower PCO_2 should point to additional respiratory alkalosis.

Osmol gap is a useful test to determine accumulation of osmotically active solutes. The normal osmol gap is calculated with the equation 2 × Na + (Glucose/18) + (BUN/2.8). This calculated osmolality is less than the measured osmolarity (the so-called osmol gap) and should be less than 10 mOsm/L. Alcohols of any kind increase the osmol gap, and blood levels can be estimated by multiplying the osmol gap with the molecular weight of the alcohol (46 for ethanol) and dividing the result by a factor of 10.

Urine testing for salicylates is important and can be done with a 10% ferric chloride solution, which turns urine purple if salicylates are present. Urine should be tested for ketones. Ketones in combination with a marked anion gap immediately suggest salicylate poisoning, but this combination can also be observed in alcohol- or diabetes-induced ketoacidosis. The absence of ketones in a patient with anion gap metabolic acidosis suggests ingestion of methanol or ethylene glycol. Urinalysis is also important, specifically in looking for calcium oxalate crystals associated with ethylene glycol (antifreeze) ingestion. The use of Wood's lamp (if available) may be important, because fluorescein is added to many antifreeze products.

Table 1.10. Blood Gas Abnormalities Due to Toxins

Metabolic acidosis (anion gap)	**Respiratory acidosis**
Methanol	Barbiturates
Ethanol	Benzodiazepines
Paraldehyde	Botulism toxin
Isoniazid	Opioids
Ethylene glycol	Organophosphates
Salicylates (other combined)	Strychnine
	Tetrodotoxin
Metabolic alkalosis	**Respiratory alkalosis**
Diuretics	Salicylates
Hyperglycemic nonketotic coma	Amphetamines
Lithium	Anticholinergics
	Cocaine
	Cyanide
	Paraldehyde
	Theophylline
	Carbon monoxide

Many hospitals have laboratories that can provide "drug screens."[73,74] Their value often lies in the demonstration of the toxin rather than quantification. The blood levels of many sedatives and alcohol correlate poorly with depth of coma, duration of mechanical ventilation, and time in the intensive care unit. This lack of correlation applies particularly to patients who attempt suicide with a medication they have taken long enough to cause tolerance.

Many smaller hospitals use thin-layer chromatography, which is less reliable, operator dependent, and unable to quantitate the toxin.[73] Most academic centers can measure with gas chromatography and mass spectrometry. This laboratory investigative tool is powerful and quantitates the toxin. The spectrum of drugs measured in serum is depicted in Appendix 1.1. Physicians assessing patients with poisoning and drug abuse should be well informed about the hospital laboratory practices available. Laboratory confirmation of the clinical diagnosis is often very desirable and may also serve a medicolegal purpose. Delay in the performance of these tests remains a major limitation, and

Table 1.11. Essential Laboratory Tests in the Evaluation of Coma

Hematocrit, white blood cell count
Electrolytes (Na, K, Cl, CO_2, Ca, PO_4)
Glucose
Urea, creatinine
Aspartate transaminase (AST) and γ-glutamyltransferase (GGT)
Osmolality
Arterial blood gases (pH, PCO_2, PO_2, HCO_3, Hb CO) (optional)
Platelets, smear, fibrinogen degeneration products, activated partial thromboplastin time, prothrombin time (optional)
Plasma thyroid-stimulating hormone (optional)
Blood and cerebrospinal fluid cultures (optional)
Toxic screen in blood and urine (optional)
Cerebrospinal fluid (protein, cells, glucose, India ink stain, and cryptococcal antigen, viral titers) (optional)

often the information becomes available too late to be useful in guiding treatment in daily practice.

Blood tests that should be performed include a full hematologic screen and differential cell count, blood glucose, serum osmolality, liver function panel, electrolytes, and renal function tests (Table 1.11). Arterial blood gas measurements further assist in categorizing the major classes of acid-base imbalance, if present. Inspection of blood during arterial puncture is important, because a chocolate brown discoloration indicates methemoglobinemia, usually caused by nitrites (frequently due to contaminated well water), dyes, and topical anesthetics.

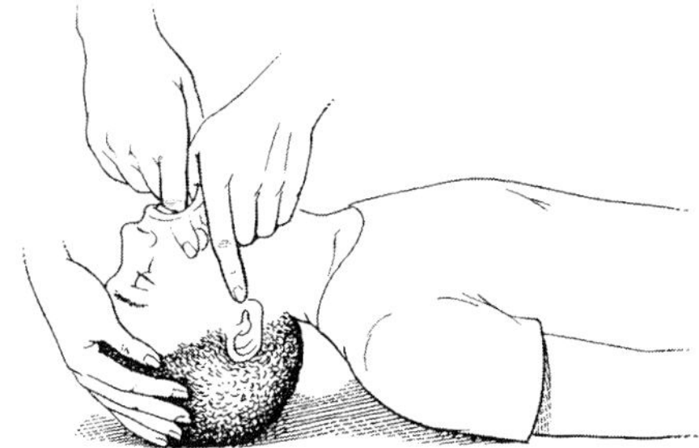

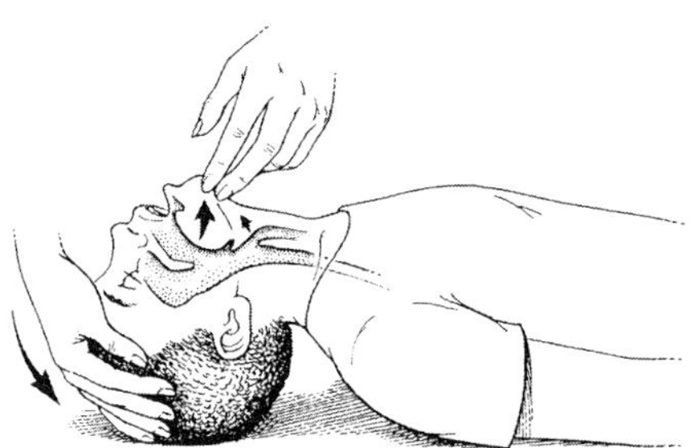

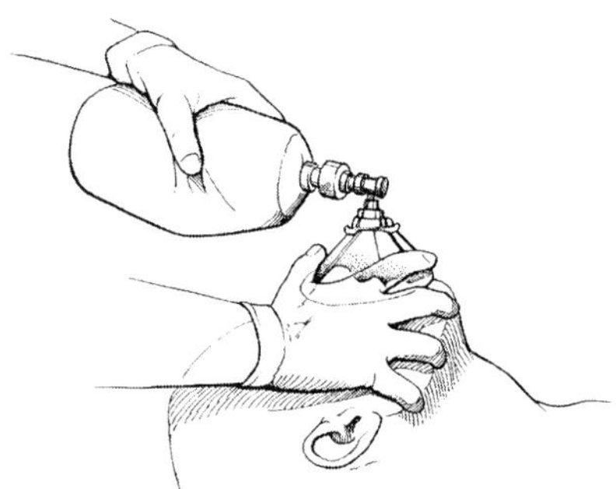

Figure 1.12. Techniques of airway management (see text for description). (From EFM Wijdicks, CO Borel. Respiratory management in acute neurologic illness. Neurology 1998;50:11. By permission of Mayo Foundation.)

Initial Management of Vital Signs in Coma

One of the fundamental responsibilities of the physician faced with the care of a comatose patient is to maintain or correct the vital signs, such as oxygenation, gas exchange, blood pressure, pulse rate, cardiac rhythm, and temperature.

Airway Assessment and Gas Exchange

Obstruction of the airway occurs in comatose patients for several reasons. First, muscles of the floor of the mouth and tongue become reduced in tone, and this changes the anatomical relationships. The tongue is repositioned to the back wall of the oropharynx and obstructs the airway. This position is even more exaggerated when the head is flexed. Therefore, with a simple technique the airway can be reopened. This so-called head-tilt/chin-lift (Figure 1.12) tilts the head backward to what is often called the "sniffing position." In this position, the trachea and pharynx angulation is minimal, allowing for air transport. Also, the index and middle fingers of the examiner's hand lift the mandible and bring the tongue forward.

Another technique is the so-called jaw-thrust/head-tilt. The examiner places the ring, middle, and little fingers underneath the patient's jaw and lifts the chin forward. The examiner's index finger and thumb are free to fit a mask snug to the face, with the other hand free to operate a resuscitation bag.

When the airway appears blocked by foreign material or dentures, this technique is modified by placing the thumb in the mouth, grasping the chin, and pulling it upward, leaving the other hand to clear any obstructing material from the airway (see Figure 1.12).

The adequacy of ventilation with this method can be gauged by movement of the chest, bilateral breath sounds, and oxygenation saturation measured with a pulse oximeter or arterial blood gas sampling.[75]

An oropharyngeal airway should be placed and is essential in patients who recently had a seizure, because it prevents further tongue biting. The placement of this oral airway device is simple. The mouth is opened, a wooden tongue depressor is placed at the base of the tongue, and downward pressure is applied to displace the tongue from the posterior pharyngeal wall. The oropharyngeal tube is then placed close to the posterior wall of the oropharynx and is moved toward the tongue until the teeth are at the bite-block section. Alternatively, the jaw is thrust forward and the device is placed concave toward the palate and then rotated.[75] Dental injury, most commonly in patients who have significant dental or periodontal disease, rarely occurs.

Jaw thrust and mask ventilation securely maintain an open airway but must be followed by endotracheal intubation done by an experienced physician. Endotracheal intubation may be complicated in a traumatized patient with possible cervical spine injury. The ideal solution in these patients is to use fiberoptic bronchoscopy, because with this procedure the risk of further neck trauma from neck movement is very low. Immediate endotracheal intubation is required in patients with penetrating neck trauma or significant intraoral bleeding. Temporarily, a cricothyrotomy can be made. A 14-gauge needle is inserted through the cricothyroid membrane, followed by insertion of a cannula. (The cricothyroid membrane is located just under the thyroid.) A formal tracheostomy should follow because ventilation through this small, highly flow resistant tube is compromised.

The need for endotracheal intubation should be assessed in any patient with a decreased level of consciousness. As a general rule, patients who are unable to rapidly localize a pain stimulus and open their eyes to pain are unlikely to be able to protect the airway from an obstructing tongue and thus require endotracheal intubation.

Hypoxemia is often encountered, and oxygen administration has a high priority in patients with impaired consciousness. The reasons for hypoxemia are not always clear, but abnormal breathing patterns (e.g., Cheyne-Stokes), aspiration, and pulmonary edema are putative mechanisms. Nasal prongs are inefficient, because they provide only 30% oxygen concentrations and often dislodge. Nasopharyngeal catheters provide 60% oxygen concentrations (but only when the tip of the catheter is visible above the soft palate) and are a better alternative. Resuscitation bags are an optimal source of oxygen, and they can deliver FIO_2 above 0.9 when the oxygen flow in the bag is 10 mL/minute. Oxygenation should be monitored with a pulse oximeter (O_2 saturation should exceed 90%) or measurement of an arterial blood gas sample (PaO_2 >100 mm Hg).

Assessment of Circulation and Blood Pressure

Dehydration resulting in reduced intravascular volume is often a cause of hypotension. Hypotension should be corrected by placing the patient in the Trendelenburg position and infusing isotonic saline or blood when indicated in traumatized patients. If blood pressure is not reversed with these measures, hypotension may indicate that the patient has (1) toxic effects from ingestion of a drug that produces vasodilation or myocardial depression, (2) major abdominal trauma, or (3) a life-threatening illness, such as myocardial infarction, pulmonary embolus, or sepsis. It is a misconception to attribute hypotension to catastrophic damage to the brain, which occurs only in patients who are brain dead or who have severe spinal cord injury. Vasoparalysis in brain death results in marked hypotension and may be noted acutely in a rapidly progressing catastrophe. Hypertension, on the other hand, is very common in a patient with an acute structural lesion in the central nervous system. Usually, hypertension is caused by a sympathoadrenal discharge or is part of the Cushing response, particularly when the brain stem is distorted. Acute severe hypertension (>140 mm Hg) may also have its origin in poisoning caused by such agents as amphetamines, cocaine, phencyclidine, and cyclic antidepressants. Often, hypertension in these types of intoxications is associated with significant tachycardia.

The management of acute hypertension in comatose patients is complex. At least theoretically, untreated hypertension may exacerbate cerebral edema in injured areas from increased cerebral blood flow. Too rapid correction of blood pressure may introduce ischemic areas surrounding acute mass lesions from reduction of cerebral perfusion pressure. In patients with longstanding hypertension, the autoregulation curve has shifted to the right, and this further increases the risk of decreased cerebral blood flow with a decrease in blood pressure at this juncture. One should probably avoid extremes, and persistent surges of blood pressure (>120 mm Hg) can be treated with a short-acting α- and β-adrenergic blocking drug, such as labetalol (1 to 2 mg/kg intravenously [IV]; additional 40 mg at 10-minute intervals).

Miscellaneous Care

Patients with hypothermia (defined as core temperature below 34°C) should be gradually warmed. Physicians should be aware that noxious stimuli applied to patients with moderate hypothermia to assess responsiveness can potentially trigger ventricular fibrillation. Virtually all brain stem reflexes are lost when the core temperature reaches 27°C, and they can entirely return after rewarming.

Patients with a core temperature of 32°C to 35°C need to be warmed with blankets, those with a core temperature of 30°C to 32°C are warmed with intravenous infusions, and those with a core temperature below 30°C may need peritoneal lavage with heated dialysate.

All patients in coma for whom the diagnosis is very unclear should receive concentrated dextrose (50% dextrose, 50 mL, 25 g IV). The well-known adrenergic symptoms from the counterregulating hormone epinephrine, such as sweating, tremor, and tachycardia, may not be present when hypoglycemia has developed more or less gradually. However, its use in patients in whom the proximate cause of coma is known is ill-advised.

Wernicke's encephalopathy is a rare cause of coma.[76] However, if chronic alcohol abuse or malnourishment is suspected during the physical examination, a "routine" glucose infusion may precipitate acute Wernicke's encephalopathy. To prevent this, 100 mg of thiamine should be administered IV (slowly over 5 minutes) or intramuscularly. Indiscriminate use of thiamine in comatose patients is potentially dangerous because of acute anaphylactic reactions and acute pulmonary edema.

Cardiac arrhythmias often define the severity of the intoxication in patients with an overdose of a cyclic antidepressant drug. Sodium bicarbonate, 1 to 2 mEq/kg IV, is advised when the QRS interval narrows. In patients with sympathomimetic agent intoxication resulting in tachycardia, esmolol can be used: 500 μg/kg over 1 minute followed by an infusion of 50 μg/kg per minute for 4 minutes; maximum maintenance dose is 200 μg/kg per minute. If tachycardia is caused by an anticholinergic overdose, physostigmine, 0.01 to 0.03 mg/kg IV, is used.[77] Patients with ventricular fibrillation or ventricular tachycardia associated with amphetamines or overdose should be treated with lidocaine, 1 to 3 mg/kg IV up to 300 mg in a 1-hour period.

Management in Specific Causes of Coma

Supratentorial Mass Lesions

Patients with a mass lesion that causes shift of brain structures need immediate management of increased intracranial pressure. If available, intracranial pressure monitoring should be inserted to monitor increases in intracranial pressure and possible development of plateau waves that indicate imminent decompensation of the brain compliance. Transfer to a neurologic or neurosurgical intensive care unit is imperative.

The most successful management of increased intracranial pressure is a combination of hyperventilation and osmotic diuretics. The most successful method of decreasing intracranial pressure is the brief use of hyperventilation (aiming at a $PaCO_2$ of

30 mm Hg) and equally effective use of osmotic diuretics, such as mannitol (aiming at an increase in plasma osmolality of 310 mOsm/L). Hyperventilation results in profound vasoconstriction from hypocapnea and reduces cerebral blood flow, thus contributing to reduction of the intracranial volume. One may expect cerebral blood flow to decrease 40% in 30 minutes if the PCO_2 is reduced by 15 to 20 mm Hg.[78] However, the physiologic effects of hyperventilation are less significant after several hours, because efficient buffering systems rapidly correct changes in cerebrospinal fluid pH. Its effect is short, probably hours.[79]

Hyperventilation can be easily instituted by changing the respiratory rate on the mechanical ventilator. The respiratory rate should be increased to approximately 20 breaths/minute while a normal tidal volume is maintained. Increasing minute ventilation by changing both components is ill-advised, because it may lead to high airway pressures and increases the risk of barotrauma.

In addition, hyperosmolar agents, preferably mannitol, should be administered, starting with a 20% solution at a dose of 1 g/kg.[80] The effect on intracranial pressure is rapid and may last for at least 4 hours. Mannitol essentially decreases brain volume by extracting water from brain tissue.[81] This influx to the intravascular compartment is generated by an osmotic gradient. Mannitol, therefore, expands the blood volume just before its diuretic action, hence the name "osmotic diuretic." First, a bolus of 1 g/kg of body weight is given. If no effect is seen after 15 minutes, a double dose is administered. The effect of mannitol is at least twofold. First, infusion of mannitol produces an osmotic gradient between the intravascular component and the brain. Second, a more complex mechanism of mannitol is a possible rheologic effect.[82] Mannitol reduces hematocrit and blood viscosity, thereby increasing cerebral blood flow. Vasoconstriction becomes a compensatory reflex and reduces cerebral blood volume. This mechanism rather than diuresis, which usually is seen at a later stage, may be the prime means by which mannitol causes a rapid response.

Failure of the patient to improve with hyperventilation and mannitol indicates that surgical evacuation of the mass should be considered. When swelling of one hemisphere is prominent, decompressive craniotomy with duraplasty can be considered. Preliminary studies in patients with encephalitis and a large hemispheric infarction have shown promise.

Table 1.12. Management of Acute Supratentorial Mass with Brain Shift

Stabilizing measures
Protect airway: intubate
Correct hypoxemia with O_2 nasal catheter or face mask, 3–4 L/min
Elevate head to 30°
Treat extreme agitation with lorazepam, 2 mg intravenously
Correct coagulopathy with fresh-frozen plasma, vitamin K (if applicable)
Specific medical measures
Hyperventilation: increase respiratory rate to 20 breaths/min, aim at PCO_2 of 25–30 mm Hg
Mannitol 20%, 1 g/kg; if no effect, 2 g/kg; aim at plasma osmolality of 310 mOsm/L
Dexamethasone, 100 mg intravenously (in tumors only)
Specific surgical measures
Evacuation of hematoma
Placement of drain in abscess
Decompressive craniotomy in brain swelling of one hemisphere

Corticosteroids should be considered in patients who have edema surrounding a cerebral metastatic lesion or primary brain tumor. There is no proof that corticosteroids improve outcome in patients with other mass lesions, such as intracranial hematoma, closed head injury, infarction, and cerebral abscess.[83,84] Corticosteroid therapy is usually initiated with a single 100-mg dose of dexamethasone given IV, and this is followed by a 16-mg daily dose.

The management of acute supratentorial mass lesions is summarized in Table 1.12.

Subtentorial Lesions

Acute posterior fossa lesions that evolve into coma from a compressive brain stem lesion need immediate neurosurgical evacuation. Only occasionally does decreased level of consciousness result from an evolving hydrocephalus, and then ventriculostomy improves the degree of responsiveness. A cerebellar hematoma or cerebellar infarct is a neurosurgical emergency, and posterior craniotomy is necessary to remove the hematoma or necrotic tissue.

Table 1.13. Management of Acute Subtentorial Mass or Brain Stem Lesion

Stabilizing measures
- Intubation and mechanical ventilation
- Correct hypoxemia with 3 L of O_2/min
- Flat body position (in acute basilar artery occlusion)

Specific medical measures
- Intra-arterial urokinase (in basilar artery occlusion)
- Mannitol 20%, 1 g/kg (in acute cerebellar mass)
- Hyperventilation to PCO_2 of 25–50 mm Hg (in acute cerebellar mass)

Specific surgical measures
- Ventriculostomy
- Suboccipital craniotomy

An intrinsic lesion of the brain stem is usually best initially treated medically with endotracheal intubation and mechanical ventilation. Patients with acute basilar artery occlusion should be placed in a flat body position to augment blood pressure, and intra-arterial thrombolysis, if available, should be considered. Although this therapy is evolving, we have been able to reverse a virtually locked-in syndrome in acute basilar occlusion by using intra-arterial thrombolysis with urokinase. Specific management in subtentorial lesions is summarized in Table 1.13.

Infectious Disorders

Comatose patients with infectious disease have fever and meningeal irritation at presentation. If focal neurologic signs are present, the three steps to take are (1) an immediate intravenous infusion with antibiotics, (2) a CT scan to exclude an abscess, and (3) a lumbar puncture for final culture of the offending organism.

Patients with acute viral encephalitis may be in a coma at presentation without any other localizing neurologic signs. The history obtained from family members may reveal fluctuating aphasia, seizures, or significant confusion before the lapse into unresponsiveness. It is important to immediately start an infusion of acyclovir. In herpes simplex encephalitis, outcome is largely determined by early treatment; however, the prospects for full recovery remain small in patients in stupor or coma.

With the emergence of immunosuppression (particularly in the human immunodeficiency virus population), toxoplasma encephalitis should be considered. Initial treatment remains empiric and includes pyrimethamine and sulfadiazine, particularly in patients with multiple abscesses. In endemic areas, patients in coma may have cysticercosis associated with *Taenia solium* infestation, and immediate treatment with praziquantel is required. It is important to start these treatments early, after consulting an infectious disease specialist. The initial management in these acute inflammatory conditions of the central nervous system is summarized in Table 1.14.

Table 1.14. Empirical Antibiotic and Antiviral Therapy in Patients in Coma Associated with Inflammatory Conditions

Antibacterial	Cefotaxime, 1–2 g every 6 hours
	Vancomycin, 2 g every 12 hours
Antiviral	Acyclovir, 10 mg/kg every 8 hours
Antiparasitic	Pyrimethamine, 75 mg p.o.
	Sulfadiazine, 2–8 g p.o. divided every 6 hours
	Praziquantel, 75 mg/kg/day

See also Chapters 9 and 10.

Acute Metabolic Derangements and Poisoning

No harm is done if patients with a high likelihood of hypoglycemia are given 50 mL of a 50% glucose solution. Immediate awakening during infusion is highly indicative of severe hypoglycemia. Failure to awaken, however, may indicate that coma is not caused by hypoglycemia (in fact, in many situations) or that hypoglycemia has been lengthy and has caused significant brain damage leading to prolonged or no recovery.

Management of severe hyponatremia involves hypertonic saline and furosemide (3% hypertonic saline, 0.5 mL/kg per hour) with frequent serum sodium surveillance. Overcorrection (≥140 μg/L) and rapid correction (within 12 hours) have been linked to the development of central pontine myelinolysis.

Hypercalcemia is adequately corrected by saline rehydration infusion (3 to 4 L) followed by parenteral biphosphonate pamidronate (infused at 60 mg over 24 hours).

The use of a "coma cocktail" in assessing and managing coma of undetermined cause must be questioned.[85] Usually, this "cocktail" consists of a combination of hypertonic dextrose, thiamine hydrochloride, naloxone hydrochloride, and, recently, flumazenil.[86] Its use must be discouraged simply because of the possible side effects of naloxone and flumazenil. Naloxone has great efficacy but also potentially serious side effects, such as aspiration from rapid arousal and development of a florid withdrawal syndrome[87] characterized by agitation, diaphoresis, hypertension, dysrhythmias, and pulmonary edema.[87,88] In addition, after 30 minutes, the patient may again lapse into coma, which if unwitnessed may cause significant respiratory depression and respiratory arrest. A more prudent approach is to prophylactically intubate the patient and to gradually reverse the overdose of opiates by use of naloxone, 0.4 to 2 mg every 3 minutes by incremental doubling. At the first sign of relapse, 0.4 to 4 mg of naloxone can be given IV[89] or an infusion of 0.8 mg/kg per hour started. Failure to reverse coma from alleged opiate overdose has many causes, and they are summarized in Table 1.15.

Flumazenil reverses the effect of any benzodiazepine but has the same major disadvantages as naloxone—rapid arousal and risk of life-threatening aspiration pneumonitis. In addition, when high doses of flumazenil are administered, seizures may occur.[90,91] Therefore, flumazenil is contraindicated in patients with a seizure disorder and in patients in whom concomitant tricyclic antidepressant intoxication is suspected.[9,90] When flumazenil is administered, cardiac arrhythmias may occur, and status epilepticus has been reported in patients who had an overdose of tricyclic antidepressants and received treatment with flumazenil.[90] The recommended dose of flumazenil, by slow intravenous administration, is 0.2 mg/minute up to a total dose of 1 mg.[28] We seldom use flumazenil to reverse coma. Benzodiazepine overdose, in general, is not life-threatening and can be managed by supportive care only.

Inducing emesis in a patient who is stuporous from poisoning may be a mistake because of the significant danger of aspiration. Gastric lavage, which is possible if a comatose patient is protected by endotracheal intubation, should be done if the suspicion of a massive overdose is great. Also, activated charcoal (60 to 100 g) can be delivered through the gastric tube. Placement of the tube in

Table 1.15. Differential Diagnosis in Failure to Reverse Coma from Alleged Opiate Overdose

Head injury, traumatic intracerebral hematoma
Hypoglycemia
Anoxic-ischemic encephalopathy
Mixed overdose with drug in another category (e.g., cocaine, ethanol)
Central nervous system infection, systemic infection, sepsis
Seizures, nonconvulsive status epilepticus (rare)

Data from Goldfrank et al.[30]

the stomach before administration of charcoal should be confirmed by radiography, because charcoal deposition in the lung is often fatal. The technique of gastric lavage includes placement of the patient in the left lateral decubitus position after intubation of the trachea with a cuffed endotracheal tube. This position greatly facilitates drainage. The largest possible gastric tube should be inserted through the nose or mouth into the stomach and checked often with air insufflation while the physician listens over the stomach. The stomach aspirate should be investigated for possible toxins, and activated charcoal should be administered before lavage is started. Charcoal absorbs material that cannot be removed by active suctioning and that may enter the intestine. Lukewarm tap water or saline in 200-mL aliquots up to a total of 2 L is infused and aspirated until no pills or toxic material is observed.

Elimination of the toxin can also be enhanced by hemodialysis and hemoperfusion, and many drugs and toxins can be cleared (the most common are acetaminophen, amitriptyline, lithium, and salicylates).

Coma of Unknown Origin

The management of coma of undetermined cause is full intensive care support and observation over time while a more detailed history and laboratory test results are awaited. When no cause of decreased arousal or coma is found and results of laboratory tests including CT scan or MRI and cerebrospinal fluid examination are negative, unidentified toxin exposure or poisoning should be considered. However, toxin exposure may have resulted in significant hypoxemic-ischemic damage, which may cause persistent coma.[92] Electroencephalography may be helpful to exclude nonconvulsive status epilepticus or prolonged postictal state despite no documentation of a seizure.

Basilar artery migraine may produce drowsiness, confusion, and prolonged amnesia and may progress to coma.[93] Typically, a strong family history of common migraine exists. Of the patients originally reported by Bickerstaff,[93] about 80% had a positive family history. Basilar artery migraine is more prevalent in children but may persist through adulthood, often converting later into common migraine. The clinical presentation is impressive. Visual hallucinations, bilateral zigzag forms or photopsia, and even sudden blindness or grayouts may occur as a result of hypoperfusion of the occipital lobes. Most of the time, patients present with vertigo, ataxia, diplopia, dysarthria, and tinnitus from ischemia to the brain stem. Bilateral throbbing headache may last for hours, commonly with vomiting, after resolution of the neurologic deficits. Coma remains uncommon in basilar migraine. More commonly, patients with migraine become drowsy or stuporous from overmedication, particularly with narcotics. A retrospective review in a large series of patients noted stupor or coma in 24% of 49 patients and more often "somnolence."[93] Bickerstaff's original descriptions highlight gradual onset of a dreamlike state. Seizures may occur and can be documented on electroencephalograms at the time of a full-blown attack. The precise nature of the disorder is unresolved. Unfortunately, brain stem infarcts may occur, with a fatal outcome.[94]

A recently reported disorder characterized by spells of sudden coma has been linked to increased endogenous production of benzodiazepines ("endozepine stupor").[95] Patients may awaken immediately after administration of flumazenil. The prevalence of this disorder, recently termed "idiopathic recurrent stupor," is unknown.

Psychogenic unresponsiveness should always be considered after all laboratory test results are negative. Unfortunately, many of these patients have already received a battery of laboratory tests even though the discrepancies with detailed clinical examination are very obvious. Most often, psychogenic unresponsiveness lasts for only 1 or 2 days, with characteristic sudden unexpected "awakening" and often complete amnesia for the episode and also for events during many months preceding hospital admission.

Malignant neuroleptic syndrome and catatonia may produce decreased responsiveness and are fatal if untreated. Profound rigidity and continuous autonomic storm with impressive tachycardia, hypertension, and profuse sweating may result in cardiac arrest (from subendocardial and myocardial hemorrhages) or renal failure (due to severe acidosis from massive rhabdomyolysis). Immediate therapy with dantrolene is needed (2 mg/kg every 5 minutes to a total dose of 10 mg/kg). Electroshock is preferred in lethal catatonia, and only after multiple series can improvement become clinically apparent.

Hereditary metabolic disorders may be manifested by impaired consciousness during adolescence. These disorders are exceptionally uncommon but should be excluded when the cause of coma is unknown. These disorders are acute porphyria (psychosis rather than coma and seizures in some), mitochondrial encephalopathies, and necrotizing encephalopathy of Leigh. Acute porphyria often has resulted in earlier visits to the emergency room because of "abdominal colic" or a chronic pain syndrome. It can be diagnosed by demonstrating increased δ-aminolevulinic acid and porphobilinogen in the urine.

The mitochondrial encephalopathies include MELAS syndrome (mitochondrial encephalopathy, lactic acidosis, and stroke-like episodes), Kearns-Sayre syndrome, and Leigh's disease. Lactic acidosis with increased lactate and pyruvate as well as typical MRI abnormalities (MELAS: cortical T2-weighted hyperintensities in both cerebral hemispheres and cerebellum; Leigh: bilateral putamen lesions) should suggest the diagnosis. Evaluation is very complex and outside the scope of this book.

References

1. Dunn C, Held JL, Spitz J, et al. Coma blisters: report and review. Cutis 1990;45:423.
2. Bauby J-D. The Diving Bell and the Butterfly. (English translation by J Leggatt.) New York: Alfred A Knopf, 1997.
3. Teasdale G, Jennett B. Assessment of coma and impaired consciousness. A practical scale. Lancet 1974;2:81.
4. Teasdale G, Knill-Jones R, van der Sande J. Observer

variability in assessing impaired consciousness and coma. J Neurol Neurosurg Psychiatry 1978;41:603.
5. Rush C. The history of the Glasgow coma scale: an interview with professor Bryan Jennett. Int J Trauma Nurs 1997;3:114.
6. Wijdicks EFM. Temporomandibular joint compression in coma. Neurology 1996;46:1774.
7. Wijdicks EFM, Kokmen E, O'Brien PC. Measurement of impaired consciousness in the neurological intensive care unit: a new test. J Neurol Neurosurg Psychiatry 1998;64:117.
8. Wijdicks EFM. Determining brain death in adults. Neurology 1995;45:1003.
9. Chern TL, Hu SC, Lee CH, et al. Diagnostic and therapeutic utility of flumazenil in comatose patients with drug overdose. Am J Emerg Med 1993;11:122.
10. Plum F, Posner JB. The Diagnosis of Stupor or Coma, 3rd ed. Philadelphia: FA Davis Company, 1982.
11. Wijdicks EFM. Intracranial Hemorrhage. In GB Young, AH Ropper, CF Bolton (eds). Coma and Impaired Consciousness: A Clinical Perspective. New York: McGraw-Hill, 1998;131.
12. Ropper AH. A preliminary MRI study of the geometry of brain displacement and level of consciousness with acute intracranial masses. Neurology 1989;39:622.
13. Ropper AH, Gress D. Computerized tomography and clinical features of large cerebral hemorrhages. Cerebrovasc Dis 1991;1:38.
14. Wijdicks EFM, Miller GM. MR imaging of progressive downward herniation of the diencephalon. Neurology 1997;48:1456.
15. Wijdicks EFM, Miller GM. Transient locked-in syndrome after uncal herniation. Neurology 1999;52:1296.
16. Wijdicks EFM, Maus TP, Piepgras DG. Cerebellar swelling and massive brain stem distortion: spontaneous resolution documented by MRI. J Neurol Neurosurg Psychiatry 1998;65:400.
17. Nice A, Leikin JB, Maturen A, et al. Toxidrome recognition to improve efficiency of emergency urine drug screens. Ann Emerg Med 1988;17:676.
18. Charness ME, Simon RP, Greenberg DA. Ethanol and the nervous system. N Engl J Med 1989;321:442.
19. Klatsky AL, Friedman GD, Siegelaub AB. Alcohol and mortality. A ten-year Kaiser-Permanente experience. Ann Intern Med 1981;95:139.
20. Reed CE, Driggs MF, Foote CC. Acute barbiturate intoxication: a study of 300 cases based on a physiologic system of classification of the severity of the intoxication. Ann Intern Med 1952;37:290.
21. Henderson A, Wright M, Pond SM. Experience with 732 acute overdose patients admitted to an intensive care unit over six years. Med J Aust 1993;158:28.
22. White A. Overdose of tricyclic antidepressants associated with absent brain-stem reflexes. CMAJ 1988; 139:133.
23. Hultén BA, Heath A. Clinical aspects of tricyclic antidepressant poisoning. Acta Med Scand 1983;213:275.
24. Boehnert MT, Lovejoy FH Jr. Value of the QRS duration versus the serum drug level in predicting seizures and ventricular arrhythmias after an acute overdose of tricyclic antidepressants. N Engl J Med 1985; 313:474.
25. Sansone ME, Ziegler DK. Lithium toxicity: a review of neurologic complications. Clin Neuropharmacol 1985; 8:242.
26. Greenblatt DJ, Allen MD, Noel BJ, Shader RI. Acute overdosage with benzodiazepine derivatives. Clin Pharmacol Ther 1977;21:497.
27. Greenblatt DJ, Shader RI, Abernethy DR. Drug therapy. Current status of benzodiazepines. N Engl J Med 1983;309:354.
28. Weinbroum A, Rudick V, Sorkine P, Nevo Y, et al. Use of flumazenil in the treatment of drug overdose: a double-blind and open clinical study in 110 patients. Crit Care Med 1996;24:199.
29. Haddad LM, Roberts JR. A General Approach to the Emergency Management of Poisoning. In LM Haddad, JF Winchester (eds). Clinical Management of Poisoning and Drug Overdose, 2nd ed. Philadelphia: WB Saunders Company, 1990; 2.
30. Goldfrank LR, Flomenbaum NE, Lewin NA, Weisman RS, et al. Goldfrank's Toxicologic Emergencies, 6th ed. Norwalk, CT: Appleton & Lange, 1998.
31. Brust JCM. Neurological Aspects of Substance Abuse. Boston: Butterworth–Heinemann, 1993.
32. Aniline O, Pitts FN Jr. Phencyclidine (PCP): a review and perspectives. Crit Rev Toxicol 1982;10:145.
33. McCarron MM. Phencyclidine intoxication. NIDA Res Monogr 1986;64:209.
34. Gawin FH, Ellinwood EH Jr. Cocaine and other stimulants. Actions, abuse, and treatment. N Engl J Med 1988;318:1173.
35. Dhuna A, Pascual-Leone A, Langendorf F, Anderson DC. Epileptogenic properties of cocaine in humans. Neurotoxicology 1991;12:621.
36. Choy-Kwong M, Lipton RB. Seizures in hospitalized cocaine users. Neurology 1989;39:425.
37. Lowenstein DH, Massa SM, Rowbotham MC, Collins SD, et al. Acute neurologic and psychiatric complications associated with cocaine abuse. Am J Med 1987;83:841.
38. Golbe LI, Merkin MD. Cerebral infarction in a user of free-base cocaine ("crack"). Neurology 1986;36:1602.
39. Levine SR, Brust JC, Futrell N, Ho KL, et al. Cerebrovascular complications of the use of the "crack" form of alkaloidal cocaine. N Engl J Med 1990; 323:699.
40. Wojak JC, Flamm ES. Intracranial hemorrhage and cocaine use. Stroke 1987;18:712.
41. Storen E, Wijdicks EFM, Crum B, Schultz G. Chronic occlusive cerebral arterial disease from cocaine use (abstract). Ann Neurol (in press).

42. Pasternak GW. Pharmacological mechanisms of opioid analgesics. Clin Neuropharmacol 1993;16:1.
43. Ginsberg MD. Carbon monoxide intoxication: clinical features, neuropathology and mechanisms of injury. J Toxicol Clin Toxicol 1985;23:281.
44. Krantz T, Thisted B, Strom J, Sorensen MB. Acute carbon monoxide poisoning. Acta Anaesthesiol Scand 1988;32:278.
45. Miura T, Mitomo M, Kawai R, Harada K. CT of the brain in acute carbon monoxide intoxication: characteristic features and prognosis. AJNR Am J Neuroradiol 1985;6:739.
46. Carrazana EJ, Rossitch E Jr, Morris J. Isolated central nervous system aspergillosis in the acquired immunodeficiency syndrome. Clin Neurol Neurosurg 1991; 93:227.
47. Sawada Y, Takahashi M, Ohashi N, Fusamoto H, et al. Computerised tomography as an indication of long-term outcome after acute carbon monoxide poisoning. Lancet 1980;1:783.
48. Horowitz AL, Kaplan R, Sarpel G. Carbon monoxide toxicity: MR imaging in the brain. Radiology 1987;162:787.
49. Ziser A, Shupak A, Halpern P, Gozal D, et al. Delayed hyperbaric oxygen treatment for acute carbon monoxide poisoning. BMJ 1984;289:960.
50. Losek JD, Rock AL, Boldt RR. Cyanide poisoning from a cosmetic nail remover. Pediatrics 1991;88:337.
51. Vogel SN, Sultan TR, Ten Eyck RP. Cyanide poisoning. Clin Toxicol 1981;18:367.
52. Carella F, Grassi MP, Savoiardo M, Contri P, et al. Dystonic-Parkinsonian syndrome after cyanide poisoning: clinical and MRI findings. J Neurol Neurosurg Psychiatry 1988;51:1345.
53. Rosenberg NL, Myers JA, Martin WR. Cyanide-induced parkinsonism: clinical, MRI, and 6-fluorodopa PET studies. Neurology 1989;39:142.
54. Peterson CD, Collins AJ, Himes JM, Bullock ML, et al. Ethylene glycol poisoning: pharmacokinetics during therapy with ethanol and hemodialysis. N Engl J Med 1981;304:21.
55. Rubinstein D, Escott E, Kelly JP. Methanol intoxication with putaminal and white matter necrosis: MR and CT findings. AJNR Am J Neuroradiol 1995;16:1492.
56. Guggenheim MA, Couch JR, Weinberg W. Motor dysfunction as a permanent complication of methanol ingestion. Presentation of a case with a beneficial response to levodopa treatment. Arch Neurol 1971;24:550.
57. Jacobsen D, Hewlett TP, Webb R, et al. Ethylene glycol intoxication: evaluation of kinetics and crystalluria. Am J Med 1988;84:145.
58. Brent J, McMartin K, Phillips S, et al. Fomepizole for the treatment of ethylene glycol poisoning. N Engl J Med 1999;340:832.
59. Hill JB. Salicylate intoxication. N Engl J Med 1973;288:1110.
60. Needs CJ, Brooks PM. Clinical pharmacokinetics of the salicylates. Clin Pharmacokinet 1985;10:164.
61. Flanagan RJ, Mant TG. Coma and metabolic acidosis early in severe acute paracetamol poisoning. Hum Toxicol 1986;5:179.
62. Bray GP, Harrison PM, O'Grady JG, et al. Long-term anticonvulsant therapy worsens outcome in paracetamol-induced fulminant hepatic failure. Hum Exp Toxicol 1992;11:265.
63. Lauterburg BH, Velez ME. Glutathione deficiency in alcoholics: risk factor for paracetamol hepatotoxicity. Gut 1988;29:1153.
64. Stilman N, Masdeu JC. Incidence of seizures with phenytoin toxicity. Neurology 1985;35:1769.
65. Schmidt S, Schmitz-Buhl M. Signs and symptoms of carbamazepine overdose. J Neurol 1995;242:169.
66. Sullivan JB Jr, Rumack BH, Peterson RG. Acute carbamazepine toxicity resulting from overdose. Neurology 1981;31:621.
67. Weaver DF, Camfield P, Fraser A. Massive carbamazepine overdose: clinical and pharmacologic observations in five episodes. Neurology 1988;38:755.
68. Spiller HA, Krenzelok EP, Cookson E. Carbamazepine overdose: a prospective study of serum levels and toxicity. J Toxicol Clin Toxicol 1990;28:445.
69. Dreifuss FE, Langer DH, Moline KA, Maxwell JE. Valproic acid hepatic fatalities. II. US experience since 1984. Neurology 1989;39:201.
70. Osborn AG. Diagnosis of descending transtentorial herniation by cranial computed tomography. Radiology 1977;123:93.
71. Rodriguez JC, Gutierrez RA, Valdes OD, Dorfsman JF. The role of computed axial tomography in the diagnosis and treatment of brain inflammatory and parasitic lesions: our experience in Mexico. Neuroradiology 1978;16:458.
72. Sotelo J, Guerrero V, Rubio F. Neurocysticercosis: a new classification based on active and inactive forms. A study of 753 cases. Arch Intern Med 1985;145:442.
73. Helliwell M, Hampel G, Sinclair E, et al. Value of emergency toxicological investigations in differential diagnosis of coma. BMJ 1979;2:819.
74. Hepler BR, Sutheimer CA, Sunshine I. The role of the toxicology laboratory in emergency medicine. II. Study of an integrated approach. J Toxicol Clin Toxicol 1984;22:503.
75. Wijdicks EFM, Borel CO. Respiratory management in acute neurologic illness. Neurology 1998;50:11.
76. Kearsley JH, Musso AF. Hypothermia and coma in the Wernicke-Korsakoff syndrome. Med J Aust 1980; 2:504.
77. Nattel S, Bayne L, Ruedy J. Physostigmine in coma due to drug overdose. Clin Pharmacol Ther 1979;25:96.
78. Raichle ME, Posner JB, Plum F. Cerebral blood flow during and after hyperventilation. Arch Neurol 1970;23:394.
79. Muizelaar JP, van der Poel HG, Li ZC, Kontos HA, et al. Pial arteriolar vessel diameter and CO_2 reactivity during prolonged hyperventilation in the rabbit. J Neurosurg 1988;69:923.

80. Marshall LF, Smith RW, Rauscher LA, Shapiro HM. Mannitol dose requirements in brain-injured patients. J Neurosurg 1978;48:169.
81. Nath F, Galbraith S. The effect of mannitol on cerebral white matter water content. J Neurosurg 1986;65:41.
82. Muizelaar JP, Wei EP, Kontos HA, Becker DP. Mannitol causes compensatory cerebral vasoconstriction and vasodilation in response to blood viscosity changes. J Neurosurg 1983;59:822.
83. Braakman R, Schouten HJ, Blaauw-van Dishoeck M, Minderhoud JM. Megadose steroids in severe head injury. Results of a prospective double-blind clinical trial. J Neurosurg 1983;58:326.
84. Dearden NM, Gibson JS, McDowall DG, et al. Effect of high-dose dexamethasone on outcome from severe head injury. J Neurosurg 1986;64:81.
85. Hoffman RS, Goldfrank LR. The poisoned patient with altered consciousness. Controversies in the use of a 'coma cocktail.' JAMA 1995;274:562.
86. Votey SR, Bosse GM, Bayer MJ, Hoffman JR. Flumazenil: a new benzodiazepine antagonist. Ann Emerg Med 1991;20:181.
87. Hoffman JR, Schriger DL, Luo JS. The empiric use of naloxone in patients with altered mental status: a reappraisal. Ann Emerg Med 1991;20:246.
88. Prough DS, Roy R, Bumgarner J, Shannon G. Acute pulmonary edema in healthy teenagers following conservative doses of intravenous naloxone. Anesthesiology 1984;60:485.
89. Goldfrank L, Weisman RS, Errick JK, Lo MW. A dosing nomogram for continuous infusion intravenous naloxone. Ann Emerg Med 1986;15:566.
90. Gueye PN, Hoffman JR, Taboulet P, et al. Empiric use of flumazenil in comatose patients: limited applicability of criteria to define low risk. Ann Emerg Med 1996;27:730.
91. Spivey WH. Flumazenil and seizures: analysis of 43 cases. Clin Ther 1992;14:292.
92. Auerbach PS. Wilderness Medicine: Management of Wilderness and Environment Emergencies, 3rd ed. St Louis: Mosby, 1995.
93. Bickerstaff ER. Basilar artery migraine. Handbook Clin Neurol 1986;48:135.
94. Caplan LR. Migraine and vertebrobasilar ischemia. Neurology 1991;41:55.
95. Lugaresi E, Montagna P, Tinuper P, et al. Endozepine stupor: recurring stupor linked to endozepine-4 accumulation. Brain 1998;121:127.

Appendix 1.1

Drug Screening Tests (Chromatographic Techniques)

Analgesics

Acetaminophen*
Acetylsalicylate
Chlorzoxazone
Codeine
Dicyclomine
Fenoprofen
Flurbiprofen
Hydrocodone
Ibuprofen
Indomethacin
Ketoprofen
Meperidine
Methaqualone
Morphine
Naproxen*
Pentazocine
Propoxyphene*
Salicylate*
Tramadol

Antidepressants

Amitriptyline*
Bupropion
Clomipramine*
Desipramine*
Doxepin*
Fluoxetine*
Imipramine*
Maprotiline
Nortriptyline*
Sertraline*
Trazodone*
Trimipramine
Venlafaxine*

Stimulants

Amphetamine
Benzoylecgonine
Benztropine
Caffeine
Cocaine
Cyclobenzaprine
Ethyl-benzoylecgonine
Methamphetamine
Phencyclidine
Phentermine
Strychnine

Sympathomimetics

Brompheniramine
Chlorpheniramine
Diphenhydramine*

If serum is submitted for analysis, quantitative reports often are issued for the drugs marked by an asterisk (*), with a therapeutic, toxic, or potentially lethal range referenced on the report. *Drugs in italics* can be detected only in urine. If serum is submitted for analysis, these drugs will not be detected, even at toxic levels. Data from WH Porter, TP Moyer. Clinical Toxicology. In CA Burtis, ER Ashwood (eds). Tietz Textbook of Clinical Chemistry, 2nd ed. Philadelphia: WB Saunders Company, 1994;1155.

Doxylamine
Ephedrine
Hydroxyzine
Phenylephrine
Phenylpropanolamine
Phenyltoloxamine
Pseudoephedrine

Antiepileptics

Carbamazepine*
N-desmethyl-methsuximide
Ethosuximide*
Felbamate*
Lamotrigine
Mephobarbital*
Methsuximide*
Phenobarbital*
Phenytoin*
Primidone*
Valproic acid*

Cardioactive agents

Diltiazem
Lidocaine*
Quinidine*
Verapamil

Tranquilizers

Chlordiazepoxide*
Chlorpromazine
Clozapine
Desalkyl flurazepam
Diazepam*
Flunitrazepam
Flurazepam
Hydroxyethyl flurazepam
Lorazepam
Midazolam
Nordiazepam
Oxazepam
Prochlorperazine
Promethazine
Temazepam
Thioridazine*
Trifluoperazine

Hypoglycemics

Acetohexamide
Chlorpropamide
Tolazamide
Tolbutamide

Sedatives and hypnotics

Allobarbital
Amobarbital*
Aprobarbital
Barbital
Butabarbital*
Butalbital*
Carisoprodol
Ethchlorvynol
Glutethimide
Meprobamate*
Metharbital
Methyprylon
Pentobarbital*
Secobarbital*
Thiopental
Zolpidem

Other

Dextromethorphan
Gemfibrozil
Methadone
Metoclopramide
Metronidazole
Pentoxifylline
Phenylbutazone
Sulfadiazine
Sulfamethoxazole
Sulfapyridine
Sulfisoxazole
Theophylline*
Ticlopidine

Chapter 2
Brain Edema

Brain edema at its core, particularly when profound and widespread, displaces brain tissue and results in impairment of consciousness. Diffuse brain edema results in buckling of the diencephalic structures and, finally, downward shift. Typical examples of diffuse brain edema are acute metabolic derangements and encephalitis.

Edema may also occur in one hemisphere and be proportionally more severe than the primary lesion (e.g., brain metastasis). In contrast, brain edema may be rather inconsequential, as in postanoxic-ischemic brain swelling, and an inevitable consequence of widespread brain damage. The complexity of acute cerebral edema warrants a separate discussion. Outcome in many instances is sinister because of the rapid emergence of irreversible damage to the brain stem.

Classification of Brain Edema

The structure and workings of the blood-brain barrier are complex and partly elucidated. A brief discussion is found in Capsule 2.1.

Brain edema has been conveniently classified, but the types are clinically indistinguishable. For comparative purposes, the different types are summarized in Table 2.1.[1] Brain edema has been classified by Klatzo[2] into (1) vasogenic edema, which is a consequence of an insult to the blood-brain barrier leading to increased capillary permeability, and (2) cytotoxic edema, which is a consequence of a direct cellular insult leading to swelling without abnormalities in the capillary permeability. An additional category has been proposed by Fishman,[1] who includes interstitial or hydrocephalic edema caused by obstruction of the cerebrospinal fluid pathways (Figure 2.1).

Milhorat[3] suggested an alternative classification, categorizing specific compartmental increases causing enlargement of brain bulk. Enlargement of brain bulk is an increase in brain volume that may take place in one of three major compartments: the vascular compartment (by arterial dilatation or venous obstruction), the astrocytes (by ischemia or intoxication), or the interstitium, including the cerebrospinal fluid compartment (by tumors, infections, trauma, or obstructive hydrocephalus).[3]

Any classification of brain edema suffers from the fact that many acute insults to the brain involve multiple compartments. In addition, the clinical manifestations are a consequence of brain tissue shift, and neither the initial presentation nor the evolution of clinical signs is much different among the different categories. The pathophysiology of brain edema is discussed in Capsule 2.2.

Diffuse cerebral edema commonly is rapid in onset and results in coma; focal cerebral edema can go largely unnoticed.

Clinical manifestations of brain edema in fulminant hepatic failure are dramatic.[14] Often, patients rather suddenly lapse into coma and may exhibit significant extensor responses with sparing of most of the brain stem reflexes unless progression to brain death occurs. When intracranial pressure is moni-

Capsule 2.1. The Blood-Brain Barrier

The exchange of fluids and solute between blood and brain in both directions is governed by multiple mechanisms. Exchange is determined by an anatomical restriction (in the true sense, a barrier), transport systems to rapidly provide the main energy source (e.g., facilitated glucose transport system), and osmolality. Breakdown of the blood-brain barrier, therefore, may not be an anatomical defect but may involve any of these control systems.

The blood-brain barrier is located at the capillary level, and its morphology is unique. A characteristic feature is the crowding of the capillary with astrocyte processes. These astrocyte feet initially appeared to define the barrier, but electron microscopy studies clearly demonstrated an open intercellular space. The physiologic function of these astrocyte foot processes is not entirely known, and their influence on the barrier may be only to moderate permeability rather than to define it anatomically. The capillary consists of a single layer of endothelial cells with a well-organized basement membrane. The endothelial cells are continuous, connected with tight junctions, and without true gaps. Structures that appear to be gaps are in fact very thin layers suggesting an opening, but the membranes are intact, securing impermeability.

tored, extreme increases with reduction in cerebral perfusion pressure are typical.

Cerebral edema in diabetic ketoacidosis usually is a devastating complication with high mortality, more often, unfortunately, in children and adolescents with juvenile diabetes. The clinical presentation is often without warning; rapidly developing stupor is soon followed by extensor posturing and fixed, dilated pupils. Many patients fulfill the clinical criteria for brain death in a matter of hours.[15–17]

Focal cerebral hemisphere edema is manifested by one of the herniation syndromes (Chapter 1) or, in less severe cases, only with more obvious drowsiness. Notably, edema surrounding neoplasms can be clinically silent. In general, degree of impaired consciousness and degree of focal edema may be very poorly related.

Cerebellar softening and swelling may quickly compress the upper brain stem, leading to sudden pontomedullary dysfunction and respiratory arrest. However, the critical threshold of tolerable swelling is not known, and we have observed dramatic swelling with spontaneous resolution.[18]

Different types of edema can be visualized by computed tomography (CT) scanning or magnetic resonance imaging (MRI). CT is not very sensitive

Table 2.1. Types of Brain Edema

	Vasogenic	Cytotoxic (cellular)	Interstitial
Pathophysiologic mechanism	Proteinaceous plasma filtrate in extracellular space	Cellular swelling from influx of water and sodium	Cerebrospinal fluid migration from increased ventricular pressure
Location	Preferentially white matter (often sparing gray matter)	Preferentially gray matter (often adjacent white matter)	Preferentially periventricular white matter
Disorders	Primary or metastatic brain tumor Inflammation Head injury	Cerebrovascular disorders Global anoxic-ischemic insult Fulminant hepatic failure Water intoxication, dysequilibrium syndrome	Obstructive hydrocephalus
Capillary permeability	Increased	Normal	Normal

Modified from Fishman.[1] By permission of WB Saunders Company.

to global cerebral edema in early stages, but the severity of edema can be graded by a simple grading system that characterizes different areas of involvement (Table 2.2). Most difficult in the evaluation of edema is the absence of sulci. This often becomes an issue in young persons who have a catastrophic illness that may produce edema but that may be difficult to appreciate because of an age-related lack of sulci (Figure 2.2).

Vasogenic edema produces increased signal intensity on T2-weighted images, particularly in the white matter. Cytotoxic edema in stroke increases the T2 signal as well but often is found in the boundary zone of the infarct between the central area of infarction and the surrounding normal brain tissue.

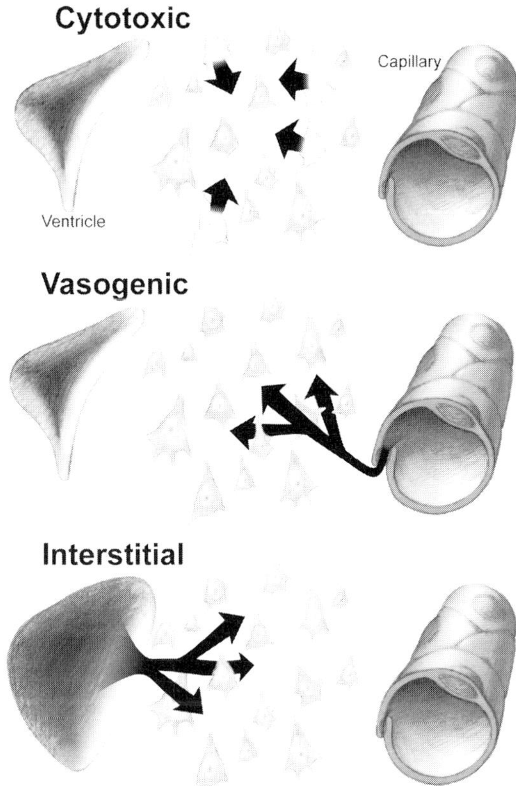

Figure 2.1. Changes in brain tissue with cytotoxic edema, vasogenic edema, and interstitial edema.

Specific Clinical Circumstances of Brain Edema

Brain Edema in Postanoxic-Ischemic Encephalopathy

Brain edema usually affects both hemispheres and invariably is present in comatose patients. Brain edema in anoxic-ischemic insults is a global astroglial swelling involving the entire hemisphere. Tissue necrosis results in the development of brain edema several days later, and its appearance is not associated with a significant increase in intracranial pressure. Therefore, brain edema in postanoxic-ischemic encephalopathy, whether from cardiac arrest or asphyxia, is a measure of the severity of the insult and implies a poor prognosis.[19]

Brain edema in survivors of cardiopulmonary resuscitation is noted only when CT scanning is performed several days after the event. Brain edema on CT scans is more common in patients with absent motor responses or extensor posturing responses, abnormal cranial nerve reflexes, and generalized myoclonus. These patients are often in cardiogenic shock and need progressively higher doses of vasopressors.

Brain edema in postanoxic-ischemic encephalopathy does not result in further clinical deterioration in these already ravaged patients. However, further progression to brain death may occur and is accompanied by further worsening of brain edema revealed by CT scans or at autopsy. CT scanning often shows loss of definition of cortical sulci, lack of gray and white matter differentiation, and, in the most severe cases, obliteration of the basal cisterns (Figure 2.3).[20] In some patients, the initial CT scans may show hypodensities of the basal ganglia (caudate and putamen), which are fields of terminal vascular supply, or of the thalamus.

Brain Edema from Acute Metabolic Derangements and Organ Failure

The water content of the brain may increase significantly as a result of changes in plasma osmolality. Brain edema may also occur as a result of an increased osmotic effect of a toxic intermediate, as in acute liver failure.[21,22] Fulminant hepatic failure has been associated with the development of brain edema, and its emergence has been linked to early mortality.[23]

Experimental evidence in hepatectomized rats found that an increase in cortical glutamine may act

Capsule 2.2. Brain Edema: Physiology and Pathology

In vasogenic edema, the breakdown of the barrier results in fluid accumulation into the white matter. Myelin sheets are swollen and filled with vacuoles, which may further result in myelin breakdown, and cysts appear in the white matter. The astrocytes are swollen at a later stage. The breakdown of the blood-brain barrier is most illustrative in vasogenic edema. Whatever disorder triggers the insult, the result is transudation of plasma into the extracellular white matter space. With this flooding of the white matter, however, cerebral blood flow remains unaffected, and cellular mechanisms remain intact.[4]

In cellular or cytotoxic edema, however, a preferential astrocyte swelling (gemistocyte) is observed, often maximal in the astrocyte foot processes. Because cytotoxic edema represents intracellular swelling, gray matter is more involved than white matter.

The mechanisms of cytotoxic edema are more complex than opening of the blood-brain barrier. Experimental studies have indicated that compounds blocking the release of excitatory amino acids reduce the water content of the brain, an indirect suggestion that glutamate has a potential role. Free radicals, prostaglandins, arachidonic acid, and, possibly, leukotrienes, may potentiate cerebral swelling.[5–7] Other evidence indicates that initial cellular acidity could activate ion antiport channels, such as Na^+/H^- and Cl^-/HCO_3^-, to extrude H^+ but at the expense of an increase in osmolarity.

Clearing of brain edema occurs predominantly through the cerebrospinal fluid. Clearance of extravasated proteins by the glial cells is also closely linked to resolution of edema fluid; this suggests a major role for colloid osmotic pressure generated by the proteins.[8,9] Edema spreads through bulk flow and a downhill pressure gradient between the white matter and the cerebrospinal fluid compartment, a mechanism that may be further facilitated when cerebrospinal fluid pressure is reduced.[10] A centrally located atrial natriuretic factor has been found to moderate the brain water content, and it might decrease edema formation.[11–13]

as an osmolyte, increase brain water, and result in astrocyte swelling. The increase in astrocyte content of glutamine in hepatic failure correlates with an increase in arterial ammonia. An increase in glutamine may therefore reflect an attempt by astrocytes to detoxify themselves from ammonia by producing glutamine, nevertheless creating an osmotically active molecule (osmolyte). The development of brain edema may be further amplified by changes in cerebral blood flow. Increased arterial ammonia may induce vasodilatation, and a relative increase in cerebral blood flow despite the decreased metabolic demand from encephalopathy (so-called luxury perfusion) may increase the development of vasogenic edema.[24,25] Other potential mechanisms are inhibition of Na^+, K^+–adenosinetriphosphatase, which may result in astrocyte swelling. This explanation is supported by one study in which serum from patients with fulminant hepatic failure inhibited this pump.[26]

CT scans may demonstrate disappearance of the sylvian fissures, and later, complete compression of

Table 2.2. Calculation of Brain Edema Severity Score on the Basis of Computed Tomographic Findings in Patients with Fulminant Hepatic Failure*

Feature	Score
Visibility of cortical sulci	
3 CT scan slices of upper cerebral area (L/R)	6
Visibility of white matter	
Internal capsule (L/R)	2
Centrum semiovale (L/R)	2
Vertex (L/R)	2
Visibility of basal cisterns	
Sylvian fissure (horizontal-vertical, L/R)	4
Frontal interhemispheric fissure	1
Quadrigeminal cistern	1
Paired suprasellar cisterns (L/R)	2
Ambient cistern (L/R)	2
Maximal total*	22

(CT = computed tomography; L/R = left and right cerebral hemispheres.)
*In CT scan with normal findings.
From Wijdicks et al.[14] By permission of Mayo Foundation for Medical Education and Research.

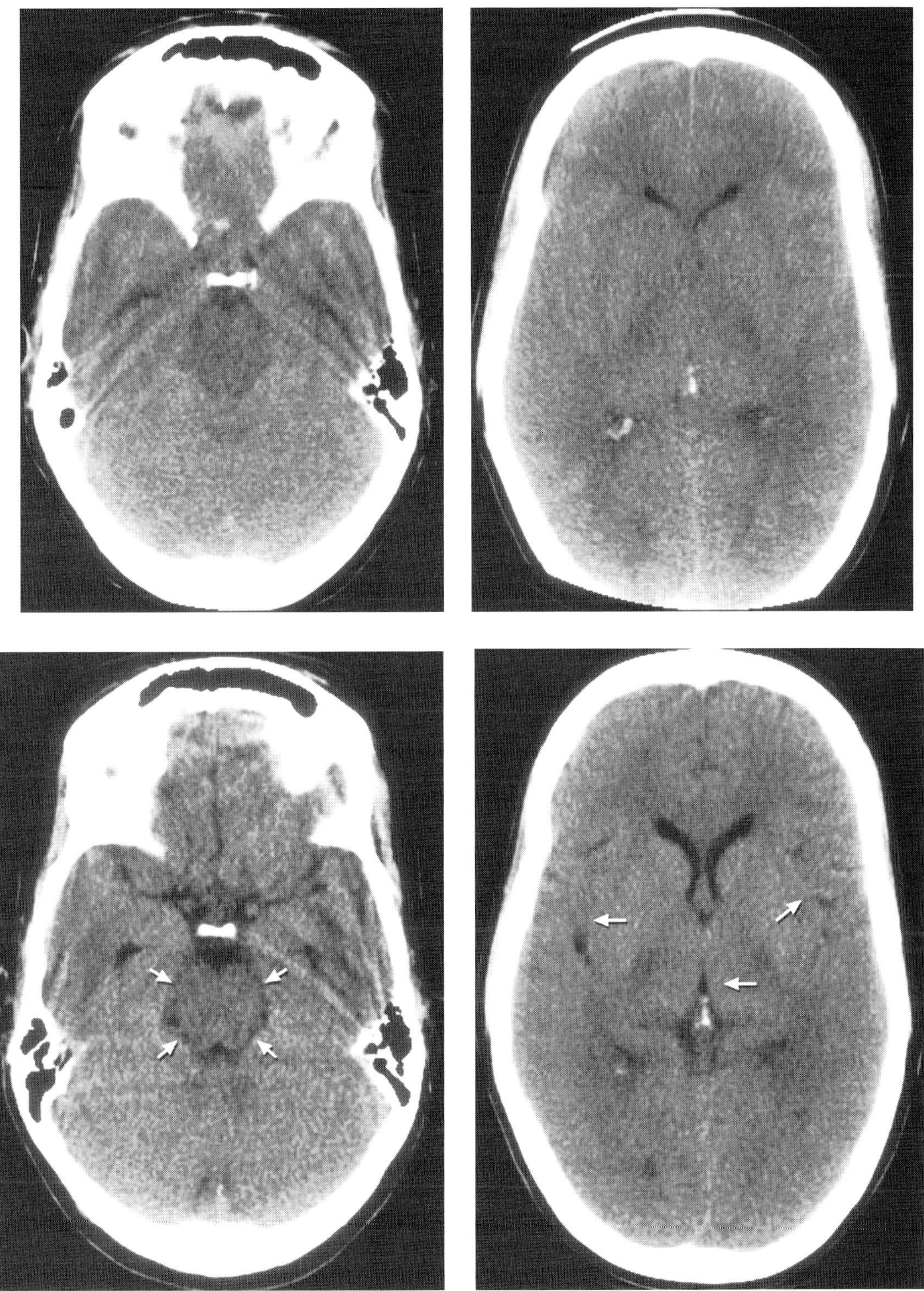

Figure 2.2. Resolving brain edema in encephalitis. Virtual lack of sulci and sylvian fissures, poor white-gray matter differentiation, and effacement of basal cistern and third ventricle with improvement (*arrows*).

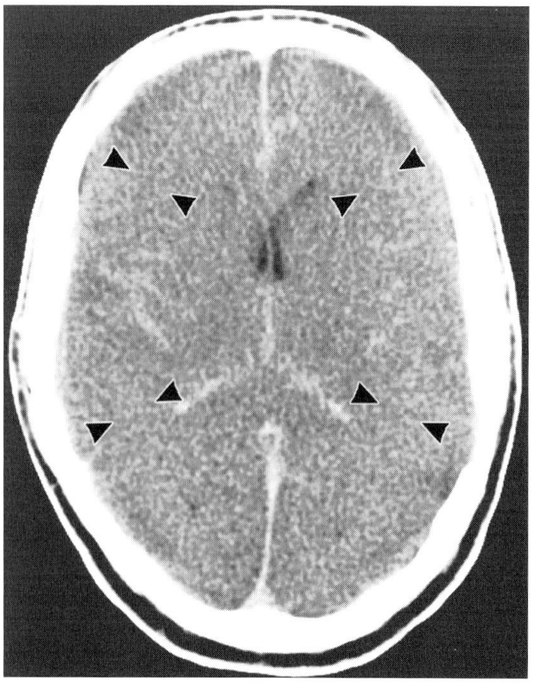
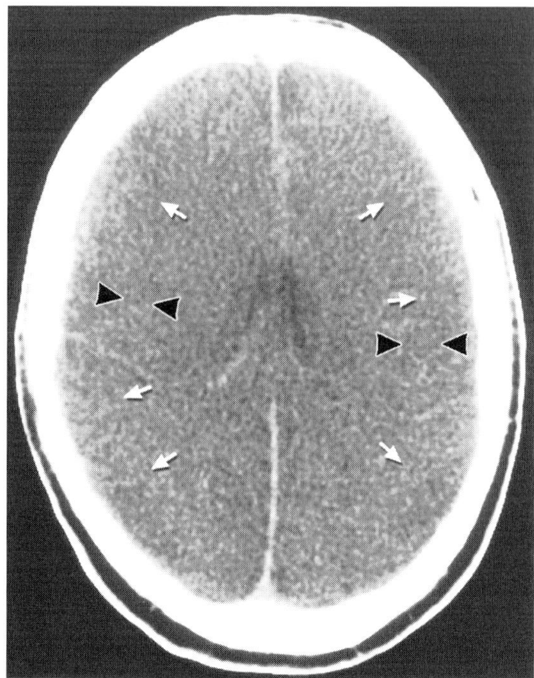

Figure 2.3. Anoxic-ischemic encephalopathy with generalized brain edema. *Arrowheads* indicate loss of gray-white matter definition. *Arrows* point to absence of sulci.

the basal cisterns and loss of white-gray matter differentiation may be seen (Figure 2.4). These abnormalities may reverse entirely with control of intracranial pressure and after liver transplantation.[20]

Brain edema is rarely present in patients with fluctuating drowsiness; it is usually not visualized on CT until patients become stuporous. A linear relationship between the severity of cerebral edema and the degree of hepatic encephalopathy has been found[14] and implies that brain edema is the final common pathway by which coma occurs.

Cerebral edema may develop in acute, often dramatic, sodium and glucose derangements. Hyperosmolality can be brought on by severe dehydration or from infusion of hypertonic solutions. This may lead to shrinkage of the endothelial cells, causing gaps and possible rupture of the interendothelial connection that result in increased permeability. Its effect is brief and reversed in a matter of hours.[27]

Acutely induced hypo-osmolality or hyponatremia of a sufficient degree (usually 100 mmol/L or less) may induce significant cerebral edema. Cerebral edema in this hypo-osmolar state has been noted either in young healthy women after general anesthesia or in patients with polydipsia, predominantly in schizophrenia. Excessive administration of free water results in acute onset of massive brain edema,[28] rapid displacement of the diencephalon, and respiratory arrest.

Nonetheless, brain edema is uncommon after acute severe hyponatremia and may be explained by a corrective mechanism due to rapid loss of organic osmolytes. Loss of osmolytes permits transport of potassium outside the cell and leads to reduction in the content of intracellular solute, minimizing the risk of cell swelling induced by this rapid osmotic change. A linear correlation between the degree of hyponatremia and the loss of important osmolytes, such as taurine, glutamate, and aspartame, by the brain has been documented.[29] Reduction in the number of osmolytes was already detectable 3 hours after the onset of hyponatremia, decreasing to a minimal concentration in 24 hours.

The mechanism of brain edema in diabetic ketoacidosis may be related to rapid fluid management to correct the ketoacidosis and dehydration, but this is not clear. At least theoretically, rapid administration of fluid may lead to intracellular

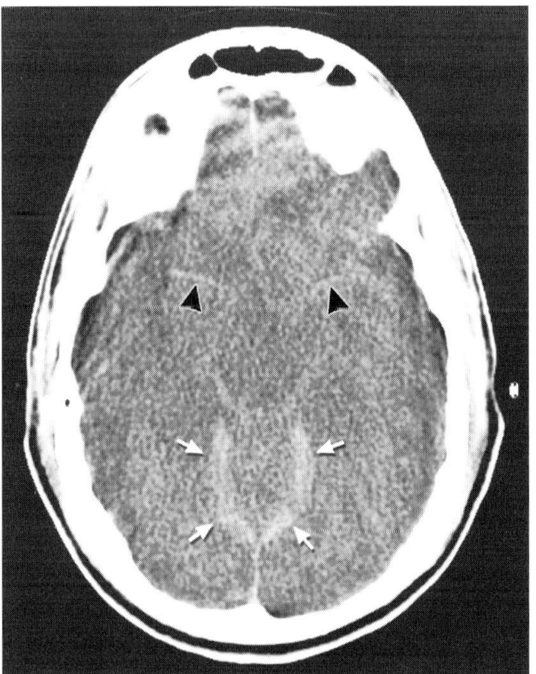

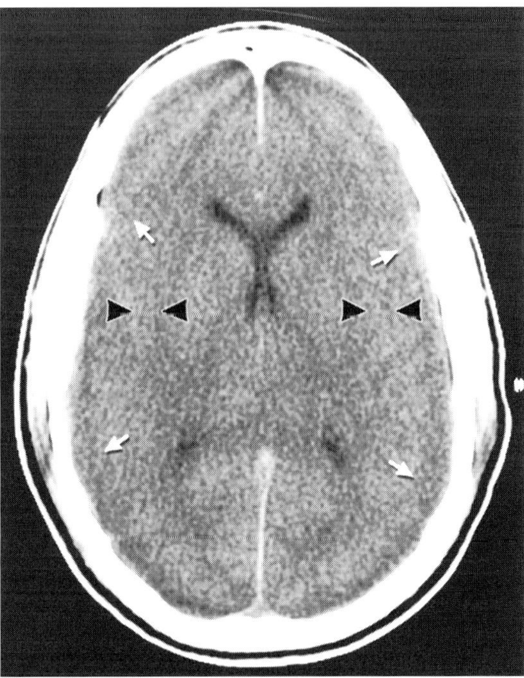

Figure 2.4. Cerebral edema in fulminant hepatic failure. *Left*, Pseudo-subarachnoid hemorrhage, which occurs when the brain tissue becomes very low in attenuation and the dura and blood vessels appear comparatively hyperdense. *Arrowheads* point to the basal cisterns and *arrows* to the tentorium region, areas typically filled with blood in true subarachnoid hemorrhage. *Right*, Loss of sylvian fissures (*arrowheads*) and loss of cortical sulci (*arrows*).

shift of water because of osmotically active molecules that are intrinsically present to protect the brain from excessive shrinkage. Rapid administration of fluid may override the washout of osmolytes when plasma osmolality rapidly corrects itself. Alternatively, insulin administration may activate the Na^+/H^+ pump, enhancing sodium and water influx.[30] Cerebral edema may be more prevalent than appreciated, and serial CT scan studies have shown the development of clinically unrecognizable cerebral edema.[31,32] In clinical practice, brain edema may also be related to anoxic damage from acidosis-related cardiopulmonary arrest.

Treatment with osmotic diuretic agents is often unsuccessful, evidence that massive cerebral edema has resulted in rapid deterioration with herniation.

Brain Edema and Acute Bacterial Meningitis

Brain edema in acute bacterial meningitis and viral encephalitis may complicate the clinical course and almost certainly increases mortality.

The true prevalence of brain edema in bacterial meningitis is not known, and reported series have been biased toward autopsy material. Brain edema occurs early in the course of bacterial meningitis but is not invariably the cause of early death. In a series of 29 patients with bacterial meningitis, 15 patients had pathologic evidence of cerebral edema by the appearance of tonsillar herniation at autopsy.[33]

There may be several mechanisms of brain edema in inflammatory disorders. It has been proposed that granulocyte ("granulocytic brain edema") products may induce edema.[34] Cytokines originating from leukocytes may cause endothelial alterations that can lead to vasogenic edema.[34,35] In addition, it has been documented that high doses of these chemotactically active agents administered intrathecally increased brain water content, but it is not clear whether this experiment, which used very high doses, reflected the changes in vivo.[36,37] The cytokine-endothelium leukocyte interaction is currently an active field of research, and recent studies have shown that both dexamethasone and monoclonal antibodies against leukocyte adhesion receptors attenuate meningeal inflammation and brain edema in rats inoculated with *Haemophilus influenzae*.[38]

CT scanning of brain edema in acute bacterial meningitis typically shows generalized edema, with edematous white matter and cortical effacement. The ventricles may become extremely small. In contrast-enhanced CT scans, enhancement of the basal cisterns due to hypervascularity or gyral configurations in cortical zones may represent extensive meningitis. MRI may document pus (see Chapter 9).

Brain Edema Associated with Hemispheric Mass

Brain edema often only surrounds a hemispheric mass irrespective of whether it is an intraparenchymal hematoma, a large territorial infarct, or a tumor.

Intracranial hematomas, when located in the basal ganglia, often have a perihematoma rim of edema that invariably represents vasogenic edema. Its significance is unknown, and an increase in the volume of edema is less common than enlargement of the hematoma within the first 12 hours after the ictus. In our experience, secondary clinical deterioration from progressive perihematoma swelling more commonly occurs in lobar hematomas.

Brain edema from a cerebral arteriovenous malformation most commonly is associated with recent hemorrhage. Brain edema may also be correlated with increased pressure on the draining veins and marked dilatation or varices of the draining veins. Acute venous occlusion may be another mechanism of venous outflow.[39] However, brain edema can be explained by seizures and is most often seen on MRI. The hyperintensity on T2-weighted images may disappear after control of seizures.

Large hemispheric infarcts may swell, usually after 3 to 5 days. In many patients, brain swelling is heralded by increasing headache[40] and a fluctuating level of consciousness (e.g., sleepy in the morning). Outcome in patients with brain stem involvement from herniation is invariably poor (Figure 2.5). Tumor-associated edema most likely involves multiple mechanisms (Capsule 2.3 and Figure 2.6).

Brain Edema Associated with Head Injury

Diffuse brain swelling is more common in children than in adults. Brain swelling is present commonly in comatose patients with closed head injury and rarely in patients who remain alert. Subsequent deterioration from diffuse brain swelling in a previously alert patient is uncommon (less than 5%). It has been reported after repeated brain injury—"the second impact syndrome"—but its mechanism remains controversial, and risk factors are not known.[47] Brain swelling occurs more often in patients who suffered a systemic insult, such as hypotension or prehospital hypoxemia. Brain swelling often is evident on CT scans and may involve absence of the third ventricle and basal cisterns in most cases. Intracranial pressure is almost always significantly increased.[48] Brain swelling in adults with closed head injury is often associated with multiple parenchymal contusions, shearing lesions, and traumatic subarachnoid hemorrhage.[48–52]

Management of Brain Edema

Acute brain edema is associated with high morbidity and mortality, and results of aggressive intervention have not been encouraging. In the course of several hours, brain shift may be extensive, resulting in permanent damage even after the water content of the brain has been ameliorated.

Osmotic diuretics, such as mannitol (1 g/kg) or hypertonic saline, may be useful initially while the true value of intracranial pressure is determined by placement of a monitor. Continuous infusion with 3% hypertonic saline should be considered if a bolus of mannitol is unsuccessful in head trauma, intracranial hematoma, or cerebral infarct. The dose is increased until serum sodium concentrations are between 145 and 155 mmol/L.[53] A recent pilot study suggested an effect from intravenous bolus administration of 23.4% saline in refractory increased intracranial pressure. Cerebral perfusion pressure was augmented as well, and intravascular volume was not depleted.[54]

Corticosteroids are useful only in metastasis or glioma with mass effect from perilesional edema. Corticosteroids (10 mg of dexamethasone intravenously) should be considered in brain edema from fulminant bacterial meningitis (Chapter 9). The major beneficial effect is improvement of cerebrospinal fluid dynamics, predominantly the cerebrospinal fluid outflow tract over the convexity. Corticosteroids have no documented value in

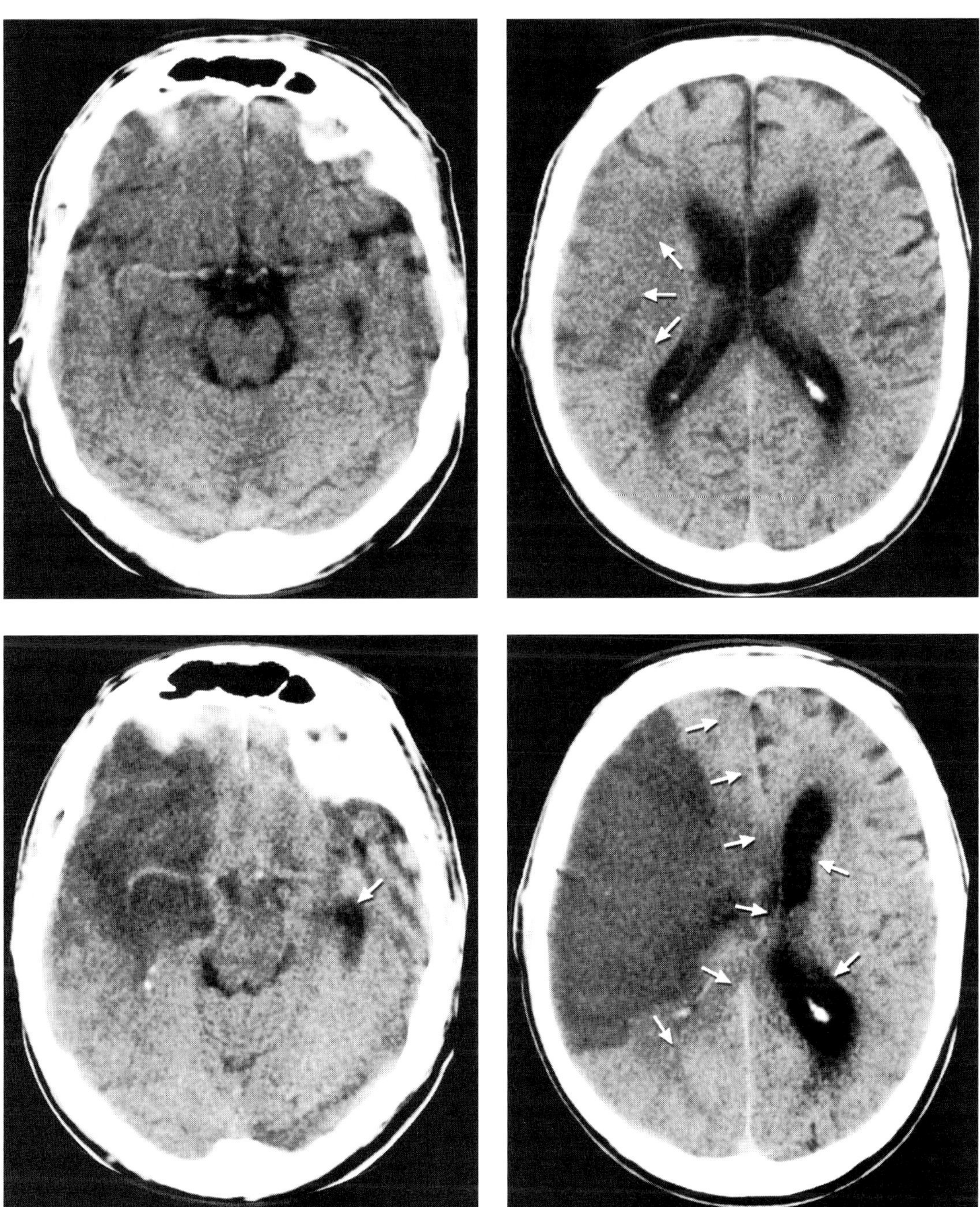

Figure 2.5. Cerebral swelling associated with middle cerebral artery territory infarct. *Top row*, Initial scan with hypodensity and loss of sulci in the middle cerebral artery territory (*arrows*). *Bottom row*, Massive edema and shift with contralateral hydrocephalus and enlargement of temporal horn (*arrows*).

Capsule 2.3. Edema in Brain Tumors

Four processes have been suggested that may be related to edema associated with primary brain tumors or metastasis[41]: (1) tumor angiogenesis of vessels with defective blood-brain barrier, characterized by large interendothelial gaps[42]; (2) increased microvascular permeability from production of mediators, such as prostaglandin E_2 and thromboxane B_2, in this process[43]; (3) an immunologic mechanism such as interleukin-2, which when injected has resulted in brain edema in experimental studies[44]; and (4) less likely, an inflammatory mechanism through substances, such as platelet-activating factor, released from polynuclear leukocytes surrounding the tumor-associated edema. Other factors that may potentiate tumor-associated edema are seizures, chemotherapeutic agents, and therapeutic radiation.[45] Plasma osmolality may play an important role, and one experimental study found a direct relation between plasma osmolality and formation of brain edema.[46]

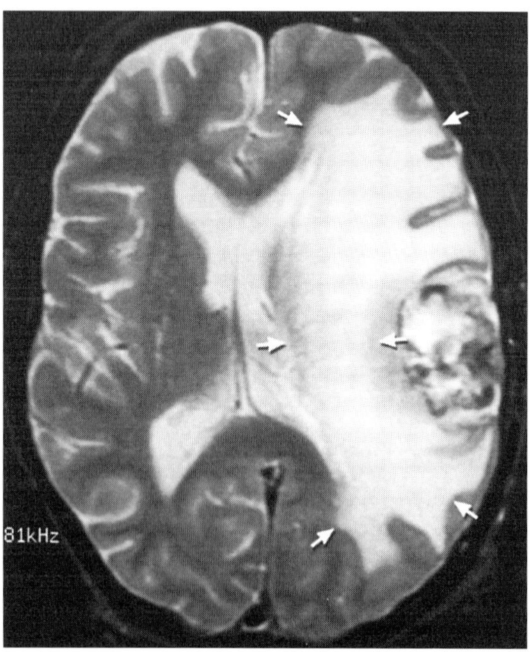

Figure 2.6. Peritumoral edema (*arrows*) in mass lesion (glioma).

brain edema from endocrine or hepatic disturbances.

Focal hemispheric edema is more difficult to manage, and craniectomy with duraplasty greatly increases the possibility for swelling outside the skull. Removal of additional swollen brain tissue (anterior temporal lobectomy or frontal lobectomy) is optional but only considered if the primary lesion is in this location (e.g., temporal lobe swelling from herpes simplex encephalitis,[55] metastasis with malignant edema).

References

1. Fishman RA. Cerebrospinal Fluid in Diseases of the Nervous System, 2nd ed. Philadelphia: WB Saunders Company, 1992.
2. Klatzo I. Presidential address. Neuropathological aspects of brain edema. J Neuropathol Exp Neurol 1967;26:1.
3. Milhorat TH. Cerebrospinal Fluid and the Brain Edemas. New York: Neuroscience Society of New York, 1987.
4. Sutton LN, Barranco D, Greenberg J, et al. Cerebral blood flow and glucose metabolism in experimental brain edema. J Neurosurg 1989;71:868.
5. Ikeda Y, Long DM. The molecular basis of brain injury and brain edema: the role of oxygen free radicals. Neurosurgery 1990;27:1.
6. Ito U, Baethmann A, Hossmann KA, et al. Brain edema IX. Acta Neurochir 1993;60:1.
7. Kimelberg HK. Current concepts of brain edema. Review of laboratory investigations. J Neurosurg 1995;83:1051.
8. Marmarou A, Hochwald G, Nakamura T, et al. Brain edema resolution by CSF pathways and brain vasculature in cats. Am J Physiol 1994;267:H514.
9. Marmarou A, Nakamura T, Tanaka K. The kinetics of fluid movement through brain tissue. Semin Neurol 1984;4:439.
10. Reulen HJ, Graham R, Spatz M, Klatzo I. Role of pressure gradients and bulk flow in dynamics of vasogenic brain edema. J Neurosurg 1977;46:24.
11. Doczi T, Joó F, Szerdahelyi P, Bodosi M. Regulation of brain water and electrolyte contents: the possible involvement of central atrial natriuretic factor. Neurosurgery 1987;21:454.

12. Nakao N, Itakura T, Yokote H, et al. Effect of atrial natriuretic peptide on ischemic brain edema: changes in brain water and electrolytes. Neurosurgery 1990;27:39.
13. Rosenberg GA, Estrada EY. Atrial natriuretic peptide blocks hemorrhagic brain edema after 4-hour delay in rats. Stroke 1995;26:874.
14. Wijdicks EFM, Plevak DJ, Rakela J, Wiesner RH. Clinical and radiologic features of cerebral edema in fulminant hepatic failure. Mayo Clin Proc 1995;70:119.
15. Clements RS Jr, Prockop LD, Winegrad AI. Acute cerebral oedema during treatment of hyperglycaemia. An experimental model. Lancet 1968;2:384.
16. FitzGerald MG, O'Sullivan DJ, Malins JM. Fatal diabetic ketosis. BMJ 1961;2:247.
17. Young E, Bradley RF. Cerebral edema with irreversible coma in severe diabetic ketoacidosis. N Engl J Med 1967;276:665.
18. Wijdicks EFM, Maus TP, Piepgras DG. Cerebellar swelling and massive brain stem distortion: spontaneous resolution documented by MRI. J Neurol Neurosurg Psychiatry 1998;65:400.
19. Lupton BA, Hill A, Roland EH, et al. Brain swelling in the asphyxiated term newborn: pathogenesis and outcome. Pediatrics 1988;82:139.
20. Wijdicks EFM, Parisi JE, Sharbrough FW. Prognostic value of myoclonus status in comatose survivors of cardiac arrest. Ann Neurol 1994;35:239.
21. Hilgier W, Olson JE. Brain ion and amino acid contents during edema development in hepatic encephalopathy. J Neurochem 1994;62:197.
22. Olafsson S, Gottstein J, Blei AT. Brain edema and intracranial hypertension in rats after total hepatectomy. Gastroenterology 1995;108:1097.
23. Blei AT, Olafsson S, Therrien G, Butterworth RF. Ammonia-induced brain edema and intracranial hypertension in rats after portacaval anastomosis. Hepatology 1994;19:1437.
24. Butterworth RF. Hepatic encephalopathy and brain edema in acute hepatic failure: does glutamate play a role? Hepatology 1997;25:1032.
25. Durham S, Yonas H, Aggarwal S, et al. Regional cerebral blood flow and CO_2 reactivity in fulminant hepatic failure. J Cereb Blood Flow Metab 1995;15:329.
26. Seda HW, Hughes RD, Gove CD, Williams R. Inhibition of rat brain Na^+, K^+-ATPase activity by serum from patients with fulminant hepatic failure. Hepatology 1984;4:74.
27. Cserr HF, DePasquale M, Patlak CS. Volume regulatory influx of electrolytes from plasma to brain during acute hyperosmolality. Am J Physiol 1987;253:F530.
28. Arieff AI. Hyponatremia, convulsions, respiratory arrest, and permanent brain damage after elective surgery in healthy women. N Engl J Med 1986; 314:1529.
29. Sterns RH, Baer J, Ebersold S, et al. Organic osmolytes in acute hyponatremia. Am J Physiol 1993;264:F833.
30. Van der Meulen JA, Klip A, Grinstein S. Possible mechanism for cerebral oedema in diabetic ketoacidosis. Lancet 1987;2:306.
31. Hoffman WH, Steinhart CM, el Gammal T, et al. Cranial CT in children and adolescents with diabetic ketoacidosis. AJNR Am J Neuroradiol 1988;9:733.
32. Krane EJ, Rockoff MA, Wallman JK, Wolfsdorf JI. Subclinical brain swelling in children during treatment of diabetic ketoacidosis. N Engl J Med 1985;312.1147.
33. Dodge PR, Swartz MN. Bacterial meningitis—a review of selected aspects. II. Special neurologic problems, postmeningitic complications and clinicopathological correlations. N Engl J Med 1965;272:954.
34. Fishman RA, Sligar K, Hake RB. Effects of leukocytes on brain metabolism in granulocytic brain edema. Ann Neurol 1977;2:89.
35. Montesano R, Orci L, Vassalli P. Human endothelial cell cultures: phenotypic modulation by leukocyte interleukins. J Cell Physiol 1985;122:424.
36. Niemöller UM, Täuber MG. Brain edema and increased intracranial pressure in the pathophysiology of bacterial meningitis. Eur J Clin Microbiol Infect Dis 1989;8:109.
37. Täuber MG, Borschberg U, Sande MA. Influence of granulocytes on brain edema, intracranial pressure, and cerebrospinal fluid concentrations of lactate and protein in experimental meningitis. J Infect Dis 1988;157:456.
38. Sáez-Llorens X, Jafari HS, Severien C, et al. Enhanced attenuation of meningeal inflammation and brain edema by concomitant administration of anti-CD18 monoclonal antibodies and dexamethasone in experimental *Haemophilus* meningitis. J Clin Invest 1991;88:2003.
39. Miyasaka Y, Kurata A, Tanaka R, et al. Mass effect caused by clinically unruptured cerebral arteriovenous malformations. Neurosurgery 1997;41:1060.
40. Wijdicks EFM, Diringer MN. Middle cerebral artery territory infarction and early brain swelling: progression and effect of age on outcome. Mayo Clin Proc 1998;73:829.
41. Del Maestro RF, Megyesi JF, Farrell CL. Mechanisms of tumor-associated edema: a review. Can J Neurol Sci 1990;17:177.
42. Coomber BL, Stewart PA, Hayakawa K, et al. Quantitative morphology of human glioblastoma multiforme microvessels: structural basis of blood-brain barrier defect. J Neurooncol 1987;5:299.
43. Cooper C, Jones HG, Weller RO, Walker V. Production of prostaglandins and thromboxane by isolated cells from intracranial tumours. J Neurol Neurosurg Psychiatry 1984;47:579.
44. Saris SC, Patronas NJ, Rosenberg SA, et al. The effect of intravenous interleukin-2 on brain water content. J Neurosurg 1989;71:169.
45. Posner JB. Neurologic Complications of Cancer. Philadelphia: FA Davis, 1995.
46. Hansen TD, Warner DS, Traynelis VC, Todd MM. Plasma osmolality and brain water content in a rat glioma model. Neurosurgery 1994;34:505.

47. McCrory PR, Berkovic SF. Second impact syndrome. Neurology 1998;50:677.
48. Eisenberg HM, Gary HE Jr, Aldrich EF, et al. Initial CT findings in 753 patients with severe head injury. A report from the NIH Traumatic Coma Data Bank. J Neurosurg 1990;73:688.
49. Lang DA, Teasdale GM, Macpherson P, Lawrence A. Diffuse brain swelling after head injury: more often malignant in adults than children? J Neurosurg 1994;80:675.
50. Pearl GS. Traumatic neuropathology. Clin Lab Med 1998;18:39.
51. Feldman Z, Zachari S, Reichenthal E, et al. Brain edema and neurological status with rapid infusion of lactated Ringer's or 5% dextrose solution following head trauma. J Neurosurg 1995;83:1060.
52. Shapira Y, Artru AA, Cotev S, et al. Brain edema and neurologic status following head trauma in the rat. No effect from large volumes of isotonic or hypertonic intravenous fluids, with or without glucose. Anesthesiology 1992;77:79.
53. Qureshi AI, Suarez JI, Bhardwaj A, et al. Use of hypertonic (3%) saline/acetate infusion in the treatment of cerebral edema: effect on intracranial pressure and lateral displacement of the brain. Crit Care Med 1998;26:440.
54. Suarez JI, Qureshi AI, Bhardwaj A, et al. Treatment of refractory intracranial hypertension with 23.4% saline. Crit Care Med 1998;26:1118.
55. Ebel H, Kuchta J, Balogh A, Klug N. Operative treatment of tentorial herniation in herpes encephalitis. Childs Nerv Syst 1999;15:84.

Chapter 3
Status Epilepticus and Recurrent Seizures

Status epilepticus can be a multifaceted neurologic emergency. Status epilepticus may occur de novo but also may be associated with clinical neurologic conditions (e.g., acute bacterial meningitis and herpes simplex encephalitis) for which therapeutic interventions are urgently indicated. The tasks at hand need to be well executed, because longstanding morbidity in many patients has been linked to lapses in aggressive control of seizure activity. Thus, rapid termination of seizures and simultaneous treatment of the underlying illness are of utmost priority in tonic-clonic status epilepticus, and this undisputed urgency must be appreciated by any physician faced with this illness. Status epilepticus lasting 1 hour or more increases morbidity tenfold. Furthermore, death may be a consequence of status epilepticus soon after acute presentation. Neurogenic pulmonary edema or life-threatening cardiac arrhythmia[1] may occur, but more likely prolonged apnea and anoxia may result in a catastrophic ischemic-anoxic insult and persistent coma, emphasizing the need for early intubation and airway control.

Concurrent destructive brain lesions are common in adult status epilepticus and thus in most are responsible for morbidity and mortality. Regrettably, outcome studies in status epilepticus include patients with myoclonus status epilepticus, a phenomenon indicative of profound brain anoxia, associated with cardiac arrest. These causes may account for 30% to 40% of the cases, thus skewing the results toward an unfavorable outcome.[1–3] Conversely, albeit uncommonly, unprovoked status epilepticus may have an excellent neurologic outcome.

Status epilepticus can be distinguished in several forms, each of which is discussed in detail. In this chapter, an approach to this catastrophic illness is presented that is based on the integration of position papers.[4–6]

Classification and Presentation of Status Epilepticus

Convulsive status epilepticus can be divided into four major categories, and nonconvulsive status epilepticus can be further divided into complex partial and absence types (Figure 3.1). The distinction has relevance because the initial choice of antiepileptic agents may be different, management may not involve antiepileptic agents (as in myoclonus status epilepticus and psychogenic seizures), and outcome may differ from category to category.

Persistence of seizure activity is the most important discriminating factor in recurrent seizures, because it is directly linked to cumulative development of medical complications. The risk of neuronal dropout resulting in morbidity is related not only to the duration of status epilepticus but also to age and systemic complications, such as severe hypoxemia from aspiration. Autonomic storm resulting in tachyarrhythmias and

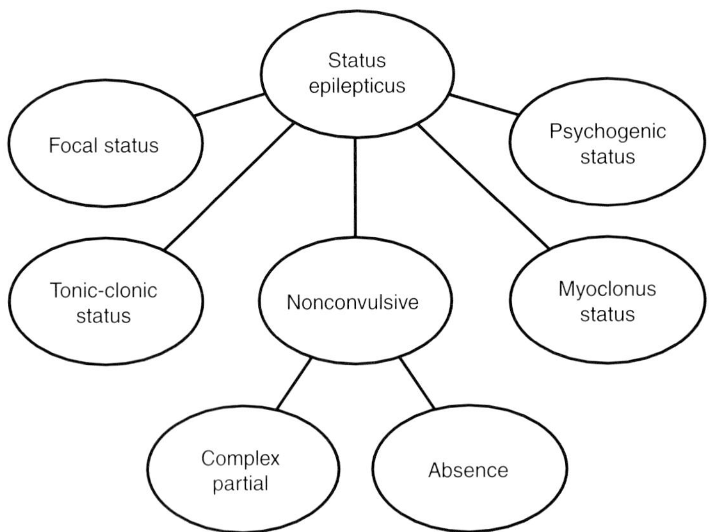

Figure 3.1. Classification of status epilepticus.

hyperthermia probably does not directly contribute to brain damage.

Tonic-Clonic Status Epilepticus

Tonic-clonic status epilepticus has typically been defined as repetitive generalized tonic-clonic seizures lasting 30 minutes or longer or seizures without full return of consciousness between episodes. The evolution of seizures into status epilepticus often becomes clear within 10 to 15 minutes, and the time criterion should not be applied rigorously.

The tonic phase involves flexion of the axial muscles, upward gaze, and marked widening of the pupil diameter with sluggish light responses. Flexion occurs in the arms and legs and is soon followed by extension, clenching of teeth, and forced expiration for several seconds. Sweating may be profuse, with an increase in blood pressure and pulse. The clonic phase begins with a tremor or shivering but gives way to uninterrupted jerking, which dies out gradually and may result in urinary and fecal incontinence after the sphincter muscles relax from a forceful contraction during the clonic phase. Usually, a generalized tonic-clonic seizure lasts 1 to 2 minutes and is followed for up to 5 minutes by a dazed state or agitation resulting in labored breathing and deep sleep. Most patients gradually awaken but never to a point that conversation is understood or simple commands are followed. Then, tonic spasm may occur again with a similar pattern of jerking and resolution.

Electrographic recordings, if available, typically show rhythmic spike- or sharp-wave complexes or sharp- and slow-wave discharges with a generalized distribution. Clinically, the distinction between a postictal confusional state emerging from a generalized tonic-clonic seizure and convulsive status epilepticus is difficult in the emergency room. Subtle eyelid or limb twitching in a stuporous patient may indicate continuous epileptic activity, but the distinction may require electroencephalographic recording.

Typical clinical findings are tongue bite (large purple hematoma or erosion at the lateral border of the tongue that should be carefully inspected while the tongue is pushed sideways with a tongue depressor) (Color Plates 5 and 6) and, occasionally, petechial hemorrhages in the conjunctiva, chest, and neck. Other complications are tachycardia, hyperglycemia, bone fractures, posterior shoulder dislocation, pulmonary aspiration, and, rarely if ever, neurogenic pulmonary edema. Prolonged status epilepticus may produce fever (up to 42°C), even on the day after presentation. The most common causes of status epilepticus are shown in Table 3.1. Withdrawal of antiepileptic agents in patients with established seizure disorder is most common.[7-9] In de novo status epilepticus, no overriding cause is apparent, but an acute brain lesion is common. In one urban hospital study, the most common causes for status epilepticus were alcohol-related.[8,10]

Nonconvulsive Status Epilepticus

Delayed diagnosis is commonplace, because behavioral abnormalities are mistaken for a postictal state or psychiatric disorder.[11] Nonconvulsive status epilepticus is further divided into complex partial status and absence status.[12] Complex partial status epilepticus is most prevalent in adults between 20 and 40 years of age.[4,13]

Clinical presentation is diverse, but clinical signs are not always suggestive and may be diagnostically confusing. Consciousness is always impaired. Nonconvulsive status epilepticus results in blank staring, sometimes with tremulousness and subtle periorbital, facial, or limb myoclonus. Patients have decreased or rambling speech output or are mute, and thus the distinction with aphasia from a structural lesion can be difficult. Aggressive behavior is uncommon,[12] and more often patients are mildly agitated and easy to restrain. A waxing and waning state alternating between agitation and obtundation is characteristic. Inappropriate laughing, crying, or even singing may occur. Some patients express a feeling of imminent death. Absence status epilepticus is additionally characterized by reduction in vigilance rather than drowsiness. Attention is absent, and automatisms may occur. Complex status epilepticus can be characterized by hallucinations and a complete amnesia for the attacks.[13]

Focal Status Epilepticus

Focal status epilepticus can be simple (normal level of consciousness) or complex (impaired consciousness but no overt jerking). Focal status epilepticus is probably similar to epilepsia partialis continua. Focal status epilepticus involves continuous clonic movements of one or two extremities. Jerking of one arm or leg can be directly observed by the patient, who should be unable to influence its jerking frequency. A hemiparesis (which may last for days) may result if the condition is treated late. Lack of treatment often is due to mistakenly attributing the continuous movement to psychogenic seizures. The disorder often is related to an acute hemispheric lesion (e.g., hemorrhage in cavernous hemangioma or metastasis, spontaneous lobar hematoma).

Table 3.1. Causes of Status Epilepticus

Change in antiepileptic drugs
Withdrawal of benzodiazepines (NCSE)
Drugs or alcohol
Bacterial meningitis or intracranial abscess
Encephalitis
Intracranial tumor or metastasis
Stroke
Arteriovenous or cavernous malformation
Hyperglycemia
Hypoglycemia
Hyponatremia
Preeclampsia
Intravenous contrast agent (NCSE)
Electroconvulsive therapy (NCSE)

(NCSE = nonconvulsive status epilepticus.)

Psychogenic Status Epilepticus

Pseudoseizures can be very difficult to differentiate from true seizures and may occur comparatively frequently in patients with proven seizure disorder. The incidence was 40% in one referral hospital, but this appears inflated.[14] The assessment of psychogenic seizures can be complicated because previous indiscriminate administration of a benzodiazepine may cloud the neurologic assessment, and electroencephalography often is not immediately available to verify the psychiatric origin of the convulsions.

Several clinical characteristics should increase the likelihood of psychogenic status epilepticus.[15,16] Jerking movements are characteristically out of phase and asynchronous, with a highly typical forward thrusting of the pelvis. Screaming is common. Tongue biting is absent, pupils may be dilated but have retained light responses, and the gag reflex is present.[15–18] Jerking of the extremities may rapidly alternate in tonic-clonic-like movements, and often the arms can be positioned above the patient's face while continuously jerking without falling on the face. The head turns from side to side, and more characteristically, both eyes are consistently deviated from the examiner, occasionally switching with the examiner's position. In between the jerking movements, the patient may speak brief sentences indicating major distress.

All these manifestations, although very characteristic, may rarely be imitated by nonconvulsive status epilepticus due to a frontal epileptic focus.

Myoclonus Status Epilepticus

Myoclonus status epilepticus is common in emergency rooms admitting comatose patients after asphyxia or cardiac arrest. The clinical manifestations of myoclonus status epilepticus are vastly different, but it is still misinterpreted as tonic-clonic seizures.

Myoclonus status epilepticus often consists of synchronous brief jerking in the limbs and face and may involve the diaphragm. Touch, intubation, and placement of catheters may provoke the movements, but continuous jerking is more commonly the rule. An episodic upward gaze of both eyes during a series of myoclonic jerks is typical. Myoclonus status epilepticus is possibly seen moments after cardiac resuscitation when the pulse has returned and the patient has failed to awaken. Pathologic withdrawal or extensor motor responses are common. Its presence denotes massive laminar cortical necrosis, often in association with ischemic damage to the thalamus and spinal cord.

Other conditions that cause myoclonus status epilepticus, such as environmental injuries (e.g., electrical injury, decompression sickness), are related to severe global anoxia produced by the insult. However, profound myoclonus status epilepticus in comatose patients may be caused by drug intoxication (predominantly lithium but also haloperidol, antiepileptic agents, tricyclic antidepressants and penicillin), toxic exposure to industrial agents (pesticides) and heavy metals, renal or hepatic failure, or a degenerative condition, such as Creutzfeldt-Jakob disease, in the final stage.

Neuroimaging in Status Epilepticus

Because withdrawal of antiepileptic drugs remains a commonly recognized cause in adults with a prior seizure disorder, computed tomography (CT) scan or magnetic resonance imaging (MRI) findings are usually normal in status epilepticus. However, CT or MRI may show acute destructive lesions, such as stroke or traumatic injury, metastatic disease, and glioma. CT scanning in anoxia-related myoclonus status epilepticus may show diffuse cerebral edema and, less often, thalamic or cerebral infarcts in watershed territories. In refractory epilepsy, the rate of detection of histopathologically proven abnormalities (glioma, hippocampal sclerosis, developmental lesions) is 95% with conventional MRI and much lower with CT scan, with a sensitivity of 32%. CT scan sensitivity for temporal lobe abnormalities is very low.[19] An imaging study of cryptic seizures at the Mayo Clinic found mesial temporal sclerosis in 55%, brain tumor in 20%, nonspecific findings in 15%, and neuronal migration disorder, vascular malformation (Figure 3.2), or head-injury-associated sclerosis in 10%.[20] Focal hyperintensities on T2-weighted images in complex partial status epilepticus may be seen as a consequence of edema associated with breakdown of the blood-brain barrier. As alluded to earlier, hippocampus or neocortical dropout abnormalities may emerge later and may be a direct correlate of seizures and not of hypoxemia[21,22] (Capsule 3.1).

Miscellaneous Tests

Physiologic changes are observed in the aftermath of status epilepticus. A single generalized tonic-clonic seizure may produce similar laboratory changes if values are obtained within 1 hour of presentation. Most laboratory changes directly resulting from seizures or status epilepticus are self-limiting and rarely need intervention. However, abnormal laboratory values may suggest a competing systemic illness.

White cell counts may increase up to 30×10^9/L.[25] Neutrophils usually remain dominant, but equally common is a lymphocyte increase in the differential count. Immature neutrophils can be present. Acute phase hepatic proteins, glycoproteins, and globulins may transiently increase the erythrocyte sedimentation rate. Plasma glucose concentration may increase but remains in an indeterminate range of less than 150 mg/dL. Plasma osmolality should be normal or mildly increased in patients with dehydration but more significantly increased if recent alcohol abuse contributes to status epilepticus. Plasma osmolalities of 400 to 600 mOsm or more should point to nonketotic hyperosmolar hyperglycemia syndrome. Hyponatremia may cause status epilepticus only when values are less than 120 mmol/L or have decreased at least 20 to 30 mmol/L within several hours.

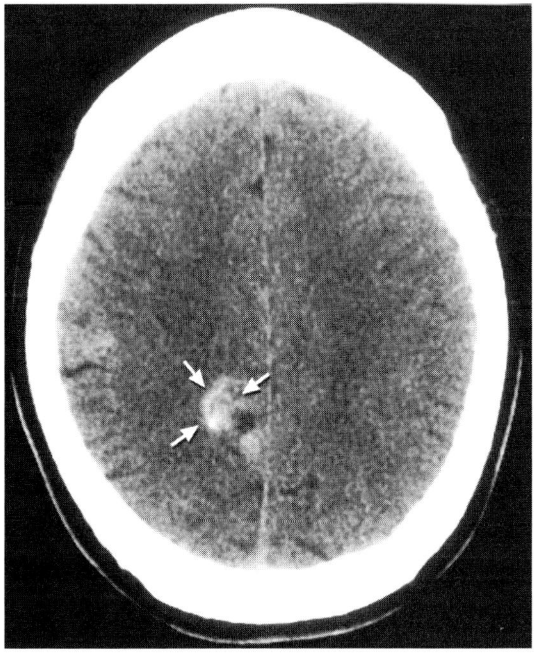
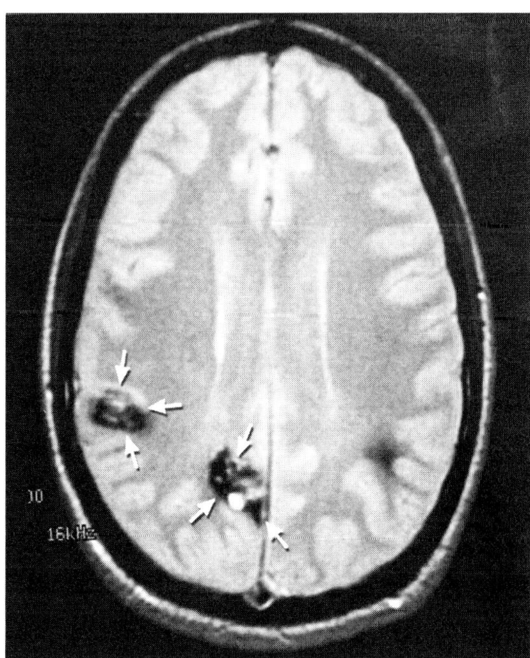

Figure 3.2. Cavernous hemangiomas (*arrows*) (computed tomography and magnetic resonance imaging) in a patient with status epilepticus at presentation.

Spontaneous hypoglycemia possibly indicates a poison (Chapter 1) or, less commonly, insulinoma. Acute renal failure should point to possible rhabdomyolysis and prompt measurement of serum creatine kinase, which may reach values in the thousands.

Arterial blood gas measurements should be done. Respiratory acidosis is as common as metabolic lactic acidosis, but the pH is rarely below 7.0[26] (Table 3.2). The abnormality is self-limiting and resolves within hours.[27] Cardiac arrhythmias, such as sinus tachycardia, bradycardia, and supraventricular tachycardia, are rarely related to changes in the blood gases. Abnormal QRS complexes are not a manifestation of status epilepticus (see Chapter 6 for comparison with subarachnoid hemorrhage).

Laboratory results may be helpful in distinguishing between status epilepticus and pseudoseizures. An entirely normal blood gas value while the patient is having convulsions supports pseudoseizures. The serum concentration of prolactin is increased (peak value 15 to 20 minutes after onset of seizure) after a single epileptic generalized seizure but seldom after pseudoseizures.[28] However, the discriminatory value in pseudo–status epilepticus has been debated,[29] and prolactin may also be increased after syncope.[30]

In any new-onset status epilepticus, cerebrospinal fluid examination should be strongly considered to exclude acute bacterial meningitis and encephalitis. White blood cell counts in the cerebrospinal fluid may increase from seizures but not above 30 mononuclear/mL, and cerebrospinal fluid protein rarely increases significantly.

Electroencephalography is particularly useful in confirmation of focal status epilepticus and detection of nonconvulsive status epilepticus. Electroencephalography may be helpful when the patient is sedated by antiepileptic drugs and clinical manifestations of electrographic discharges are difficult to detect.[31] The findings should guide further use of antiepileptic agents or an increase in dose until epileptic activity is entirely suppressed. The patterns are shown in Figure 3.4.

Management of Status Epilepticus

Not only do patients in status epilepticus urgently need antiepileptic agents to reduce morbidity from

Capsule 3.1. Neuronal Damage Associated with Status Epilepticus

Convulsive status epilepticus may greatly increase the excitatory amino acid glutamate, which in turn opens cation channels to calcium through *N*-methyl-D-aspartate receptors ("excitotoxic theory"). Whether this damage with a proclivity for the hippocampus, thalamus, cerebellum, and neocortex is also caused by additional hyperglycemia, anoxia, hyperpyrexia, or severe acidosis in humans remains unresolved. Neuronal dropout in the neocortex is predominantly apparent in inappropriately treated or unrecognized long-standing status epilepticus. It can take the form of dramatic laminar necrosis (*arrows* on illustration). Hippocampal cell damage does not occur after single seizures or nonconvulsive status epilepticus[23] (Figure 3.3). Paradoxically, a recent study found that hypoxemia protects against edema, possibly because of an early adaptive response involving stress-related transcription factors.[24]

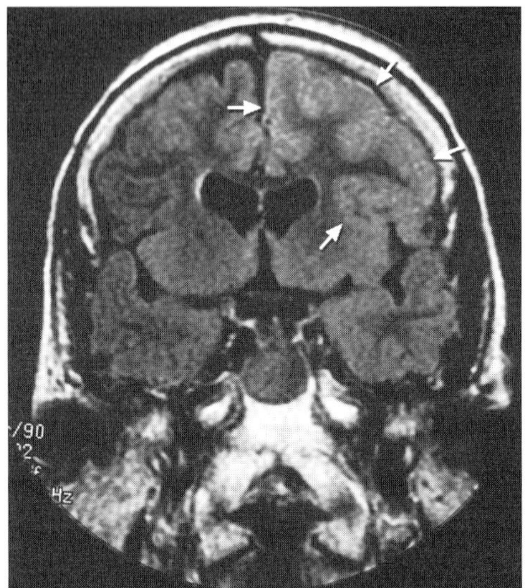

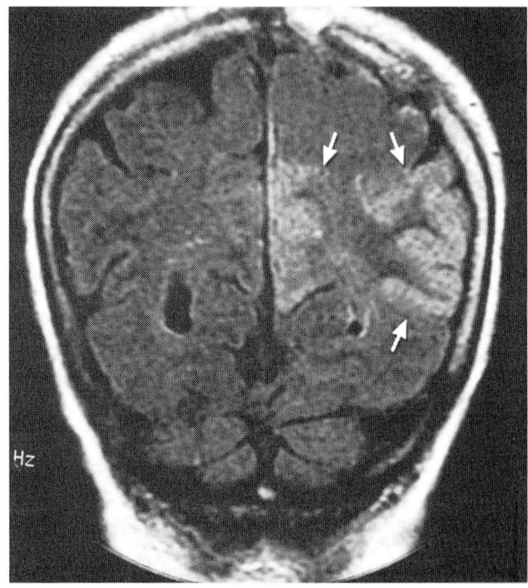

Figure 3.3.

injurious seizure activity but also the systemic effects are potentially harmful and may evolve into a complex medical emergency. It is important to immediately ventilate with oxygen, secure instruments to intubate quickly, and obtain intravenous access (Capsule 3.2).

Table 3.2. Acid-Base Disorders Associated with Status Epilepticus

Derangement	Number of patients	pH
Respiratory acidosis	10	7.10–7.25
Respiratory and metabolic acidosis	6	7.11–7.15
Metabolic acidosis	8	7.05–7.13
Respiratory alkalosis	8	7.51–7.55
Normal	6	7.35–7.45

Modified from Wijdicks and Hubmayr.[26] By permission of Mayo Foundation for Medical Education and Research.

Aspiration is very common in status epilepticus and may be the overriding cause of hypoxemia at presentation. In patients with altered pulmonary defenses, such as those with chronic obstructive pulmonary disease or alcohol abuse, pneumonia develops rapidly. Food particles may obstruct large airways and cause atelectasis and hypoxemia. Adult respiratory distress syndrome may follow rapidly and actually evolve in the emergency room. Dyspnea is profound from alveolar flooding, hypoxemia worsens within minutes, and patients with underlying chronic pulmonary disease have hypercapnia as well. These patients need intubation for airway protection and possibly fiberoptic bronchoscopy if early

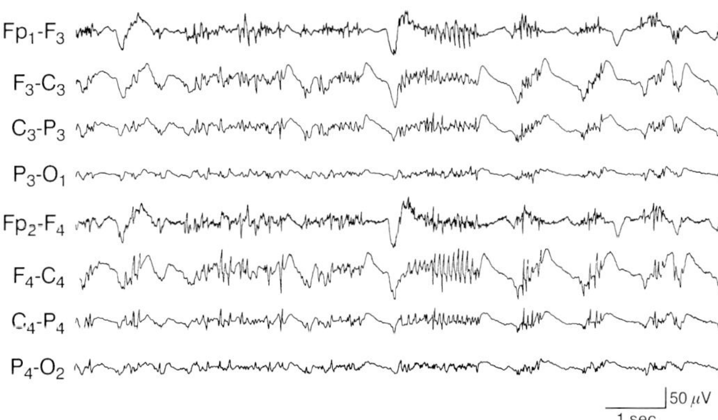

A

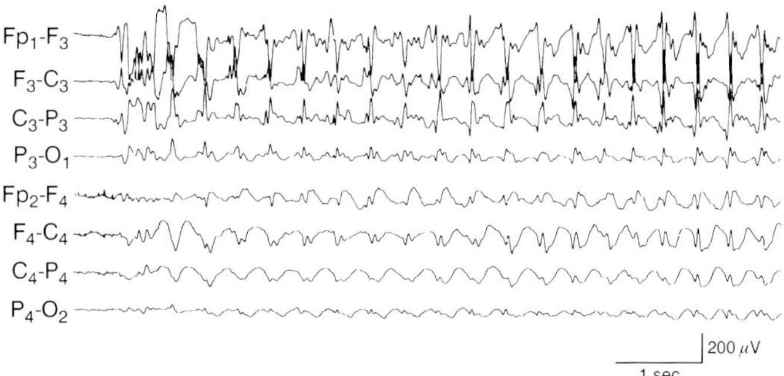

B

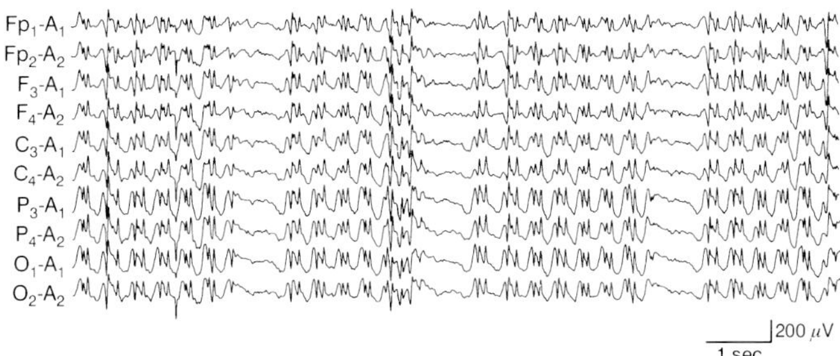

C

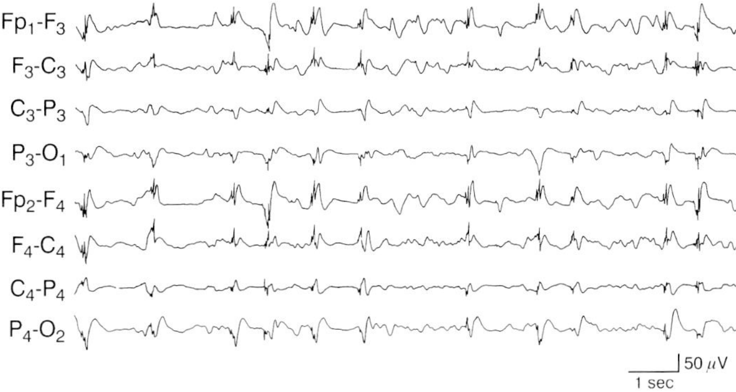

D

Figure 3.4. Electroencephalographic patterns of different types of status epilepticus. **A.** Generalized tonic-clonic seizures (generalized high-frequency spikes and spike-and-wave discharges). **B.** Focal status epilepticus (rhythmic waves and spikes in one hemisphere). **C.** Nonconvulsive status epilepticus (episodes of spike-and-wave discharges coinciding with obtundation). **D.** Myoclonic status epilepticus (continuous epileptiform discharges with a burst-suppression pattern).

Capsule 3.2. No Intravenous Access

Lack of intravenous access can be anticipated in long-term users of intravenous drugs. Intramuscular administration of fosphenytoin (12 to 20 mg/kg phenytoin equivalent) produces plasma concentrations of phenytoin equal to those with the oral dose within 30 minutes of administration, divided over different ejection sites. If intramuscular fosphenytoin is not available, diazepam should be used rectally (0.5 mg/kg) in repeated doses. Other options are intramuscular use of midazolam (5 mg) and observation for 3 minutes to allow absorption. Alternatively, the intranasal route can be considered for midazolam, with rapid absorption (within minutes) (0.1 to 0.2 mg/kg).[32–34] Probably the last resort but the most effective way to counter status epilepticus is to use inhalation anesthetic agents. This should be followed by a saphenous vein cutdown at the ankle. The superficial location of the vein and large diameter make it suitable for placement of a large-bore cannula. Phenytoin can then be administered. Administration of isoflurane is started at 0.5% inspired concentration, with a gradual increase while end-tidal concentrations are monitored until a seizure-free electroencephalogram is obtained. Blood pressure most likely requires support with fluid infusions, the Trendelenburg position, and dopamine, phenylephrine, or dobutamine.

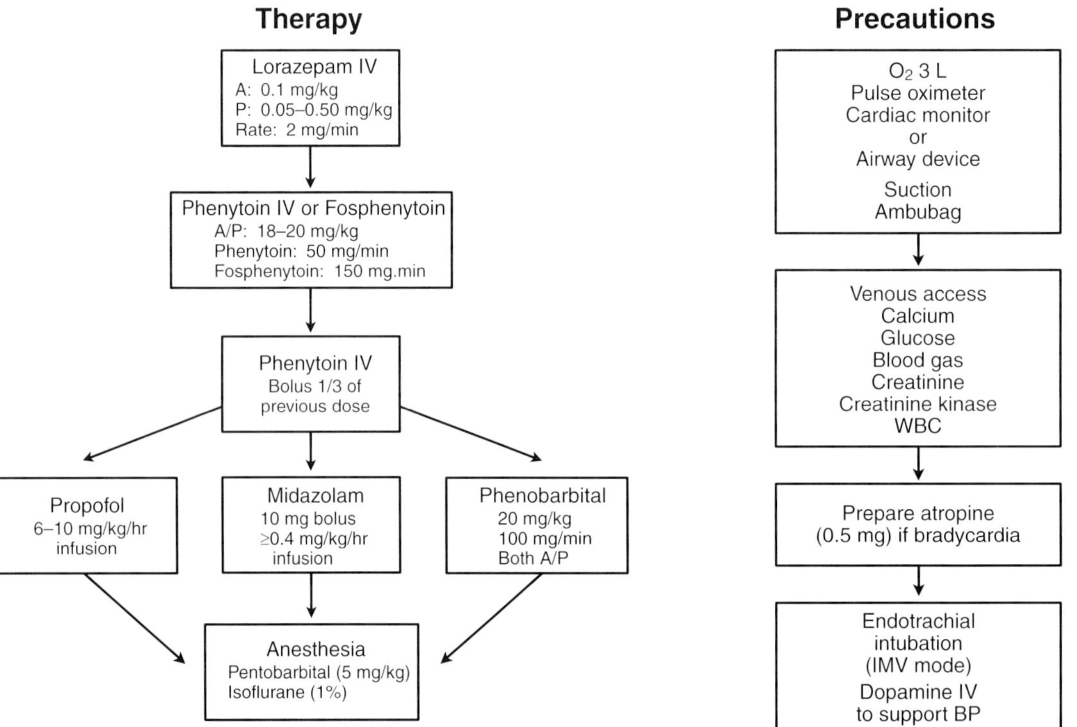

Figure 3.5. Algorithm for management of convulsive status epilepticus. (A = adult dose; BP = blood pressure; IMV = intermittent mandatory ventilation; IV = intravenous; P = pediatric dose; WBC = white blood cells.)

Capsule 3.3. Phenytoin

Phenytoin is rapidly distributed to body tissue and the brain. Respiratory depression does not occur in loading doses of 10 to 20 mg/kg. Sinus bradycardia is the most common cardiac arrhythmia. Transient diastolic pauses may occur and may worsen any heart block. Asystole has been reported. Phenytoin can be mixed only in isotonic saline, because it precipitates in glucose. Oral dosage should resume 6 to 12 hours after infusion.

chest x-ray findings so indicate. Early antibiotic therapy (penicillin G, 1 to 2 million units intravenously every 4 hours, or clindamycin, 600 to 900 mg intravenously every 8 hours) does not prevent chemical injury but may reduce the severity of pneumonitis. Neurogenic pulmonary edema from status epilepticus is uncommon but has been linked to sudden death, mostly in children and young adults. Chest x-ray findings are typical widespread "white-out" infiltrates, which rapidly resolve after several hours of positive end-expiratory pressure ventilation.

Cardiac arrhythmias may appear only if continuous seizures have resulted in prolonged significant lactic acidosis. Many patients have sinus tachycardia from the sympathetic overdrive state. Only cardiac arrhythmias causing measurable blood pressure reduction need correction with antiarrhythmic agents and bicarbonate infusion. Overzealous use of bicarbonate may cause alkalosis, which may perpetuate status epilepticus by lowering the seizure threshold.

Creatine kinase should be measured in each patient, because rhabdomyolysis may result in acute renal failure, which can be entirely prevented by liberal intake of fluids.

The sequence of use of antiepileptic agents in status epilepticus continues to evolve. An approach with additional precautionary measures is shown in Figure 3.5. Lorazepam (0.1 mg/kg) administered at a maximal rate of 2 mg/minute is more effective than phenytoin for initial therapy.[35] Up to 90% of patients are successfully managed with a combination of benzodiazepines and phenytoin.[36,37] Failure to control seizures probably is related to inappropriate phenytoin loading (the popular "1 gram of phenytoin" is almost always inadequate) and also to failure to appreciate that a second intravenous bolus of phenytoin may abort status epilepticus. A common sequence is phenytoin (Capsules 3.3 and 3.4), midazolam or propofol[38–42] (Capsules 3.5 and 3.6), and barbiturates (Capsule 3.7). Doses of the most commonly used antiepileptic drugs are shown in Table 3.3.

A particularly difficult situation is created by epilepsia partialis continua. Treatment is phenytoin loading followed by increasing doses of phenobarbital, starting with 40 mg, or in resistant cases, with intravenous administration of valproate[54] (20 mg/minute; 2.5 to 4 mg/kg every 6 hours). In

Capsule 3.4. Fosphenytoin

Fosphenytoin sodium (Cerebyx) is a prodrug of phenytoin that is rapidly (within minutes) converted by enzymes to phenytoin. Both intravenous and intramuscular administration of 15 to 20 mg/kg produce therapeutic total (≥10 μg/mL) and free (≥1 μg/mL) plasma levels. Intramuscular loading (9 to 12 mg/kg phenytoin equivalent) produces therapeutic levels in 1 hour and can be considered in status epilepticus but only if intravenous access is not available. Fosphenytoin is completely water soluble. Therefore, phlebitis, resistance to heparin, hypotension, and cardiac arrhythmias typically associated with the propylene glycol–based intravenous phenytoin are very infrequent. However, cardiac arrhythmias may still occur when fosphenytoin is infused at rates of more than 150 mg/minute. There is no pharmacokinetic drug interaction with intravenously administered diazepam or lorazepam. Major side effects are nystagmus, headache, ataxia, and drowsiness. Previously unrecognized and highly typical side effects (up to 30%) are transient but very annoying paresthesias and itching in the groin, genitalia, and head and neck.[43]

Capsule 3.5. Midazolam

It is not clear why midazolam works when benzodiazepines and phenytoin fail to control seizures. The drug is currently also being evaluated for initial management in outpatients.[44] The half-life of midazolam (1 to 12 hours) is less than that of lorazepam (10 to 12 hours), and midazolam produces sedation of short duration in status epilepticus. Infusion of 0.05 mg/kg per hour should be continued for at least 12 hours before the dose is tapered. The cost, comparable with that of lorazepam, is high, approaching $800 for 24 hours of continuous infusion. The absence of propylene glycol solution in midazolam reduces the risk of hypotension, bradycardia, and electrocardiographic changes, which are more common with diazepam and lorazepam.[45] High rates of infusion may produce cardiac depression and hypotension. Often, the mean dose to abolish seizure activity is three times the starting dose. When administration is discontinued, full consciousness is expected in 4 to 5 hours in most patients.[46–52]

Capsule 3.6. Propofol

Propofol has been considered controversial because of its association with myoclonic jerking and opisthotonos in humans. However, several studies confirmed that it inhibits seizure activity. These animal studies included lidocaine-induced seizure activity or pentylenetetrazol-induced epilepsy. Propofol has been used in anesthetic doses to control status epilepticus and has reduced the risk of prolonged seizures in electroconvulsive therapy. Seizures may be controlled with a bolus of 100 to 200 mg of propofol, but infusion (6 to 10 mg/kg per hour) is needed.

Capsule 3.7. Barbiturates

Failure to control seizures with therapeutic levels of phenytoin (≥25 μg/mL) may justify intravenous administration of phenobarbital. Phenobarbital is much more potent than pentobarbital. Its major drawbacks are direct myocardial depression and vascular dilatation, but these are not treatment-limiting. Phenobarbital also has a very long elimination half-life (24 to 140 hours) but zero-order elimination at high doses (constant amount of drug elimination per unit of time).

Intravenous barbiturate anesthesia virtually always controls status epilepticus, but relapse can be substantial, usually preceded by electrographic recurrence of seizure activity.[53] Pentobarbital and phenobarbital are equal in effectiveness. Experience with propofol and midazolam will reduce the use of barbiturates greatly, but barbiturates remain very useful also in partial status epilepticus.

our experience, control is commonly achieved without need for endotracheal intubation due to respiratory depression.

Nonconvulsive status epilepticus, when documented by electroencephalography, can be countered under electroencephalographic monitoring with benzodiazepines (lorazepam, 8 mg, or diazepam, 10 mg).

The management of seizures in patients with preeclampsia is notably different. Magnesium sulfate remains the standard in prevention and treatment of seizures or status epilepticus.[55] Magnesium sulfate is given at a beginning dose of 4 to 5 g intravenously or 10 g intramuscularly.[56] An intravenous infusion of 1 g/hour is started. Additional antiepileptic agents are not warranted and may cause respiratory depression in the newborn. Magnesium toxicity may, however, also reduce mother and child respirations. Reduced tendon reflexes may occur and may indicate imminent toxicity and thus are a useful monitoring sign during titration of treatment.

Antiepileptic therapy in myoclonus status epilepticus is usually not effective after cardiac arrest. Clonazepam has been advocated for treatment but has not been persistently effective in our experience. There is no rationale to aggressively treat these myoclonic jerks with a series of antiepileptic drugs. Neuromuscular blocking agents should be considered to eliminate the constant generalized jerks until the level of care has been assessed.

Psychogenic epilepticus typically lasts longer but may be aborted almost instantaneously with a supportive suggestion. The diagnosis can be confirmed by an electroencephalogram, but the jerking movements are often so bizarre that it is clear from the outset. A recent study found that psychogenic status epilepticus could be rapidly induced by administering saline intravenously and telling the patient (who has visited many different emergency rooms) that the saline solution will provoke seizures.[57] However, the use of these deceptive provocative techniques is ethically questionable and should be considered only as a last resort.[58]

Management of Recurrent Seizures

A clinical policy for the initial approach to patients with a seizure who are not in status epilepticus has recently been published by the American College of Emergency Physicians.[59] Four major guidelines are highlighted. First, prolonged altered consciousness should not be attributed to a postictal state. Second, patients with prior epilepsy who are alert and have normal findings on neurologic examination do not require aggressive evaluation other than measurement of antiepileptic drug levels. Third, alcohol-related seizures may indicate serious underlying morbidity. Fourth, the patient should be implicitly told that driving and operation of machines should be restricted until a reasonable observation period has passed to prevent future disasters.

Approximately three-fourths of patients with two or three unprovoked seizures have further seizures within 4 years.[60] In contrast, the risk of a second seizure is approximately 35% in the subsequent 3 to 5 years.[61] The risk of seizure recurrence is substantially increased (probably doubled) when an identifiable brain lesion is found.

Table 3.3. Common Initial Drug Dosages to Control Status Epilepticus

Agent	Dose (mg/kg)	Rate
Lorazepam	0.1	0.04 mg/kg/min
Phenytoin	20	0.3 mg/kg/min
Midazolam	0.2	0.1–0.2 mg/kg/hr
Propofol	15	6–10 mg/kg/hr
Phenobarbital	12	0.2–0.4 mg/kg/min

Before a patient is sent out of the emergency room, several diagnostic tests should be done (Table 3.4), but in many instances, admission for intravenous phenytoin loading is advised.

The recommended drugs for primary generalized tonic-clonic seizures or partial seizures with secondary generalization are phenytoin (300 mg/day in one dose; therapeutic level, 10 to 20 μg/mL), carbamazepine (300 to 1,200 mg daily; therapeutic level, 4 to 12 μg/mL), and valproate (600 to 3,000 mg/day; therapeutic level, 50 to 150 μg/mL). The first-line agent for absence seizures is ethosuximide (1 to 2 g/day; therapeutic level, 40 to 100 μg/mL).

The alternative medication, mostly if seizures occur with first-line agents at therapeutic levels, could be gabapentin (900 mg/day in three gradually increasing doses) or other second-line antiepileptic drugs (e.g., lamotrigine, topiramate, tiagabine).

Specific concerns may arise when seizures are observed during pregnancy without evidence of eclampsia. Antiepileptic drugs for brief treatment of recurrent seizures should be well tolerated when pregnancy is beyond the first trimester and the risk

Table 3.4. Diagnostic Tests in Recurrent de Novo Seizures

Computed tomography scan with contrast
Cervical spine radiograph (if trauma is suspected)
Cerebrospinal fluid (predominantly in immunosuppressed patients; human immunodeficiency virus)
Toxicologic screen, alcohol level
Electrolytes, calcium, magnesium, blood urea nitrogen, creatinine, complete blood cell count, glucose

to the infant seems unsubstantiated. Antiepileptic drugs in pregnancy double the risk of congenital malformations, including limb deformities, spina bifida (valproate), and growth retardation. Folic acid, 0.4 mg/day, should be added during pregnancy, but its effect on reducing birth defects probably takes place around conception.[62] Monitoring phenytoin levels in pregnancy is complicated by a decrease in serum albumin levels; thus, the unbound fraction should be measured to manage dosage. In addition, the increased volume of distribution and increased clearance by liver and placenta may force an increase in the total daily dose.

Discontinuation of antiepileptic therapy is considered after a 2-year seizure-free interval, and if this can be achieved, recurrence is very low except in patients with documented brain lesions (e.g., cavernous angioma, cerebral contusion). Sudden withdrawal may increase the risk of recurrence and in some instances, unfortunately, status epilepticus. Recurrence of seizures cannot be entirely excluded by a normal electroencephalogram before discontinuation is attempted.

References

1. Scholtes FB, Renier WO, Meinardi H. Generalized convulsive status epilepticus: causes, therapy, and outcome in 346 patients. Epilepsia 1994;35:1104.
2. Towne AR, Pellock JM, Ko D, DeLorenzo RJ. Determinants of mortality in status epilepticus. Epilepsia 1994;35:27.
3. Treiman DM. Generalized convulsive status epilepticus in the adult. Epilepsia 1993;34(Suppl 1):S2.
4. Cascino GD. Generalized convulsive status epilepticus. Mayo Clin Proc 1996;71:787.
5. Gemma M, Cipriani A, Mungo M. Management of status epilepticus (letter to the editor). Intensive Care Med 1994;20:611.
6. Runge JW, Allen FH. Emergency treatment of status epilepticus. Neurology 1996;46(Suppl 1):S20.
7. DeLorenzo RJ, Hauser WA, Towne AR, et al. A prospective, population-based epidemiologic study of status epilepticus in Richmond, Virginia. Neurology 1996;46:1029.
8. Lowenstein DH, Alldredge BK. Status epilepticus at an urban public hospital in the1980s. Neurology 1993;43:483.
9. Sung CY, Chu NS. Status epilepticus in the elderly: etiology, seizure type and outcome. Acta Neurol Scand 1989;80:51.
10. Alldredge BK, Lowenstein DH. Status epilepticus related to alcohol abuse. Epilepsia 1993;34:1033.
11. Fagan KJ, Lee SI. Prolonged confusion following convulsions due to generalized nonconvulsive status epilepticus. Neurology 1990;40:1689.
12. Kaplan PW. Nonconvulsive status epilepticus in the emergency room. Epilepsia 1996;37:643.
13. Cockerell OC, Walker MC, Sander JW, Shorvon SD. Complex partial status epilepticus: a recurrent problem. J Neurol Neurosurg Psychiatry 1994;57:835.
14. Howell SJ, Owen L, Chadwick DW. Pseudostatus epilepticus. Q J Med 1989;71:507.
15. Rosenberg ML. The eyes in hysterical states of unconsciousness. J Clin Neuroophthalmol 1982;2:259.
16. Shen W, Bowman ES, Markand ON. Presenting the diagnosis of pseudoseizure. Neurology 1990;40:756.
17. Jagoda A, Richey-Klein V, Riggio S. Psychogenic status epilepticus. J Emerg Med 1995;13:31.
18. King DW, Gallagher BB, Murvin AJ, et al. Pseudoseizures: diagnostic evaluation. Neurology 1982;32:18.
19. Bronen RA, Fulbright RK, Spencer DD, et al. Refractory epilepsy: comparison of MR imaging, CT, and histopathologic findings in 117 patients. Radiology 1996;201:97.
20. Jack CR Jr. Magnetic resonance imaging in epilepsy. Mayo Clin Proc 1996;71:695.
21. Meierkord H, Wieshmann U, Niehaus L, Lehmann R. Structural consequences of status epilepticus demonstrated with serial magnetic resonance imaging. Acta Neurol Scand 1997;96:127.
22. Tien RD, Felsberg GJ. The hippocampus in status epilepticus: demonstration of signal intensity and morphologic changes with sequential fast spin-echo MR imaging. Radiology 1995;194:249.
23. Bertram EH, Lothman EW, Lenn NJ. The hippocampus in experimental chronic epilepsy: a morphometric analysis. Ann Neurol 1990;27:43.
24. Emerson MR, Nelson SR, Samson FE, Pazdernik TL. Hypoxia preconditioning attenuates brain edema associated with kainic acid-induced status epilepticus in rats. Brain Res 1999;825:189.
25. Barry E, Hauser WA. Pleocytosis after status epilepticus. Arch Neurol 1994;51:190.
26. Wijdicks EFM, Hubmayr RD. Acute acid-base disorders associated with status epilepticus. Mayo Clin Proc 1994;69:1044.
27. Yaffe K, Lowenstein DH. Prognostic factors of pentobarbital therapy for refractory generalized status epilepticus. Neurology 1993;43:895.
28. Laxer KD, Mullooly JP, Howell B. Prolactin changes after seizures classified by EEG monitoring. Neurology 1985;35:31.
29. Tomson T, Lindbom U, Nilsson BY, et al. Serum prolactin during status epilepticus. J Neurol Neurosurg Psychiatry 1989;52:1435.
30. Oribe E, Amini R, Nissenbaum E, Boal B. Serum prolactin concentrations are elevated after syncope. Neurology 1996;47:60.
31. Privitera MD, Strawsburg RH. Electroencephalographic monitoring in the emergency department. Emerg Med

Clin North Am 1994;12:1089.
32. Kendall JL, Reynolds M, Goldberg R. Intranasal midazolam in patients with status epilepticus. Ann Emerg Med 1997;29:415.
33. Kofke WA, Young RS, Davis P, et al. Isoflurane for refractory status epilepticus: a clinical series. Anesthesiology 1989;71:653.
34. Rey E, Delaunay L, Pons G, et al. Pharmacokinetics of midazolam in children: comparative study of intranasal and intravenous administration. Eur J Clin Pharmacol 1991;41:355.
35. Treiman DM, Meyers PD, Walton NY, et al. A comparison of four treatments for generalized convulsive status epilepticus. N Engl J Med 1998;339:792.
36. Mitchell WG. Status epilepticus and acute repetitive seizures in children, adolescents, and young adults: etiology, outcome, and treatment. Epilepsia 1996;37(Suppl 1):S74.
37. Weise KL, Bleck TP. Status epilepticus in children and adults. Crit Care Clin 1997;13:629.
38. Borgeat A, Wilder-Smith OH, Jallon P, Suter PM. Propofol in the management of refractory status epilepticus: a case report. Intensive Care Med 1994;20:148.
39. Kuisma M, Roine RO. Propofol in prehospital treatment of convulsive status epilepticus. Epilepsia 1995;36:1241.
40. Mackenzie SJ, Kapadia F, Grant IS. Propofol infusion for control of status epilepticus. Anaesthesia 1990; 45:1043.
41. Pitt-Miller PL, Elcock BJ, Maharaj M. The management of status epilepticus with a continuous propofol infusion. Anesth Analg 1994;78:1193.
42. Stecker MM, Kramer TH, Raps EC, et al. Treatment of refractory status epilepticus with propofol: clinical and pharmacokinetic findings. Epilepsia 1998;39;18.
43. Browne TR. Fosphenytoin (Cerebyx). Clin Neuropharmacol 1997;20:1.
44. LeDuc TJ, Goellner WE, el-Sanadi N. Out-of-hospital midazolam for status epilepticus (letter to the editor). Ann Emerg Med 1996;28:377.
45. Labar DR, Ali A, Root J. High-dose intravenous lorazepam for the treatment of refractory status epilepticus. Neurology 1994;44:1400.
46. Crisp CB, Gannon R, Knauft F. Continuous infusion of midazolam hydrochloride to control status epilepticus. Clin Pharm 1988;7:322.
47. Jawad S, Oxley J, Wilson J, Richens A. A pharmacodynamic evaluation of midazolam as an antiepileptic compound. J Neurol Neurosurg Psychiatry 1986;49:1050.
48. Kumar A, Bleck TP. Intravenous midazolam for the treatment of refractory status epilepticus. Crit Care Med 1992;20:483.
49. Lal Koul R, Raj Aithala G, Chacko A, et al. Continuous midazolam infusion as treatment of status epilepticus. Arch Dis Child 1997;76:445.
50. Mayhue FE. IM midazolam for status epilepticus in the emergency department. Ann Emerg Med 1988;17:643.
51. Nordt SP, Clark RF. Midazolam: a review of therapeutic uses and toxicity. J Emerg Med 1997;15:357.
52. Parent JM, Lowenstein DH. Treatment of refractory generalized status epilepticus with continuous infusion of midazolam. Neurology 1994;44:1837.
53. Krishnamurthy KB, Drislane FW. Relapse and survival after barbiturate anesthetic treatment of refractory status epilepticus. Epilepsia 1996;37:863.
54. Kaplan PW. Intravenous valproate treatment of generalized nonconvulsive status epilepticus. Clin Electroencephalogr 1999;30:1.
55. Crowther C. Magnesium sulphate versus diazepam in the management of eclampsia: a randomized controlled trial. Br J Obstet Gynaecol 1990;97:110.
56. Lucas MJ, Leveno KJ, Cunningham FG. A comparison of magnesium sulfate with phenytoin for the prevention of eclampsia. N Engl J Med 1995;333:201.
57. Ney GC, Zimmerman C, Schaul N. Psychogenic status epilepticus induced by a provocative technique. Neurology 1996;46:546.
58. Cohen RJ, Suter C. Hysterical seizures: suggestion as a provocative EEG test. Ann Neurol 1982;11:391.
59. American College of Emergency Physicians. Clinical policy for the initial approach to patients presenting with a chief complaint of seizure who are not in status epilepticus. Ann Emerg Med 1997;29:706.
60. First Seizure Trial Group. Randomized clinical trial on the efficacy of antiepileptic drugs in reducing the risk of relapse after a first unprovoked tonic-clonic seizure. Neurology 1993;43:478.
61. Hauser WA, Rich SS, Lee JR, et al. Risk of recurrent seizures after two unprovoked seizures. N Engl J Med 1998; 338:429.
62. Lindhout D, Omtzigt JG. Teratogenic effects of antiepileptic drugs: implications for the management of epilepsy in women of childbearing age. Epilepsia 1994;35(Suppl 4):S19.

Chapter 4
Acute Obstructive Hydrocephalus

The cerebrospinal fluid (CSF) is produced in the choroid plexus in the lateral ventricle and circulated throughout a system with critical passages at the foramen of Monro, third ventricle, and aqueduct of Sylvius and absorbed through arachnoid villi. Any impingement at these locations causes increased hydrostatic pressure in a matter of hours (Capsule 4.1). Enlargement of the ventricular system may be acutely created by a mass obstructing CSF outflow or by sudden stretching and ballooning out from introduction of a jet of arterial blood. Only ventriculostomy results in an adequate diversion of flow and in fact may be lifesaving.

It is important to recognize the urgency of acute hydrocephalus in the emergency room, and this chapter describes clinical presentation, causes, and shunt placement. Definitive management, carefully planned later, implies resection or debulking of the tumor or permanent placement of a ventriculoperitoneal shunt.

Clinical Presentation

Patients with acute obstructive hydrocephalus have diminished alertness at presentation. Often in retrospect, episodes of headache have been common and frequently intense. Earlier periods of blurring of vision and obscurations (sudden grayouts or blackouts lasting seconds) associated with papilledema (due to pressure-induced relative ischemia of the optic nerve) are reported.[1] Unfortunately the diagnosis in some patients is made only after symptoms and signs referable to brain stem compression or brain stem shift have occurred. Papilledema may occur, implying long-standing increased CSF pressure, but remains an uncommon clinical finding in most intraventricular, pineal, or choroid plexus tumors.

Decrease in level of consciousness from ventricular enlargement may have several mechanisms. First, hydrocephalus may impair the ascending reticular activating system (ARAS) at the level of the periaqueduct, which pushes against relay nuclei and fibers of the ARAS when it expands. Second, displacement of the upper brain stem by a massively enlarged third ventricle may tilt it backwards and kink its structure. Third, when intracranial pressure from increased ventricular pressure rises above the cerebral perfusion pressure, and certainly when the increase in pressure occurs rapidly, global ischemic damage to both hemispheres or herniation of brain tissue bilaterally through the tentorium or foramen magnum produces an advanced stage of coma. Fourth, decreased arousal may also be caused by tumor infiltration into paramedian thalamic nuclei or the mesencephalon, which at the same time obstructs normal CSF flow (see Chapter 1).

Fifth, tumors that obstruct the ventricles may produce clinical signs from compression by the mass effect itself to the brain stem (e.g., pinealoma). These signs may combine to form Parinaud's syndrome, consisting of upward gaze palsy and impaired convergence, with a so-called light-near dissociation of the pupillary light reflex (pupil constriction to accommodation and not to light); it is typically overlooked with a cursory examination.[1] The lesion for the classic

Capsule 4.1. Pathophysiology of Acute Hydrocephalus

Acute hydrocephalus occurs when normal physiologic equilibrium is disturbed. CSF production (an ultrafiltrate from capillaries) occurs in the choroid plexus and may increase in the plexus papilloma. The circulation of CSF depends on several variables, such as rate of production (0.30 mL/minute), choroid plexus pulsations (filling of choroid plexus with each arterial pulse generates a pumping force), resistance (series of conduits, including foramina, aqueduct of Sylvius, and arachnoid villi), and sagittal sinus pressure (CSF pressure is greater, and flow depends on this pressure gradient). Absorption is linearly related to CSF pressure. Reduction in CSF therefore may be achieved by decreasing CSF production (carbonic anhydrate inhibitors; acetazolamide, which takes hours to achieve the effect), removing obstructing tumor, and improving absorption (e.g., corticosteroids to reduce inflammatory response in arachnoid villi).

findings of Parinaud's syndrome is in the dorsal midbrain (pretectum) and interrupts the supranuclear mechanisms for upward gaze. However, the dorsal midbrain can also be distorted by enlargement of the posterior third ventricle and periaqueductal structures.

Pineal gland tumors may directly compress the midbrain, and compression may persist despite CSF diversion methods. Colloid cysts are incidentally found, but they obstruct the foramen of Monro only after reaching a critical size. Intermittent headaches may precede acute deterioration, which can lead to sudden brain death.

Specific Disorders Associated with Acute Hydrocephalus

In a large proportion of patients, the cause of acute hydrocephalus in adults seen in the emergency room is ventricular dilatation associated with subarachnoid hemorrhage, lobar hematoma, primary intraventricular hemorrhage, or, much less commonly, malfunctioning ventriculolumbar or peritoneal shunts for previous hydrocephalus or associated with de novo brain tumors. The causes of acute hydrocephalus associated with masses in adults are shown in Table 4.1.

Intracranial Hematoma

Primary intraventricular hemorrhage commonly causes acute hydrocephalus, although a more delayed course has been noted. Usually, the hemorrhage is massive (Figure 4.1A) (see also Chapter 7). Intraventricular introduction of a thalamic, caudate, or large lobar hematoma produces acute ventricular enlargement. Acute hemorrhage in the cerebellum, particularly when it extends to the vermis, may rapidly block the fourth ventricle, leading to obstructive hydrocephalus (Figure 4.1B).

Hydrocephalus in supratentorial intracerebral hematoma is an independent predictor of poor outcome.[14] In addition, a recent study seriously questioned the use of ventriculostomy in parenchymal supratentorial hemorrhage.[15] Ventricular drainage controlled intracranial pressure but did not consistently improve level of consciousness, suggesting direct irreversible tissue damage from hydrocephalus. Moreover, hemorrhagic dilatation of the fourth ventricle has been identified as an important indicator of poor outcome, confirming the impression that sudden massive enlargement causes damage to the periaqueductal area.[16]

Acute hydrocephalus in pontine hemorrhage is merely a consequence of its destructive hemorrhage, and ventriculostomy will not reverse coma. Extension to the mesencephalon and occasionally bilaterally to the thalamus precludes awakening. (After several unsuccessful attempts in our patients, we categorically forgo ventriculostomy.)

Cerebellar hematoma and acute hydrocephalus can be treated by ventriculostomy when the fourth ventricle is blocked and no brain stem compression is evident on computed tomography (CT) scans. Only in this particular clinical situation can ventriculostomy

Table 4.1. Masses Causing Acute Obstructive Hydrocephalus*

Type	CT scan characteristics	Treatment
Intraventricular tumors		
Colloid cyst	Rounded, anterior 3V, widened SP, collapse of posterior 3V, ID or HYP	Surgery or stereotactic aspiration
Plexus papilloma	Oval, 4V, LV, HYP	Total excision
Subependymoma	Lobulated, 4V, LV, ID	Excision and radiotherapy
Oligodendroglioma	Lobulated, LV, HYP, C	Resection
Ganglioglioma	3V, ID, HYP	Resection
Astrocytoma	LV, HD or HYP, irregular shape	Radiation, resection
Epidermoid cyst	4V, HYP, ID	Resection
Masses in pineal region		
Pineoblastoma	Lobulated, HD at peripheral rim, C	Resection, radiation
Germinoma	ID, rounded	Radiation
Teratoma	HD or HYP, C, lipid content	Resection
Vein of Galen aneurysm	HYP, rounded, triangular	Endovascular occlusion

(C = calcifications; CT = computed tomography; HD = hypodense; HYP = hyperdense; ID = isodense; LV = lateral ventricle; SP = septum pellucidum; 3V = third ventricle; 4V = fourth ventricle.)
See references 2–13.
*Other common causes are metastasis, lymphoma, and bacterial or parasitic abscesses (see also Chapter 1, Table 1.7).

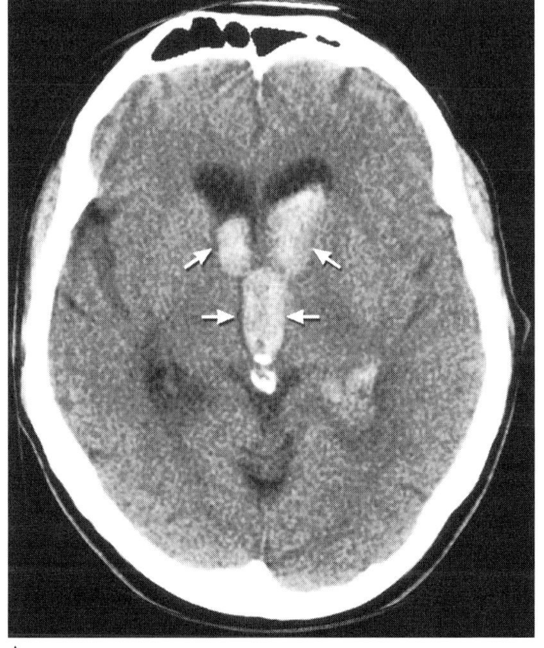

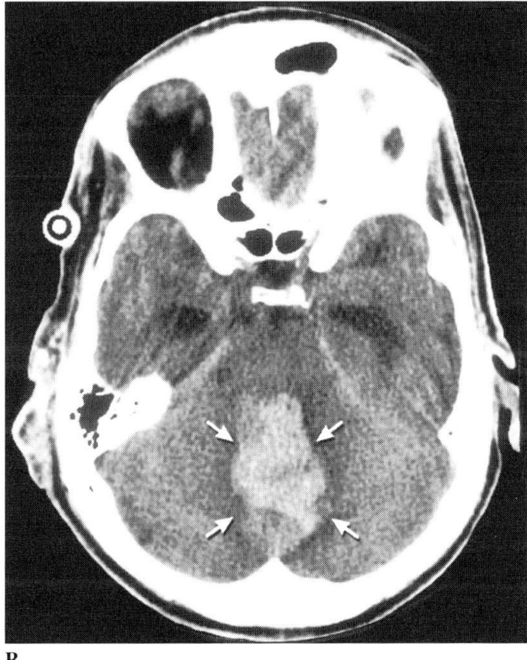

A B

Figure 4.1. A. Acute hydrocephalus in intraventricular hemorrhage due to sudden arterial jet of blood. **B.** Acute hydrocephalus associated with cerebellar hematoma effacing the fourth ventricle.

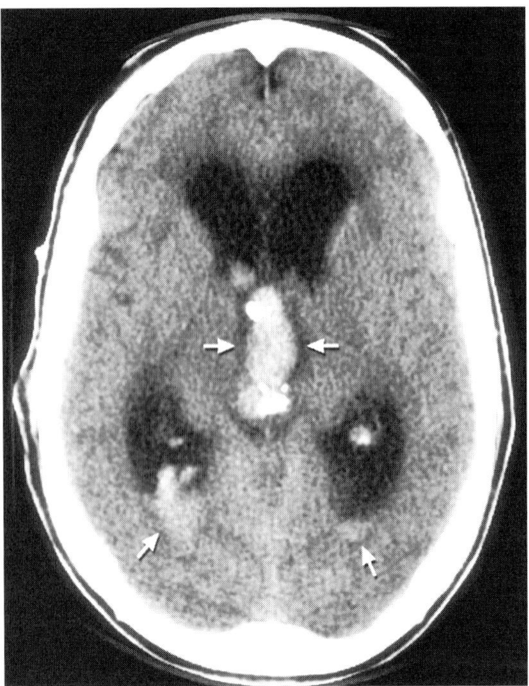

Figure 4.2. Acute hydrocephalus in subarachnoid hemorrhage with intraventricular blood (third ventricle and posterior horns) from ruptured anterior cerebral aneurysm.

be beneficial; in all other instances, decompression of the pons by occipital craniotomy is more logical.

Aneurysmal Subarachnoid Hemorrhage

CT scan evidence of acute hydrocephalus is common in aneurysmal subarachnoid hemorrhage (Figure 4.2). Acute hydrocephalus may be caused by obstruction of CSF outflow at the level of the ambient cisterns, by clogging of the arachnoid space with subarachnoid blood, or occasionally from the mass effect of a giant aneurysm obstructing the third ventricle.[17] Commonly, the temporal horns are dilated early, typically before identifiable dilatation of the third and lateral ventricles. Ventriculostomy is certainly justified when clinical worsening in level of consciousness is clearly documented, when serial CT scans unmistakably demonstrate further enlargement, or when the third ventricle has changed into a balloon-shaped structure. One may argue that early ventriculostomy is a safeguard against rebleeding in the first hours, but conversely it may be argued that reducing the CSF pressure may reduce the sealing pressures of the aneurysm and thus increase the risk of bleeding. None of these views is supported by convincing data. Some interventional neuroradiologists prefer a ventriculostomy at the time of coiling if a suitable aneurysm is found on cerebral angiography. Iatrogenic rerupture can be managed by siphoning through the ventriculostomy, particularly in anterior circulation aneurysms that rupture through the lamina terminalis into the third and lateral ventricles.

Bacterial Meningitis

Obstruction of the ventricular communication with the subarachnoid space by inflammatory exudate is the most likely mechanism. Acute obstructive hydrocephalus can occur several weeks after bacterial meningitis begins and typically appears insidiously. The ventricular system, however, can be enlarged soon after the illness but usually to a minor degree and transiently (Figure 4.3). Rarely is there a need to place a ventriculostomy tube early when hydrocephalus occurs within the first days, but late-onset hydrocephalus (10% in adult bacterial meningitis) may require placement of a drain.

Pineal Region Tumors

These tumors predominate in young adults (and children). Compression of the quadrigeminal plate depends on the size of the tumor, and compression of the cerebral aqueduct or tumor growth into the posterior third ventricle produces obstructive hydrocephalus.

Pineal parenchymal neoplasms can be divided into pineoblastoma (with histologic characteristics nearly identical to those of medulloblastoma) and pineocytoma (characteristic rosette formation).

The outcome of pineoblastoma is poor, with survival rarely extending beyond 2 years.[5] Pineocytoma with neuronal differentiation, such as large rosette formation or ganglion cells, has a much better long-term outcome—up to 3 decades after diagnosis, resection, and radiotherapy. Germinomas may arise from this location, as may other germ cell tumors, such as teratomas, embryonal carcinoma, endodermal sinus tumor, and choriocarcinoma.

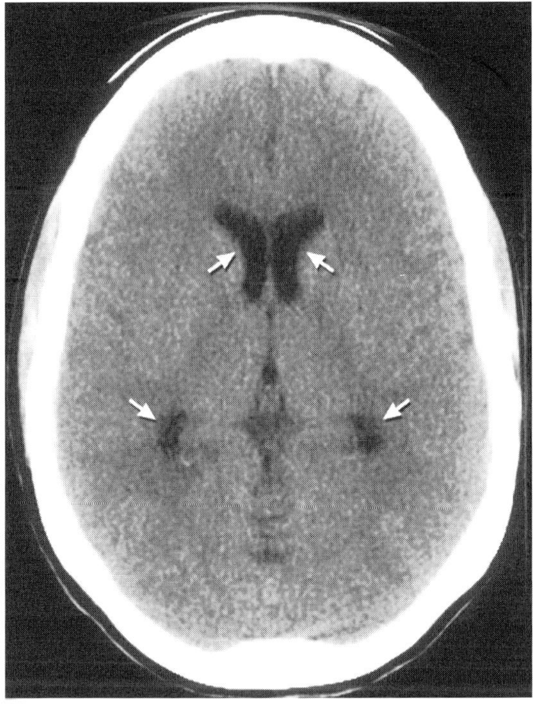

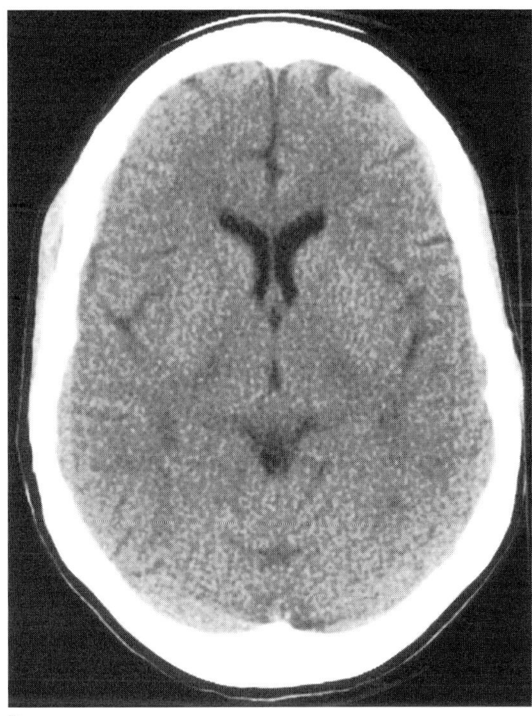

Figure 4.3. A. Acute hydrocephalus in pneumococcal meningitis. **B.** Resolution (particularly temporal horns) of the enlargement but also reappearance of sulci 4 days after antibiotic therapy.

Germinomas are very radiosensitive, and long-term survival or cure is expected after resection. CSF should be sampled at the time of ventricular shunting. Choriocarcinoma and pineal germinoma secrete human chorionic gonadotropin. Alpha-fetoprotein is increased in endodermal sinus tumors, infiltrating teratoma, embryonal carcinoma, and choriocarcinoma.[18] CSF markers may help in differentiation.

Colloid Cyst of the Third Ventricle

The incidence of colloid cyst of the third ventricle is about 0.5% to 2% of all intracranial tumors. This developmental abnormality is filled with homogeneous viscous material containing cellular debris. Its location in the third ventricle causes intermittent marked enlargement of the ventricles, and brain death may ensue if recurrent headaches are not sufficiently investigated.[4,19] Colloid cysts are a cause of sudden death in pediatric patients.[20,21]

In the Karolinska Hospital–based series of 37 consecutive patients, 5 patients were admitted to the emergency room and 2 died despite emergency ventriculostomy.[22,23]

Full resection should be planned. Unfavorable long-term results were associated with aspiration and subtotal resection.[22] However, transcallosal microsurgery produced excellent results.[22–25]

Ependymoma

Neoplastic growth of the epithelial lining on the ventricular surface is most commonly supratentorial in adults and more commonly intratentorial in children.[6,26] Seeding throughout the CSF occurs in some instances. These malignant tumors grow slowly, and outcome is determined by grade, with 5-year survival of 80% in patients with low-grade tumors. Anaplastic or poorly differentiated ependymoma with typical histologic features of high mitotic activity, vascular proliferation, and necrosis reduces survival to 50%.

Plexus Papilloma

Tumors of the choroid plexus often are papillary and highly vascularized. Intratumor hemorrhage is common. Localization is commonly in the fourth ventricle in adults.[27] These tumors do not invade and are comparatively easy to resect.

Epidermoid Cysts

Epidermoid cysts are ectodermal elements displaced during embryogenesis that become symptomatic in adults.[28] Rupture of the cyst may cause aseptic ventriculitis. Predilection is for the fourth ventricle, and because of compression of the brain stem, cranial nerve palsy, ataxia, and hemiparesis may occur. Because of its slow growth and pliable nature, however, it may only produce intermittent headaches.

Neuroimaging in Acute Hydrocephalus

Different sites of obstruction in acute hydrocephalus are shown in Figure 4.4. CT scanning clearly delineates the degree of hydrocephalus and in many instances the obstructing tumor. Usually, the largest parts of the ventricular system (the anterior horns of the lateral ventricles) enlarge first, the temporal horns next, and then the third and fourth ventricles. When hydrocephalus has developed over weeks, subependymal effusions are clear evidence of increased CSF pressure. These periventricular hypodensities may occur in up to 40% of patients with acute obstructing hydrocephalus, but this capping surrounding the ventricle may also be evident in elderly patients with long-standing hypertension and diabetes but no hydrocephalus.[29]

The degree of hydrocephalus can be carefully assessed by several measuring systems. These simple linear measurements not only determine the degree of hydrocephalus but also can be used to monitor change. The ventricular size index measures the bifrontal diameter (transverse inner diameter) and divides it by the frontal horn diameter. The bicaudate index might be more reliable, because consistent normal values have been established. This index is determined by the width of the frontal horns at the level of the caudate nuclei divided by the maximum width of the brain at the same level (Figure 4.5).

The temporal horns remain sensitive indicators for hydrocephalus on CT scans. Temporal horns, usually barely visible, become large boomerang-shaped ventricles in acute hydrocephalus. This configuration often clearly differentiates obstruction from cortical cerebral atrophy. Other features compatible with atrophy rather than hydrocephalus are widening sylvian and interhemispheric fissures, leaving marked hypodense fluid-filled spaces and prominent dilated cortical sulci.

It is important to identify tumors that may obstruct the ventricular system, particularly those located in the intraventricular compartment, which may be isodense to the brain tissue. Characteristically, colloid cysts of the third ventricle are very subtle and difficult to detect, because they blend in with brain tissue. A mass should be strongly considered if the third ventricle cannot be identified or the septum pellucidum is widened, separating the posterior medial aspects of the frontal horns. It is important to scrutinize the posterior fossa for a mass lesion that may be evident only from distortion of the fourth ventricle.

Magnetic resonance imaging, however, should disclose any obstructive mass lesion.[30] Magnetic resonance imaging also is particularly important to demonstrate meningeal enhancement (such as in sarcoidosis or carcinomatous meningitis)[31,32] and lesions typically missed on CT scanning (such as smaller pineal region cysts).

Management

Untreated obstructive hydrocephalus leads to altered arousal, coma, and in some cases brain death and thus needs urgent neurosurgical intervention irrespective of its cause. Unfortunately, the rarity and rapid progression of acute obstructive hydrocephalus often delay diagnosis and limit the ability to treat. The emphasis in the emergency room is therefore early intervention with ventriculostomy and identification of the trigger. Acute CSF diversion with placement of a ventriculostomy drain into the largest ventricle has priority and, if feasible, should be performed in the emergency department suite. The ventriculostomy tube is connected to a manometric CSF drainage system draining at 10 to 15 cm H_2O. If the CSF is bloody, drainage at 0 cm H_2O or lower should be considered to reduce clotting in the catheter (Capsule 4.2).

Ventricular clearing of blood with ventriculostomy is not optimal and may lead to obstruction of the catheter; use of intraventricular thrombolytic

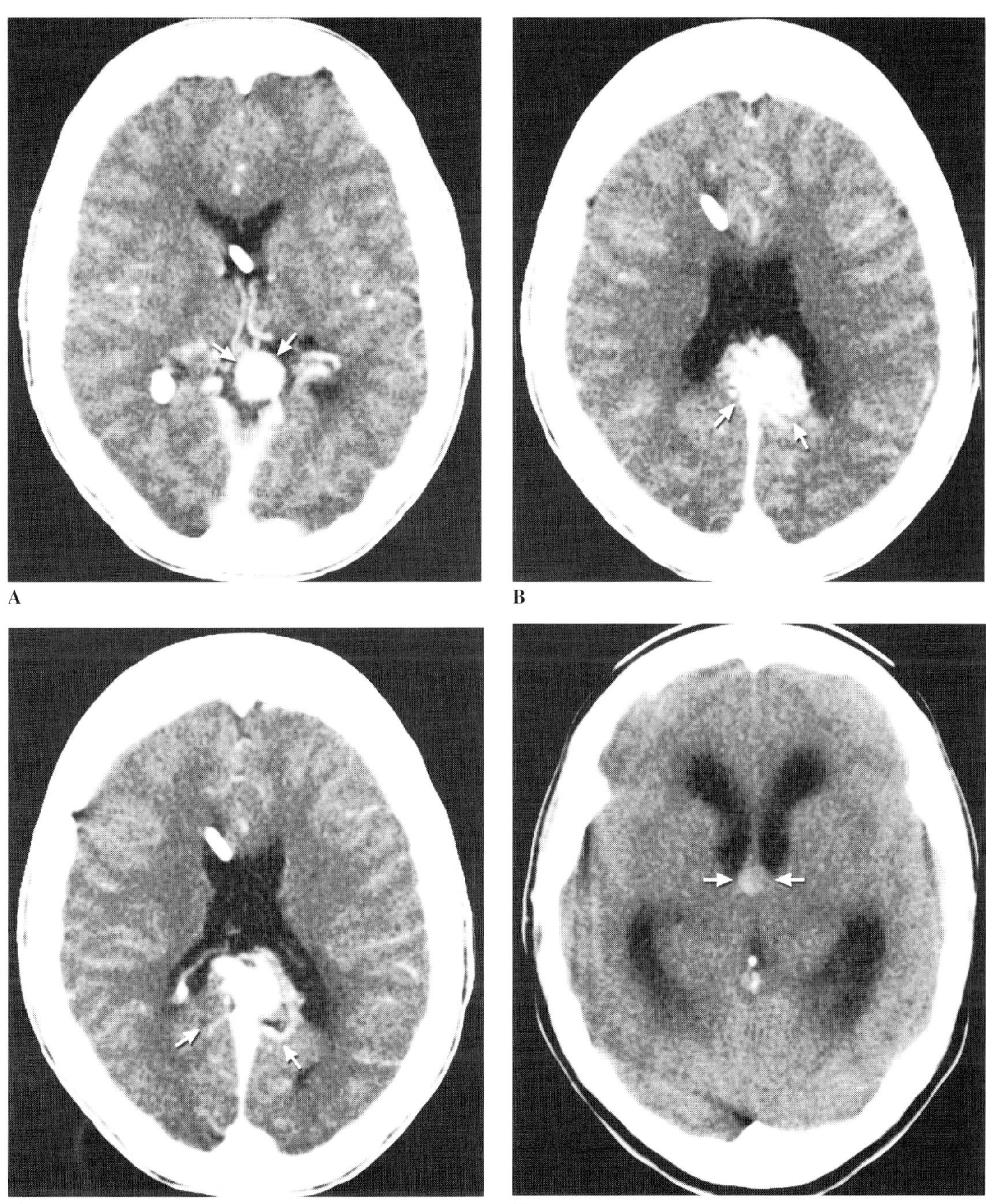

Figure 4.4. Examples of different sites of obstruction. **A–C.** Arteriovenous malformation with giant vein of Galen. **D–E.** Colloid cyst in third ventricle (note absence of third ventricle). **F.** Neurocytoma in third ventricle. **G.** Low-grade glioma in pineal region. **H.** Central nervous system lymphoma compressing fourth ventricle.

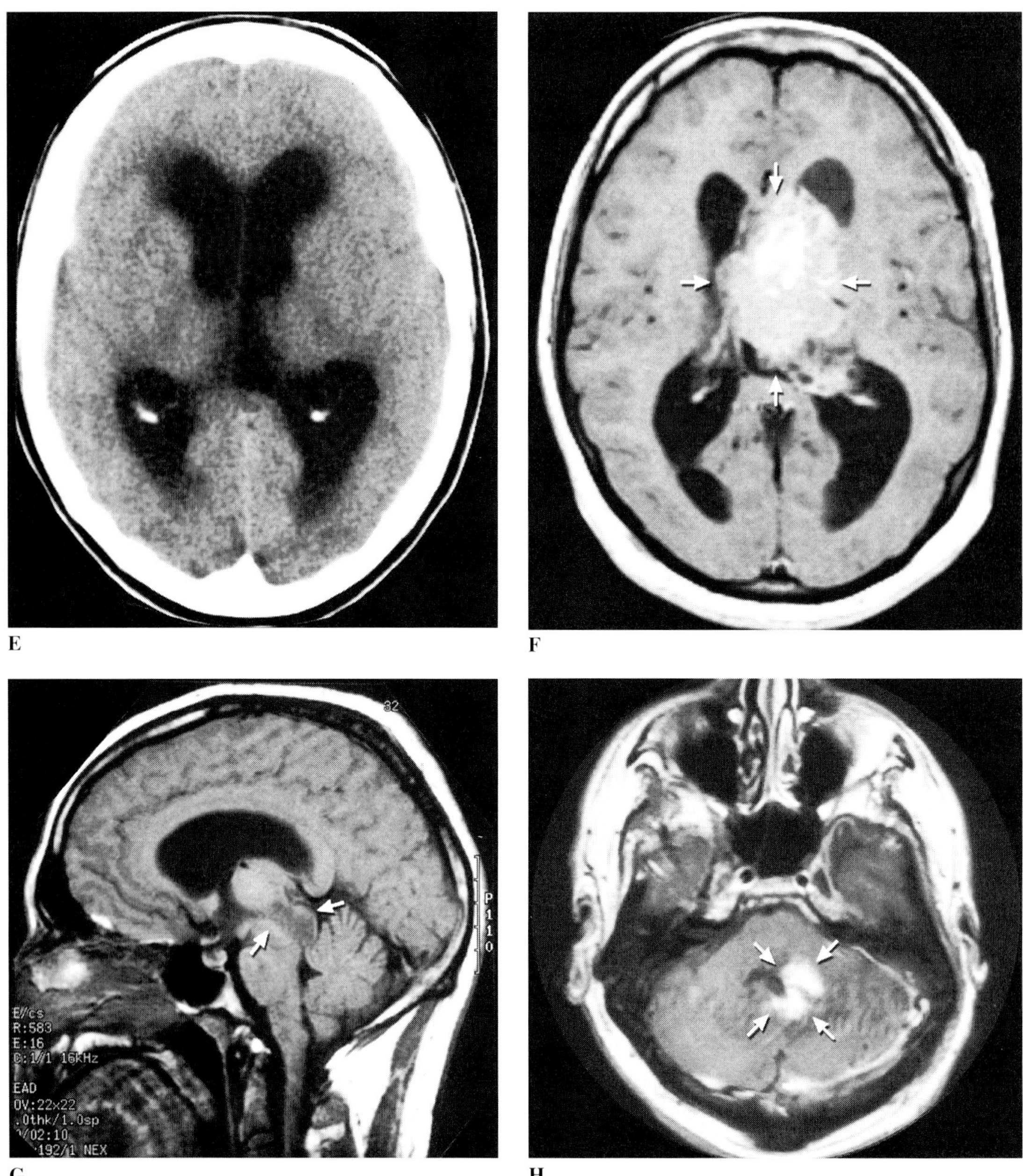

Figure 4.4. *Continued.*

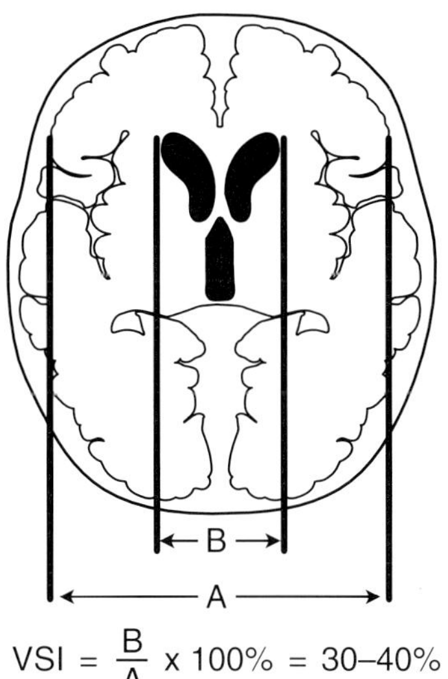

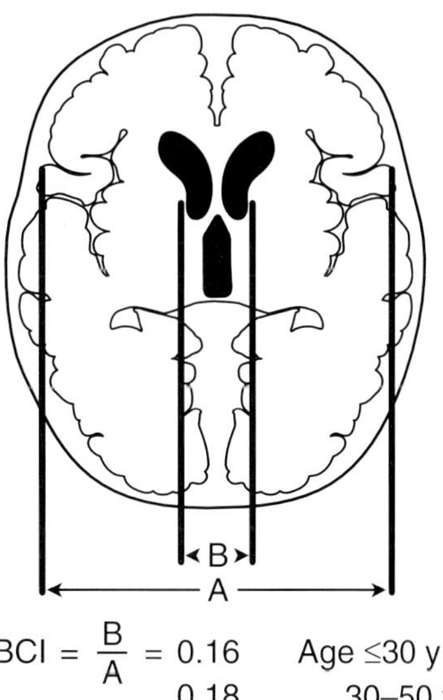

Figure 4.5. Measurement on computed tomography scan of the ventricular system in acute hydrocephalus. Numbers indicate normal values. The ventricular size index (VSI) is not corrected for age. (BCI = bicaudate index.)

Capsule 4.2. Ventriculostomy

A ventricle catheter is inserted in the right (or, better, nondominant) frontal region. The patient is fully supine. In many instances, the bur hole is placed 1 to 2 cm anterior to the coronal suture in the mid-pupillary line (see illustration). The catheter is directed to the middle of the nose. The ventricular system (particularly when dilated) is reached at 5 to 7 cm below the skin. After insertion, the tube is subcutaneously tunneled and secured. Many neurosurgeons administer antibiotics. Complications are rare. They include ventriculitis (probably reduced with antibiotic prophylaxis and subcutaneous tunneling); epidural, subdural, or intraparenchymal hematoma (mostly in patients with severe coagulopathy); malfunctioning through blood clot obstruction; and migration against the ventricular wall and rarely creation of a dural arteriovenous fistula. All are reasons to replace the catheter (Figure 4.6).

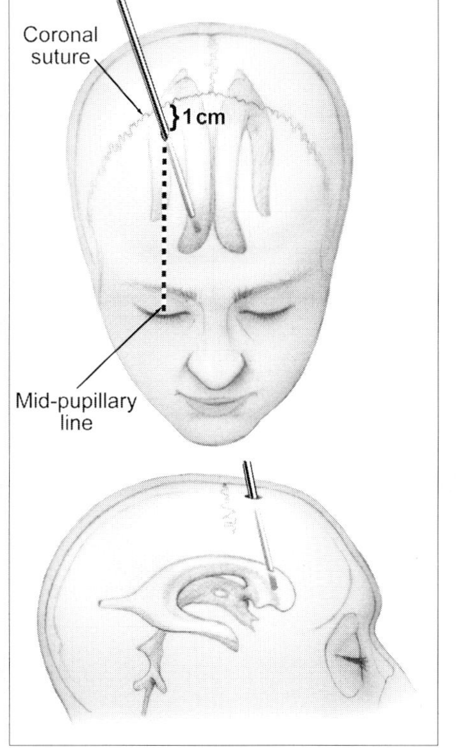

Figure 4.6.

agents is currently under investigation. Hemoventricle with hydrocephalus from primary intraventricular hemorrhage has been treated with additional instillation of urokinase.[33] One study of 22 patients treated with intraventricular urokinase found a trend toward better outcome than that in a nearly similar control group. Clearance of the third ventricle predicted better outcome, suggesting that the focus of monitoring of these patients should perhaps be clearance of third ventricle clot.[34]

Definitive treatment of the obstructing mass warrants endoscopic removal in most cases, and some patients need permanent ventriculoperitoneal shunts or fenestration of the third ventricle, accomplished by endoscopic techniques.[35–37] The lamina terminalis, septum pellucidum, and floor of the third ventricle can all be punctured and then dilated with catheters to divert CSF.

References

1. Wray SH. The Neuro-Ophthalmic and Neurologic Manifestations of Pinealomas. In HH Schmidek (ed), Pineal tumors. New York: Masson Publishing USA, 1977:21.
2. Abe T, Matsumoto K, Kiyota K, Tanaka H. Vein of Galen aneurysmal malformation in an adult: a case report. Surg Neurol 1996;45:39.
3. Case records of the Massachusetts General Hospital. Weekly clinicopathological exercises (Case 35-1983). N Engl J Med 1983;309:542.
4. Buttner A, Winkler PA, Eisenmenger W, Weis S. Colloid cysts of the third ventricle with fatal outcome: a report of two cases and review of the literature. Int J Legal Med 1997;110:260.
5. Chang SM, Lillis-Hearne PK, Larson DA, et al. Pineoblastoma in adults. Neurosurgery 1995;37:383.
6. Chiechi MV, Smirniotopoulos JG, Jones RV. Intracranial subependymomas: CT and MR imaging features in 24 cases. AJR Am J Roentgenol 1995;165:1245.
7. Chiechi MV, Smirniotopoulos JG, Mena H. Pineal parenchymal tumors: CT and MR features. J Comput Assist Tomogr 1995;19:509.
8. Dolinskas CA, Simeone FA. CT characteristics of intraventricular oligodendrogliomas. AJNR Am J Neuroradiol 1987;8:1077.
9. Duong H, Sarazin L, Bourgouin P, Vezina JL. Magnetic resonance imaging of lateral ventricular tumours. Can Assoc Radiol J 1995;46:434.
10. Johnston IH, Whittle IR, Besser M, Morgan MK. Vein of Galen malformation: diagnosis and management. Neurosurgery 1987;20:747.
11. Lasjaunias P, Ter Brugge K, Lopez Ibor L, et al. The role of dural anomalies in vein of Galen aneurysms: report of six cases and review of the literature. AJNR Am J Neuroradiol 1987;8:185.
12. Tien RD, Barkovich AJ, Edwards MS. MR imaging of pineal tumors. AJR Am J Roentgenol 1990;155:143.
13. Tomsick TA, Ernst RJ, Tew JM, et al. Adult choroidal vein of Galen malformation. AJNR Am J Neuroradiol 1995;16(Suppl): 861.
14. Diringer MN, Edwards DF, Zazulia AR. Hydrocephalus: a previously unrecognized predictor of poor outcome from supratentorial intracerebral hemorrhage. Stroke 1998;29:1352.
15. Adams RE, Diringer MN. Response to external ventricular drainage in spontaneous intracerebral hemorrhage with hydrocephalus. Neurology 1998;50:519.
16. Shapiro SA, Campbell RL, Scully T. Hemorrhagic dilation of the fourth ventricle: an ominous predictor. J Neurosurg 1994;80:805.
17. Smith KA, Kraus GE, Johnson BA, Spetzler RF. Giant posterior communicating artery aneurysm presenting as third ventricle mass with obstructive hydrocephalus. Case report. J Neurosurg 1994;81:299.
18. Allen JC, Nisselbaum J, Epstein F, et al. Alphafetoprotein and human chorionic gonadotropin determination in cerebrospinal fluid. An aid to the diagnosis and management of intracranial germ-cell tumors. J Neurosurg 1979;51:368.
19. Camacho A, Abernathey CD, Kelly PJ, Laws ER Jr. Colloid cysts: experience with the management of 84 cases since the introduction of computed tomography. Neurosurgery 1989;24: 693.
20. Ferrera PC, Kass LE. Third ventricle colloid cyst. Am J Emerg Med 1997;15:145.
21. Opeskin K, Anderson RM, Lee KA. Colloid cyst of the 3rd ventricle as a cause of acute neurological deterioration and sudden death. J Paediatr Child Health 1993;29:476.
22. Mathiesen T, Grane P, Lindgren L, Lindquist C. Third ventricle colloid cysts: a consecutive 12-year series. J Neurosurg 1997;86:5.
23. Mathiesen T, Grane P, Lindquist C, von Holst H. High recurrence rate following aspiration of colloid cysts in the third ventricle. J Neurosurg 1993;78:748.
24. Kondziolka D, Lunsford LD. Stereotactic management of colloid cysts: factors predicting success. J Neurosurg 1991;75:45.
25. Abdou MS, Cohen AR. Endoscopic treatment of colloid cysts of the third ventricle. Technical note and review of the literature. J Neurosurg 1998;89:1062.
26. Oppenheim JS, Strauss RC, Mormino J, et al. Ependymomas of the third ventricle. Neurosurgery 1994;34:350.
27. Sharma R, Rout D, Gupta AK, Radhakrishnan VV. Choroid plexus papillomas. Br J Neurosurg 1994;8:169.
28. Kendall B, Reider-Grosswasser I, Valentine A. Diagnosis of masses presenting within the ventricles on computed tomography. Neuroradiology 1983;25:11.
29. Mori K, Handa H, Murata T, Nakano Y. Periventricular lucency in computed tomography of hydrocephalus and cerebral atrophy. J Comput Assist Tomogr 1980;4:204.
30. McConachie NS, Worthington BS, Cornford EJ, et al.

Computed tomography and magnetic resonance in the diagnosis of intraventricular cerebral masses. Br J Radiol 1994;67:223.
31. Maisel JA, Lynam T. Unexpected sudden death in a young pregnant woman: unusual presentation of neurosarcoidosis. Ann Emerg Med 1996;28:94.
32. Spencer N, Ross G, Helm G, et al. Aqueductal obstruction in sarcoidosis. Clin Neuropathol 1989;8:158.
33. Todo T, Usui M, Takakura K. Treatment of severe intraventricular hemorrhage by intraventricular infusion of urokinase. J Neurosurg 1991;74:81.
34. Coplin WM, Vinas FC, Agris JM, et al. A cohort study of the safety and feasibility of intraventricular urokinase for nonaneurysmal spontaneous intraventricular hemorrhage. Stroke 1998;29:1573.
35. Veto F, Horvath Z, Doczi T. Biportal endoscopic management of third ventricle tumors in patients with occlusive hydrocephalus: technical note. Neurosurgery 1997;40:871.
36. Wisoff JH, Epstein F. Surgical management of symptomatic pineal cysts. J Neurosurg 1992;77:896.
37. Hopf NJ, Grunert P, Fries G, et al. Endoscopic third ventriculostomy: outcome analysis of 100 consecutive procedures. Neurosurgery 1999;44:795.

Chapter 5

Acute Spinal Cord Compression

An expedited evaluation in patients with acute spinal cord compression is paramount because reversal of paraparesis is time-locked.[1] Paraplegia beyond a certain interval may remain complete, with no prospect of future ambulation or bladder control. Fortunately, patients with spinal cord compression from malignant disease often have some degree of ambulation at presentation. In the Memorial Sloan-Kettering series, 50% of the patients were ambulatory, 35% paraparetic, and 15% paraplegic at the time of diagnosis.[2] In addition, it has been estimated that 30% of patients with epidural spinal cord compression from metastatic cancer become paraplegic within 1 week.[3]

A considerable number of patients with spinal cord compression are admitted to the emergency department. Typically, patients present with severe spontaneous pain and increasing difficulty supporting their weight because of leg weakness. Unfortunately, unacceptable delay in diagnosis, referral, and investigation occurs in patients with spinal cord compression.[4]

The major problems in acute management of spinal cord compression and the priorities of evaluation are discussed in this chapter. In almost all instances, magnetic resonance imaging (MRI) or cerebrospinal fluid (CSF) examination facilitates appropriate triage, and these patients should be urgently transferred to institutions that have these services available at all times. Alternative diagnostic considerations to acute spinal compression are also considered. One commonly encountered cause of acute spinal cord syndrome is acute transverse myelitis, which is covered in detail in Chapter 11. Injuries severe enough to damage the spinal cord are commonly associated with head, abdominal, or chest trauma, and management of traumatic spinal cord injury is discussed in Chapter 12.

Neurologic Assessment of Acute Spinal Cord Compression

Neurologic examination should localize the lesion in patients with acute paraplegia. Sensory abnormalities localize in the vertical plane (thoracic, lumbar, sacral) and when combined with other long tract signs, point to localization in the horizontal plane (extradural, intradural, or intramedullary).[5]

The major cord syndromes are summarized in Table 5.1. Further clinical clues helpful in localization are found in the appendix to this chapter (Appendix 5.1). All sensory modalities should be tested (pinprick, position, and vibration sense, light touch with a wisp of cotton, pressure touch, and temperature tested with a cold or hot piece of metal [e.g., warmed under running hot water]). Abnormal pinprick is usually interpreted as touch without identification of a sharp sting and is most valuable in localizing segments. When a vibration tuning fork is unavailable, at least position sense should be tested. Normally, movement of a few degrees in the position of the toe joints should be easily appreciated. Normal function suggests intact pos-

Table 5.1. Major Acute Spinal Cord Syndromes

Complete Transection	Hemisection (Brown-Séquard)
All sensory modalities and reflexes impaired below level of severance; pinprick loss most valuable	Loss of pain and temperature opposite to the lesion
Flaccid; paraplegia or tetraplegia	Sensory loss two segments below lesion
Fasciculations	Loss of proprioception on same side as lesion
Urinary or rectal sphincter dysfunction	Light touch may be normal or minimally decreased
Sweating, piloerection diminished below lesion	Weakness on same side as lesion
Genital reflexes lost; priapism	
	Anterior Horn
Central	Pain and temperature loss below lesion
Vestlike loss of pain and temperature	Proprioception spared
Initial sparing of proprioception	Flaccid, areflexia
Sacral sensation spared	Paraparesis or tetraparesis
Paraparesis or tetraparesis	Fasciculations
	Urinary or rectal sphincter dysfunction
	Dysautonomia absent

terior column tracts but also nerve root function. Tactile discrimination should be tested, and a 2- to 3-cm difference between two points should be detectable at the soles. Saddle anesthesia (S3-S5) is an indication of a conus medullaris lesion, which can be accurately delineated but may be missed with superficial examination in a supine patient. The sensory loss is often dissociated, with sparing of touch but loss of pinprick. Absence of dissociation suggests involvement of the cauda equina, not just the conus.

Sacral sparing of the sensory symptoms is an important sign, because it implies an intramedullary central cord lesion. (The representation of the sacral fibers is very peripheral in the spinothalamic tracts, so that pinprick and temperature sensation may be spared in acute central cord lesions.)

Dissociating sensory lesions may be further localized in the horizontal plane. A Brown-Séquard syndrome is strongly indicative of extramedullary compression. However, it may occur in patients with cancer after spinal radiation and indicate radiation myelopathy. Its clinical hallmark is loss of pain and temperature sensation opposite to the lesion, with loss of position and vibration and more prominent leg weakness at the level of the lesion. The patient often may be puzzled by numbness in one leg and weakness in the other. A Brown-Séquard syndrome is rarely uniform in presentation, but marked unilateral leg weakness with Babinski's sign and lack of position recognition of the toe should point to acute extramedullary compression. The classic patterns of sensory loss in myelopathies are depicted in Figure 5.1.

Muscle strength should be graded with the British Medical Research Council scale (Appendix 5.2) in the proximal (iliopsoas, gluteus, quadriceps, hamstrings) and distal (tibialis anterior and posterior, peronei, gastrocnemius, soleus, extensor and flexor of toes) index muscles. Further progression can be easily assessed by this validated grading system.

Tendon, abdominal, and anal reflexes are usually unelicitable in patients with acute paraplegia from a spinal cord lesion. The abdominal reflexes involve the T7-T12 segment, but absence of these reflexes is not particularly helpful in localization, and they are absent in most obese patients. The cremaster reflex involves the L1-L2 arc, and the anal reflexes involve the S2-S4 arc; both reflexes have localizing value in sorting out the segment of involvement in the spinal cord.

Immediate assessment of the bladder is warranted. Sensation of bladder distention may be lost, resulting in overflow incontinence. Detrusor areflexia can be expected with perianal anesthesia, absence of the bulbocavernosus reflex (a usually unpleasant but important reflex triggered when a squeeze of the glans penis is followed by contraction of the bulbocavernous muscle assessed by palpation), and poor anal tone or loss of voluntary control of the anal sphincter. Distention of the bladder should be prevented by immediate catheterization.

Pain is common in acute spinal cord compression. However, significant destructive and com-

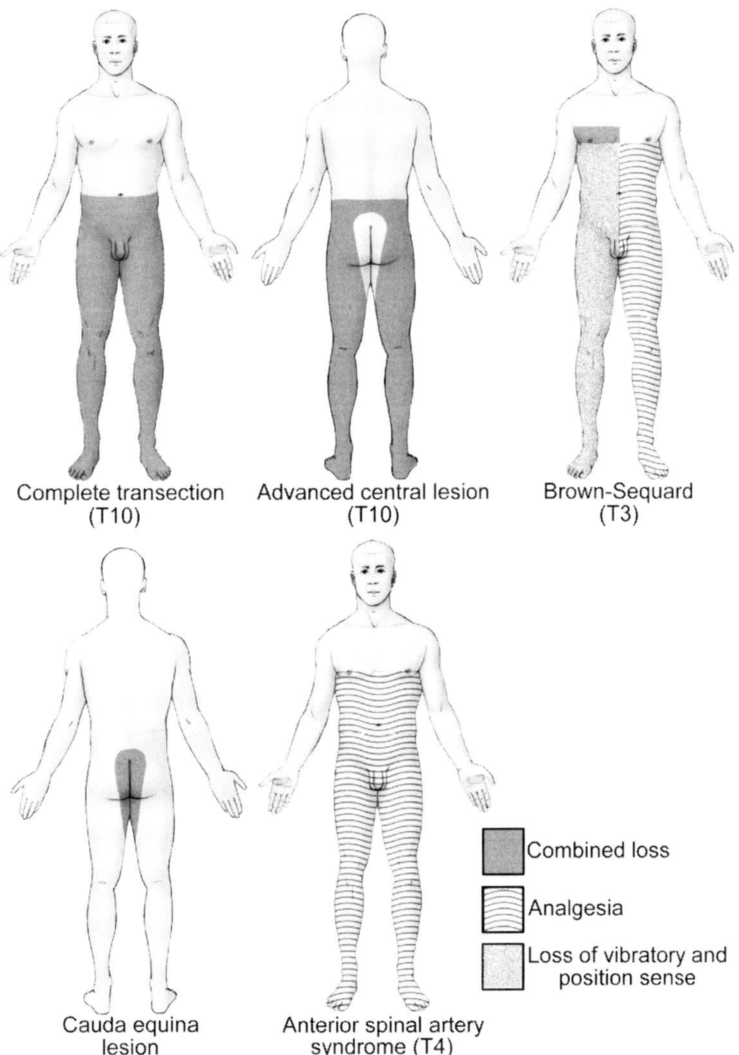

Figure 5.1. Abnormal sensory patterns in acute spinal cord disease. (Modified from TN Byrne and SG Waxman. Spinal Cord Compression: Diagnosis and Principles of Management. Philadelphia: F.A. Davis Co., 1990:39. By permission of the publisher.)

pressive spinal lesions may be virtually painless. Pain that is worse with lying down may signal an epidural spinal tumor and can be explained by additional traction from lengthening of the spine in the supine position.[6] Excruciating pain closely associated in time with acute paraplegia should suggest intramedullary, subarachnoid, or acute epidural hemorrhage, particularly in patients receiving anticoagulation, but is also suggestive of spinal epidural abscess, in which acute paraparesis can evolve in hours.

Pain should be classified as local, referred, radicular, or funicular. Local spinal percussion pain (deep, boring) in the thoracolumbar spine should be evaluated by having the patient turn to the side and by carefully tapping on the spinous processes with a reflex hammer. Pain in the lower back area may be referred from a dissecting aneurysm; it may begin in the lower lumbar spine and be followed by acute paraplegia from spinal cord infarction. In young patients, acute low back pain preceding acute paraplegia may indicate fibrocartilaginous emboli to the spinal cord from thoracic disk herniation.[7] Pain referred to the abdomen is often experienced by patients with acute spinal cord lesions, who may feel they are strapped into a corset. Acute radicular pain (sharp, stabbing) should be further confirmed by straight leg testing and a forceful cough or Valsalva

Table 5.2. Two Neurosurgical Emergencies That Mimic Disorders Common to the Emergency Department

Symptoms	Mimics	Diagnosis
Fever, neck and back pain, shock, respiratory distress	Sepsis Bacterial meningitis	Epidural abscess
Pain in the chest or back with breathing	Myocardial infarction Ruptured abdominal aortic aneurysm Pulmonary embolus	Epidural hematoma

maneuver. Funicular pain (burning, stabbing, electrical) is a less clearly characterized pain sensation of burning, jolting, and jabbing without clear localization and often occurring with sudden movements of the spine. The pain may signal intramedullary disease (e.g., tumor or demyelination).

A psychiatric disorder may be a cause of paraplegia. Surprisingly, the history may not reveal any psychologic traumatic event, and previous medical evaluations resulting in an undetermined cause or repeated visits to the emergency department may not be volunteered by the patient. True weakness can be differentiated from psychogenic weakness by decreased resistance over the entire tested range. In most patients, grimacing with a mix of smile and anger, periodic Valsalva's maneuvers, or frequent sighing is observed during muscle testing. In patients with preserved strength or clear asymmetry in leg weakness, the abduction test can be useful. In this test, abduction in the supposedly normal leg is much stronger. Lack of counterbalance in the other leg may also appear when one leg is raised. The difference becomes apparent when both hands are placed under the heels. Increasing pressure in the heel of the normal or less affected leg occurs when the abnormal leg is voluntarily lifted. Less objective measures are interpretation of the dropping of the leg at the examiner's table (which should be less rapid than gravity dictates). However, observation of a spontaneous movement during an unguarded moment may be more significant than any clever test to unmask psychogenic weakness.

Two neurosurgical emergencies need special mention not only because recognition may be difficult even for a seasoned, astute clinician but also because presentation mimics common disorders seen in the emergency department (Table 5.2). First, epidural spinal abscess is caused in 50% of the patients by *Staphylococcus aureus* infection.[8] Brittle diabetes mellitus, intravenous drug use, and chronic alcoholism predispose to diskitis and osteomyelitis, which may extend to the epidural space. Recognition is difficult because most patients have signs suggesting sepsis, confusion, and delirium. Local back tenderness may not be prominent, but paraparesis and loss of voluntary muscles and sphincters may rapidly become defining features in patients admitted to the emergency department. Blood cultures have a much higher yield in identifying the organism than CSF. CSF examination in the emergency department may also be potentially dangerous, because shifts in CSF pressure that displace the spinal cord may cause sudden worsening of paraparesis.

Second, epidural hematoma may present with acute chest pain or pain between the shoulder blades. The pain has been described as a dagger thrust ("le coup de poignard") and is rapidly followed by tingling, a sensory level, and often a Brown-Séquard syndrome. This type of pain in combination with use of warfarin or tissue plasminogen activator[9] should immediately point to this diagnosis. Spontaneous spinal subarachnoid hematoma, although rare, may lead to paralysis when located dorsally in the spinal cord. A ventral type of spinal subarachnoid hematoma[10] has a much more benign presentation and resolves spontaneously.

Many neurologic disorders can mimic spinal cord compression. Essential facts in the medical history include recent viral illness, vaccinations, illicit drug use, fever, weight loss, myalgia, severe back pain with radiation, recent tick bite, and skin rash, which may indicate acute myelitis or polyradiculopathy. It is very important to determine whether the patient is immunocompromised (e.g., cyclosporine, non-Hodgkin's lymphoma), has clinical evidence of human immunodeficiency virus (HIV) infection, or has risk factors for the acquired immunodeficiency syndrome (AIDS) virus, including previous blood or

Table 5.3. Diagnostic Considerations in Acute Paraplegia from Causes Other Than Spinal Cord Compression

Disorder	History of	Suggests
Myelitis	Vaccination	Postvaccination myelopathy
	Febrile illness	Postinfectious transverse myelitis
	Optic neuritis	Multiple sclerosis
	Travel	Schistosomiasis, cysticercosis
	Tick bite	Lyme disease
	Immunosuppression; AIDS	Tuberculosis, aspergillosis, coccidioidomycosis, syphilis
Myelopathy	Cancer	Acute necrotic myelopathy
	Aortic aneurysm or recent catheterization, low back pain	Infarction of the cord (thromboemboli, fibro-cartilaginous emboli)
	Connective tissue disease (Sjögren's, SLE)	Vasculitis
	Cancer	Radiation myelopathy Paraneoplastic myelopathy
	Anticoagulation	Epidural hematoma Intramedullary hemorrhage
	Progressive symptoms with occasional exacerbation, profound muscle wasting	Spinal AVM Dural AV fistula
Polyradiculopathy	Diarrhea, URI, CMV, HS, EBV, diabetes mellitus, leukemia, sarcoidosis	Guillain-Barré syndrome Acute diabetic polyradiculopathy Infiltrative or inflammatory polyradiculopathy
Neoplastic meningitis	Carcinoma, lymphoma, or other hematologic-oncologic disease	Leptomeningeal spread
Psychogenic paraplegia	Recent psychotraumatic event, previous unexplained admissions	Hysteria, malingering

(AIDS = acquired immunodeficiency syndrome; AV = arteriovenous; AVM = arteriovenous malformation; CMV = cytomegalovirus; EBV = Ebstein-Barr virus; HS = herpes simplex; SLE = systemic lupus erythematosus; URI = upper respiratory infection.)
See also references 5, 11–16.

blood product transfusions (the risks were higher before 1985, when regular HIV screening was not available in blood banks). Recent travel may be relevant and may suggest a myelopathy from *Schistosoma* species (endemic in Brazil) or cysticercosis (any country in Latin America).

The most common mimicking disorders are shown in Table 5.3. They are mentioned only for reference and not further discussed.

Neuroimaging in Acute Spinal Cord Compression

A plain radiograph of the spine is useful, because it quickly identifies bone destruction from metastatic disease and the consequences for stability of the spine. Plain radiographs can appear misleadingly normal in approximately 25% of patients with documented metastatic spinal cord compression; furthermore, plain radiographic abnormalities may not correspond to the location of the tumor, often showing cord compression at a much higher or lower thoracic level.

Bone scan with 99m technetium diphosphate is occasionally used for screening and as a supplementary test,[17] but MRI of the spine, with specific attention to the level determined by clinical localization, should be considered the standard in acute spinal cord compression.[18] MRI of the spine can classify abnormalities as intramedullary or extramedullary, in which the lesions are often intradural. Often more than one lesion is involved, supporting a policy of MRI of the whole spine in these patients.[18]

For reference purposes, a normal MRI of the cervical, thoracic, and lumbar regions of the spine, with T1- and T2-weighted images, is shown in Figure 5.2. An adequate MRI study of the spine should

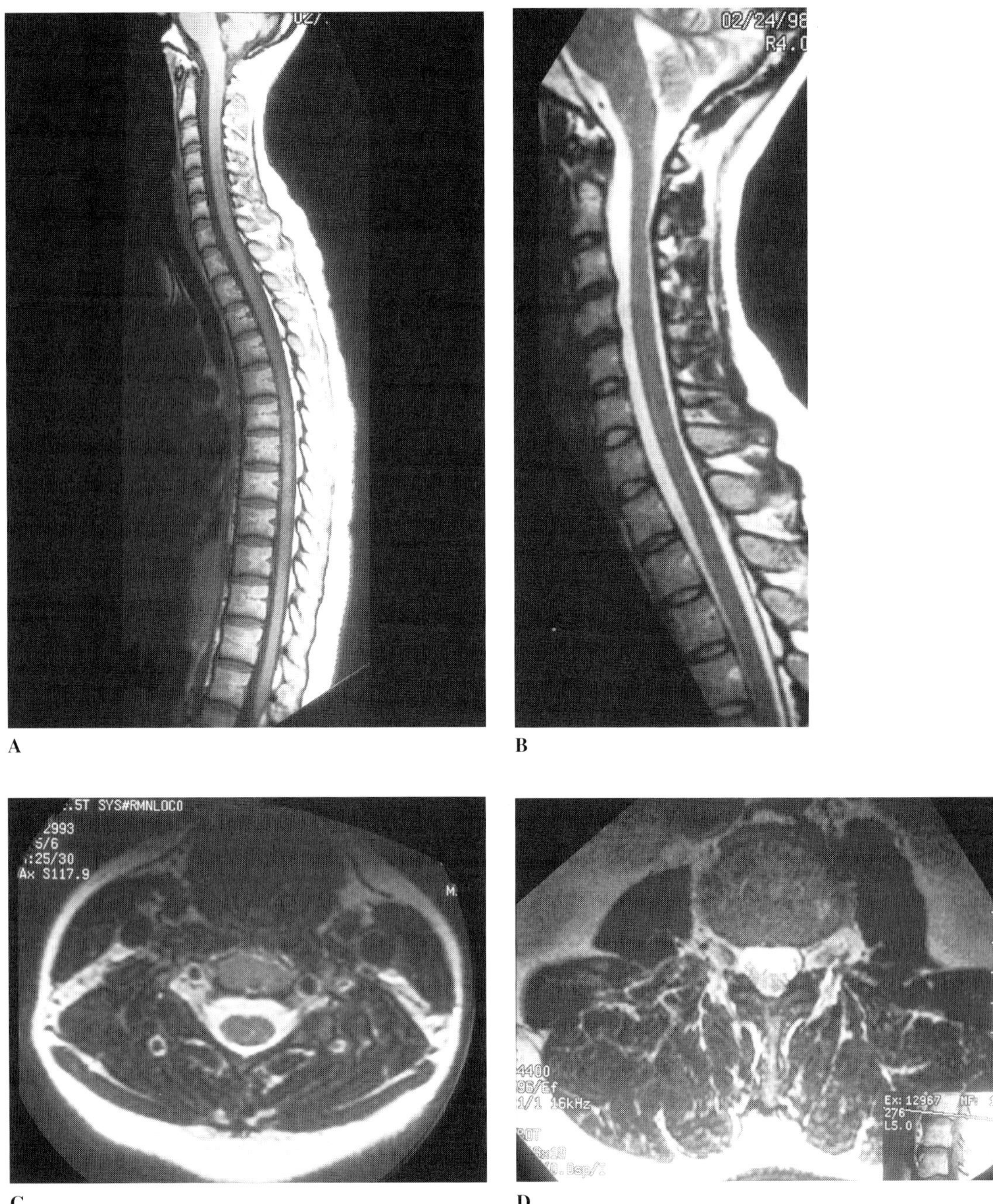

Figure 5.2. A–D. Normal T1 and T2 characteristics of sagittal and axial magnetic resonance images of the cervical, thoracic, and lumbar regions of the spine (see text for description).

have sagittal T1- and T2-weighted images with thin (4 to 5 mm) sections.

Several important features can be identified on MRI of the spine. On the *T1-weighted images*, bone marrow in the vertebral bodies produces a high intensity but a low signal of the cortical bone. T1-weighted images may underestimate the width of the spinal canal because CSF characteristics are of low signal as well. The nerve roots may emerge on axial slices against the high-intensity signal of epidural fat and low intensity of CSF. Disks also have a low T1 signal. The spinal cord signal is intermediate but higher than that of surrounding CSF.

On the *T2-weighted images*, the CSF is bright (also called "the myelographic effect"). The intravertebral disks are brighter. The nerve roots are much better appreciated on T2 images because of the distinctive bright signal of the CSF.

Motion artifacts may produce hyperintense or hypointense bands (phantom images or harmonics) suggesting a cavity in the cord or neoplasm.

Gadolinium does not penetrate the central nervous system; therefore, if the blood-brain barrier is intact, the spine should not become enhanced. T1-weighted images enhance the basivertebral veins, epidural venous plexus, and spinal ganglions caused by a venous plexus. Necrosis in the spine appears as a high signal intensity in T1-weighted images after gadolinium injection. Because tumor has a high signal enhancement, gadolinium is useful in further evaluation of intramedullary, intradural, and extramedullary lesions.

Nerve root enhancement with gadolinium ordinarily does not appear unless disease is present but occasionally is observed when a dose of very high contrast is used (0.3 mmol/kg of body weight). Enhancement of the spinal nerve roots is an important finding, and several patterns have been described.[19] Diffuse enhancement of the cauda can occur in leptomeningeal metastasis, most often associated with systemic malignant disease, such as breast, lung, or skin cancer. However, diffuse enhancement can be seen in inflammatory polyradiculopathy, such as cytomegalovirus radiculopathy in AIDS. Tuberculosis should be considered in persons from endemic areas and, more recently, in patients with AIDS. Epidural compression may be caused by granuloma formation, which is apparent as thickening of the nerve roots. Virtually any leptomeningeal infection can cause enhancement, including *Mycobacterium tuberculosis* infection and cysticercosis.[20] Sarcoidosis should be considered when enhancement is linear at the nerve roots.[21]

In spinal cord compression from cancer, vertebral compression fractures may not coexist with an epidural mass. Malignant lesions on MRI most often have a low-intensity signal on T1-weighted images and a high-intensity signal on T2-weighted images (as noted earlier, normal adult marrow has a high signal intensity on T1 and an intermediate on T2 images). Contrast enhancement increases the sensitivity of detecting malignant lesions in further defining epidural mass effect, which may not be evident on unenhanced images.[22,23]

The diagnosis of epidural hematoma has been greatly facilitated by MRI. A high signal often identifies a hematoma that may be scattered throughout the spinal canal, with various degrees of compression at different levels.

MRI is the preferred test in epidural abscess, and sometimes after gadolinium enhancement, compartmentalization becomes evident.

Acute spinal cord syndromes may be caused by infarction or an arteriovenous malformation.[24,25] Arteriovenous malformation may be located in the dura and cause significant backlogging of venous flow and a dramatic swelling of the cord.[25–27]

The characteristic MRI findings in these disorders are shown in Figures 5.3 and 5.4. Further visualization of the different compartments in the spine is demonstrated in Figure 5.5 for additional orientation.

Cerebrospinal Fluid Examination

Infectious myelitis is the most common alternative diagnosis in acute spinal cord syndromes and often involves viral infections. Viruses affecting spinal gray matter usually include herpes zoster, but other herpes viruses (cytomegalovirus, herpes simplex) may attack nerve roots. CSF in herpes zoster myelitis shows pleocytosis, increased protein levels, and normal glucose values. Viruses with a proclivity for white matter include HIV and human T-cell lymphotropic virus (type I). A viral serologic panel should be obtained in the emergency room in appropriate cases. Increased white cell count should suggest an acute transverse myelitis. A moderate lymphocytic pleocytosis is common in acute transverse myelitis and may be accompanied by increased IgG and oligoclonal bands. Cytologic examination of CSF should focus on malignant cells (only 50% positive yield), and flow cytometry is indicated if atypical lymphocytes are found. This test may demonstrate antibodies to T cells or monotypic expressions with B cells of kappa light chains compatible with lymphoma.

Oligoclonal bands in CSF suggest multiple sclerosis, particularly if other white matter lesions are

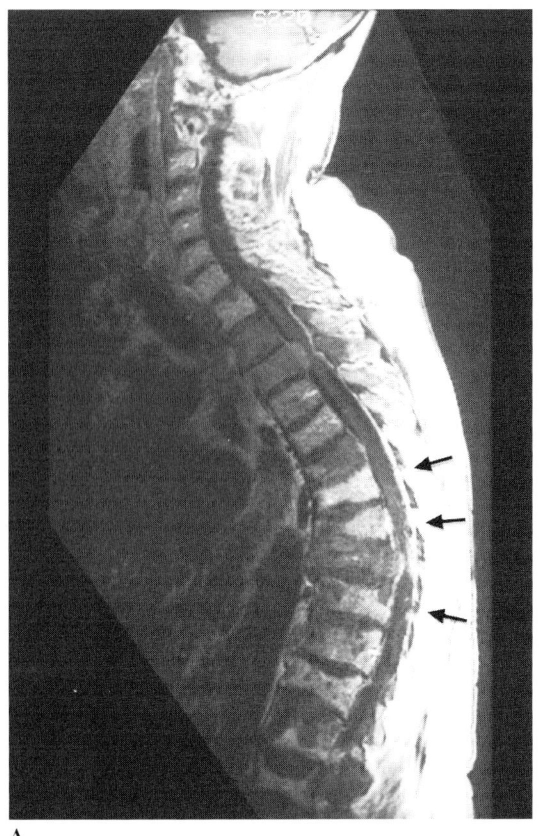

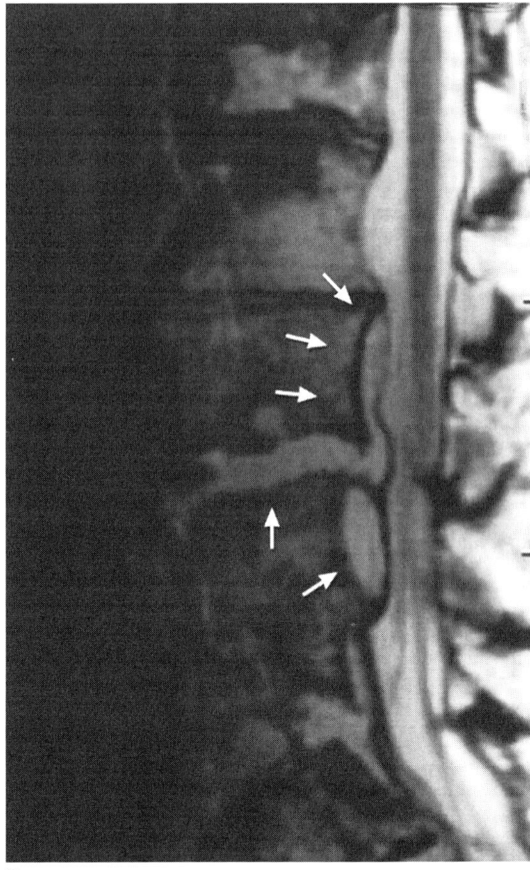

A B

Figure 5.3. Composite magnetic resonance images of the most common causes of spinal cord compression: **(A)** epidural metastasis, **(B)** epidural abscess, **(C–D)** epidural hematoma, and **(E)** granulomatous disease and thickening of nerve roots.

found (up to 80% positive predictive value). It should be noted that oligoclonal bands may also be positive in neurosarcoidosis, with increased angiotensin-converting enzyme in half the cases.[28]

Management

The pathophysiologic mechanism of cord compression is poorly understood, but recent insights may provide an avenue of treatment (Capsule 5.1).

The approach to acute spinal cord compression is determined by its cause, but immediate surgical management is an established route in patients with an epidural abscess localized in a few levels, epidural hematoma, or extradural metastasis with rapidly evolving neurologic deterioration. Its benefit lies in preservation of at least partial mobility and, equally important, complete bladder function. Outcome also depends on the ability to prevent complications and treat non-neurologic problems (pulmonary, skin, bladder) early.

Surgery should be the preferred approach when the primary tumor is unknown and histologic diagnosis is needed.[31–33] If vertebral collapse coincides with spinal cord compression, the chances for ambulation are less and the potential for further deterioration after surgery is real. Spinal stabilization techniques may overcome this situation, but experience is limited. These techniques include vertebral body resection, rod stabilization, and anterior (abdominal or thoracic) decompression. Epidural metastatic lesions often can be treated effectively only by surgery with anterior-posterior resection

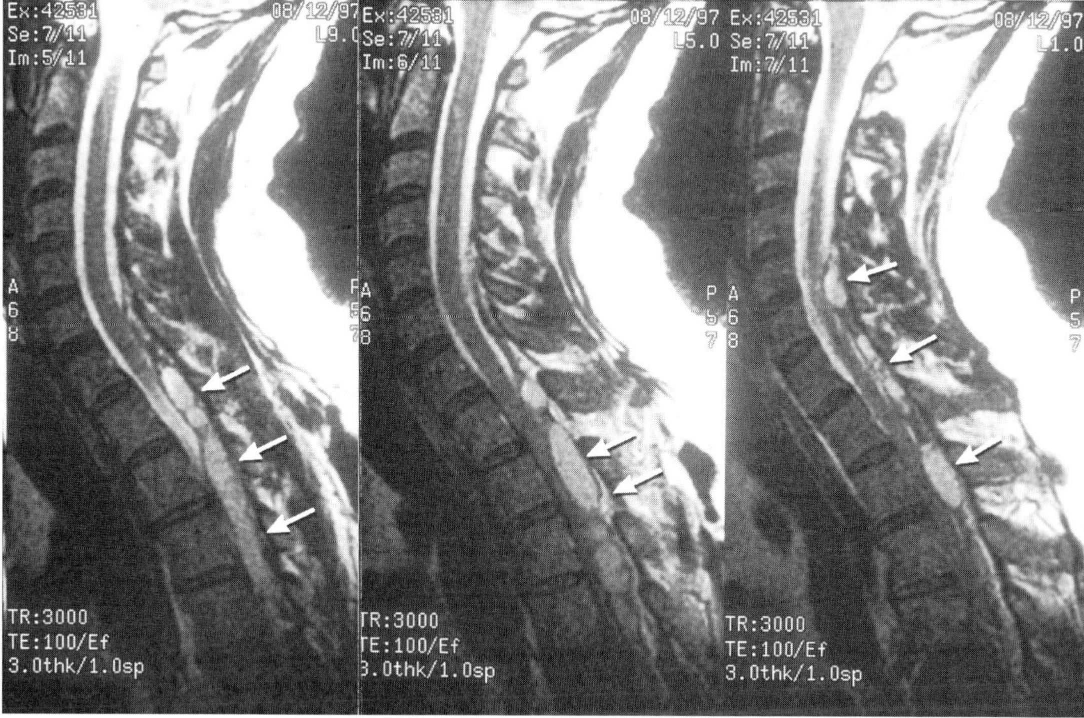

C

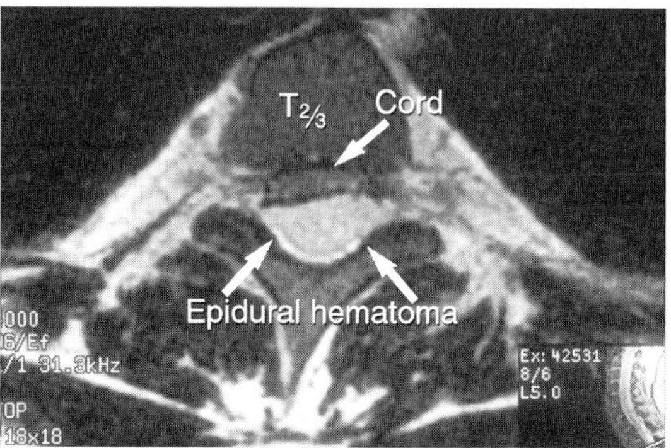

D

Figure 5.3. *Continued.*

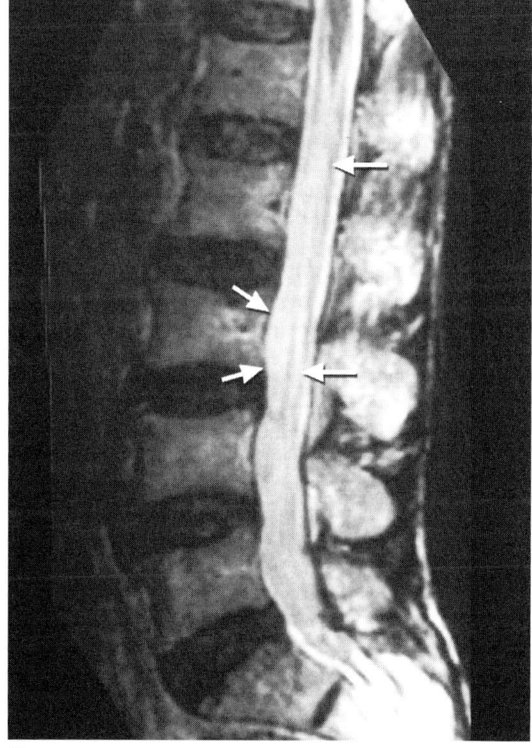

E

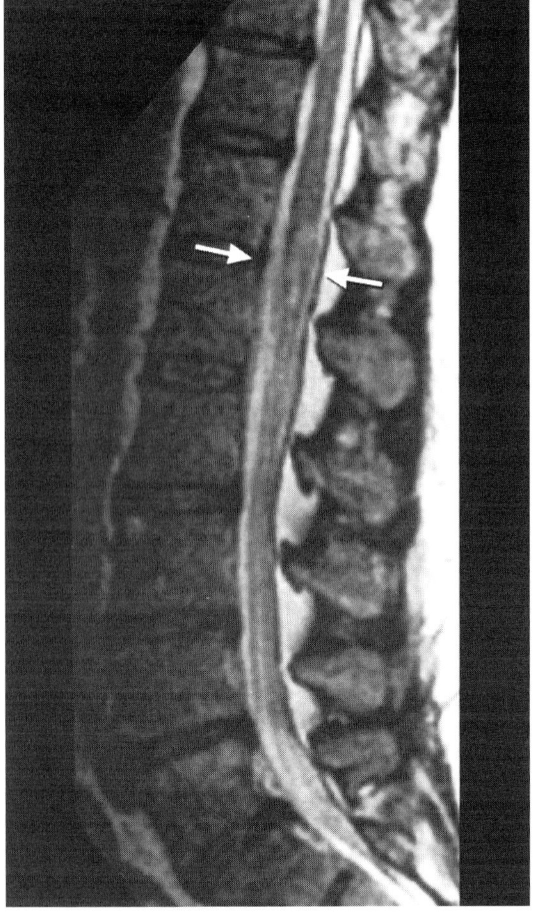

A

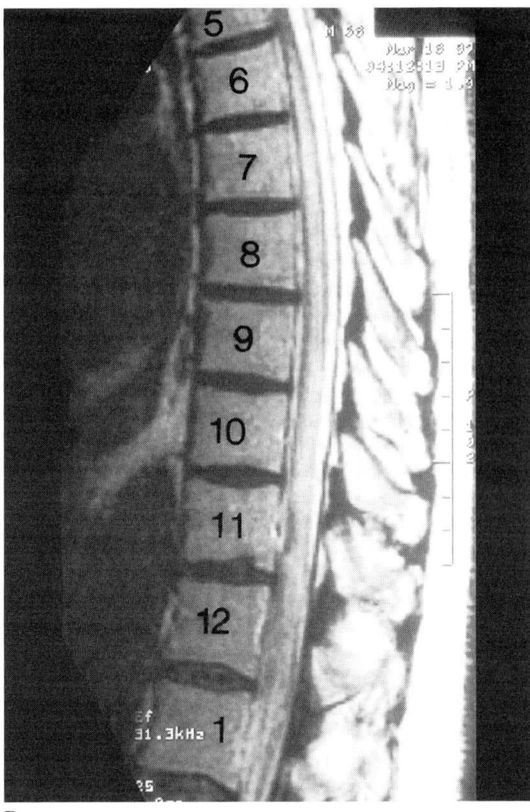

B

Figure 5.4. Common magnetic resonance images in patients with acute spinal cord syndromes but without spinal cord compression. **A.** Spinal cord infarction. **B–C.** Spinal cord swelling from dural arteriovenous malformation, with resolution after surgical extirpation.

with instrumentation.[34] Marginal life expectancy and the degree of metastasis often preclude major surgery.

Approximately 70% of patients with malignant spinal extradural compression remain or become mobile after surgical treatment.[35] Radiotherapy is preferred in patients with known radiosensitive tumors[5] (Capsule 5.2). A short fractionated course (20 to 30 Gy) in 4 to 10 sessions, often with corticosteroids, is appropriate in most patients.[36] Single-fraction therapy should be considered when the aim of treatment is palliation of pain only. Reirradiation in patients with recurrent spinal cord compression from cancer also preserves ambulation. In one study, ambulation was achieved in two-thirds of the patients, but median survival was 4 months.[37] Primary chemotherapy has been advocated for lymphoma, myeloma, and germ cell tumors but in most patients is combined with radiotherapy.

Dexamethasone (Capsule 5.3) is given to all patients with metastatic cord compression (100-mg intravenous push followed by 96 mg orally daily in divided doses) until definitive management has been determined. Patients with back pain only and normal findings on neurologic examination can be treated with 16 mg in divided doses.

Patients with an epidural hematoma need fresh-frozen plasma and vitamin K for immediate reversal of anticoagulation to international normalized ratio (INR) levels within the normal

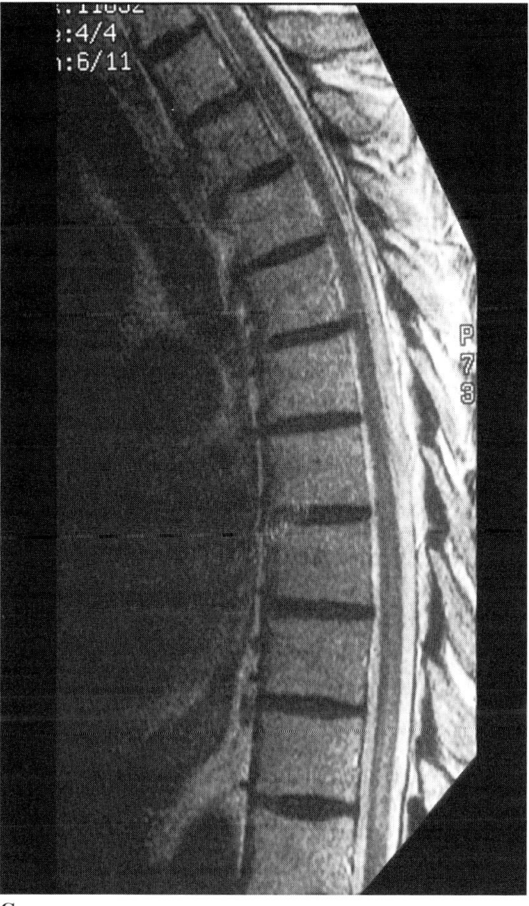

C

Figure 5.4. *Continued.*

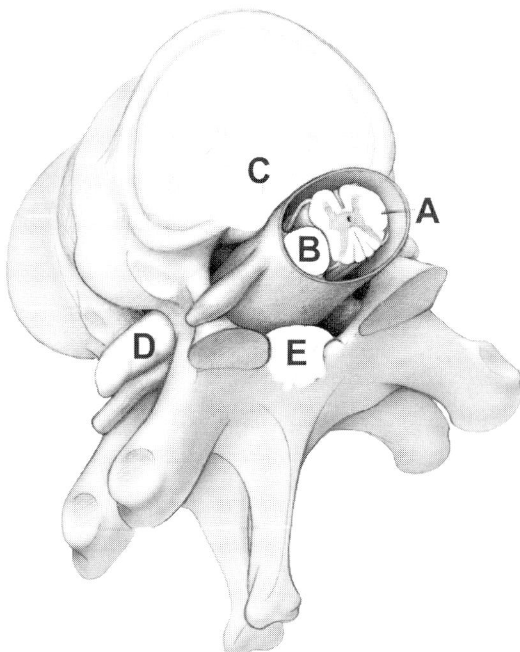

Figure 5.5. Localization of metastatic lesions in compartments inside the spinal canal: A = intramedullary process; B = leptomeningeal process; C = process in vertebral body extending into the epidural space; D = paravertebral process; and E = epidural process. (Modified from TN Byrne. Spinal cord compression from epidural metastases. N Engl J Med 1992;327:614. By permission of the Massachusetts Medical Society.)

Capsule 5.1. Pathophysiology of Metastatic Cord Compression

Spinal cord compression from metastatic disease may be caused by vascular congestion[29] due to venous occlusion of the paravertebral venous plexus in the epidural space. Vasogenic edema is an early feature, caused by a breakdown of the blood–spinal cord barrier. The following sequence of events after compression has been documented.[30] After 3 hours of cord compression, selective demyelination occurs without axonal damage. It evolves over 24 hours and is associated with production of prostaglandin. Experimental blocking of serotonin receptors not only inhibits prostaglandin production but also delays the onset of paraplegia. Prolonged compression results in irreversible cord ischemia. If the epidural mass suddenly enlarges from hemorrhage or an extensively infiltrated vertebral body suddenly collapses, acute spinal cord compression may progress very rapidly. Further spinal cord damage may occur if the tumor mass encases radicular arteries.

Capsule 5.2. Radiotherapy in Spinal Canal Tumors

The radiation field is determined by the extent of involvement and includes two vertebral levels above and below the lesion. With this extended field, early local recurrence is less likely. A common radiation dose is 30 Gy in 10 to 20 fractions administered in 2 to 4 weeks. The effect is greatest in radiosensitive tumors, such as lymphoma, seminoma, myeloma, Ewing's sarcoma, and neuroblastoma, and less in breast and prostate cancer.

If paraplegia existed for up to 9 days, recovery of ambulation can be expected 3 to 6 months later. Recovery is more rapid in patients with gradual onset of paraplegia over weeks. Reirradiation in relapsing patients ("infield" recurrence) frequently preserves ambulation. However, reirradiation in nonambulatory patients may result in the ability to ambulate in a few.

Capsule 5.3. Corticosteroids

Dexamethasone used in patients with metastatic epidural spinal cord compression decreases water content of the spinal cord, reduces epidural swelling, and reduces tumor mass in lymphoma (it may even "disappear"). However, its most dramatic clinical effect is on pain reduction, often within hours of intravenous injection. Dexamethasone has a 4-hour half-life, and repeated doses are needed. High dose (intravenous bolus of 100 mg followed by 96 mg orally for 3 days) or high dose with gradual reduction (96 mg intravenously tapered in 14 days) may not be more effective than 10 mg intravenously followed by 16 mg orally for 7 days and tapered in 2 weeks. There is good evidence to support the use of high-dose dexamethasone therapy in conjunction with radiotherapy.[38] Pain relief is more complete with higher doses. Corticosteroids significantly decrease gastric pH and may rapidly lead to pseudo-obstructive ileus from constipation. These side effects may be reduced by stool softeners, antacids, and H_2 blockers. Serious early side effects are psychosis, hyperglycemia, gastric ulcer bleeding, gastrointestinal perforation, and masking of clinical signs of infections.

range. Multiple doses are needed to reach an INR level that is satisfactory for exploration of the spinal canal (INR <2). Patients with a high risk for cardioembolization (e.g., metallic heart valve) may tolerate short-term discontinuation of anticoagulation, but experience is limited. Reinstitution of anticoagulation is usually considered 1 week after surgery.[39] Spontaneous complete resolution of spinal epidural hematoma has been reported in approximately 7 of more than 250 cases reported in the literature, but identifying these patients and accurately predicting a benign course remain very difficult.[40–42]

Three major factors predict favorable postoperative recovery in spontaneous epidural hematoma: incomplete cord syndrome, decompression within 36 hours in patients with complete cord syndrome, and decompression within 48 hours in patients with incomplete cord syndrome.[43] Rapid onset of paraplegia is not predictive of outcome and should not discourage surgical intervention.

References

1. Helweg-Larsen S. Clinical outcome in metastatic spinal cord compression. A prospective study of 153 patients. Acta Neurol Scand 1996;94:269.
2. Posner JB. Neurologic Complications of Cancer. Philadelphia: FA Davis, 1995.
3. Stark RJ, Henson RA, Evans SJ. Spinal metastases. A

retrospective survey from a general hospital. Brain 1982;105:189.
4. Husband DJ. Malignant spinal cord compression: prospective study of delays in referral and treatment. BMJ 1998;317:18.
5. Byrne TN, Waxman SG. Spinal Cord Compression: Diagnosis and Principles of Management. Philadelphia: FA Davis, 1990.
6. Nicholas JJ, Christy WC. Spinal pain made worse by recumbency: a clue to spinal cord tumors. Arch Phys Med Rehabil 1986;67:598.
7. Pal B, Johnson A. Paraplegia due to thoracic disc herniation. Postgrad Med J 1997;73:423.
8. Hoppe B. Spinal epidural abscess: the nurse's role in early detection and intervention. Heart Lung 1996;25:463.
9. Sawin PD, Traynelis VC, Follett KA. Spinal epidural hematoma following coronary thrombolysis with tissue plasminogen activator. Report of two cases. J Neurosurg 1995;83:350.
10. Komiyama M, Yasui T, Sumimoto T, Fu Y. Spontaneous spinal subarachnoid hematoma of unknown pathogenesis: case reports. Neurosurgery 1997;41:691.
11. Case records of the Massachusetts General Hospital (Case 26-1976). N Engl J Med 1976;294:1447.
12. Case records of the Massachusetts General Hospital (Case 42-1970). N Engl J Med 1970;283:806.
13. Krendel DA, Albright RE, Graham DG. Infiltrative polyneuropathy due to acute monoblastic leukemia in hematologic remission. Neurology 1987;37:474.
14. Miller DH, Ormerod IE, Rudge P, et al. The early risk of multiple sclerosis following isolated acute syndromes of the brainstem and spinal cord. Ann Neurol 1989;26:635.
15. Salonen R, Rinne JO, Halonen P, et al. Lyme borreliosis associated with complete flaccid paraplegia. J Infect 1994;28:181.
16. Case records of the Massachusetts General Hospital (Case 5-1991). N Engl J Med 1991;324:322.
17. Tryciecky EW, Gottschalk A, Ludema K. Oncologic imaging: interactions of nuclear medicine with CT and MRI using the bone scan as a model. Semin Nucl Med 1997;27:142.
18. Cook AM, Lau TN, Tomlinson MJ, et al. Magnetic resonance imaging of the whole spine in suspected malignant spinal cord compression: impact on management. Clin Oncol (R Coll Radiol) 1998;10:39.
19. Georgy BA, Snow RD, Hesselink JR. MR imaging of spinal nerve roots: techniques, enhancement patterns, and imaging findings. AJR Am J Roentgenol 1996;166:173.
20. Zee CS, Segall HD, Boswell W, et al. MR imaging of neurocysticercosis. J Comput Assist Tomogr 1988; 12:927.
21. Nesbit GM, Miller GM, Baker HL Jr, et al. Spinal cord sarcoidosis: a new finding at MR imaging with Gd-DTPA enhancement. Radiology 1989;173:839.
22. Lim V, Sobel DF, Zyroff J. Spinal cord pial metastases: MR imaging with gadopentetate dimeglumine. AJNR Am J Roentgenol 1990;11:975.
23. Sellwood RB. The radiological approach to metastatic cancer of the brain and spine. Br J Radiol 1972; 45:647.
24. Anderson NE, Willoughby EW. Infarction of the conus medullaris. Ann Neurol 1987;21:470.
25. Criscuolo GR, Oldfield EH, Doppman JL. Reversible acute and subacute myelopathy in patients with dural arteriovenous fistulas. Foix-Alajouanine syndrome reconsidered. J Neurosurg 1989;70:354.
26. Oldfield EH, Doppman JL. Spinal arteriovenous malformations. Clin Neurosurg 1988;34:161.
27. Symon L, Kuyama H, Kendall B. Dural arteriovenous malformations of the spine. Clinical features and surgical results in 55 cases. J Neurosurg 1984;60:238.
28. Oksanen V. New cerebrospinal fluid, neurophysiological and neuroradiological examinations in the diagnosis and follow-up of neurosarcoidosis. Sarcoidosis 1987;4:105.
29. Siegal T. Spinal cord compression: from laboratory to clinic. Eur J Cancer 1995;31A:1748.
30. Carlson GD, Minato Y, Okada A, et al. Early time-dependent decompression for spinal cord injury: vascular mechanisms of recovery. J Neurotrauma 1997;14:951.
31. Wiley RG. Neurological Complications of Cancer. New York: M Dekker, 1995.
32. Schiff D, Batchelor T, Wen PY. Neurologic emergencies in cancer patients. Neurol Clin 1998;16:449.
33. Gokaslan ZL. Spine surgery for cancer. Curr Opin Oncol 1996;8:178.
34. Sundaresan N, Sachdev VP, Holland JF, et al. Surgical treatment of spinal cord compression from epidural metastasis. J Clin Oncol 1995;13:2330.
35. Huddart RA, Rajan B, Law M, et al. Spinal cord compression in prostate cancer: treatment outcome and prognostic factors. Radiother Oncol 1997;44:229.
36. Maranzano E, Latini P. Effectiveness of radiation therapy without surgery in metastatic spinal cord compression: final results from a prospective trial. Int J Radiat Oncol Biol Phys 1995;32:959.
37. Schiff D, Shaw EG, Cascino TL. Outcome after spinal reirradiation for malignant epidural spinal cord compression. Ann Neurol 1995;37:583.
38. Loblaw DA, Laperriere NJ. Emergency treatment of malignant extradural spinal cord compression: an evidence-based guideline. J Clin Oncol 1998;16:1613.
39. Phoung LK, Wijdicks EFM, Sanan A. Spinal epidural hematoma and high thromboembolic risk: between Scylla and Charybdis. Mayo Clin Proc 1999;74:147.
40. Silber SH. Complete nonsurgical resolution of a spontaneous spinal epidural hematoma. Am J Emerg Med 1996;14:391.
41. Cirek B, Guven MB, Akalan N. Spontaneous spinal epidural hematoma (letter to the editor). Arch Phys Med Rehabil 1999;80:125.
42. Kumar R, Gerber C. Resolution of extensive spinal epidural haematoma with conservative treatment (letter to the editor). J Neurol Neurosurg Psychiatry 1998;65: 949.
43. Groen RJ, van Alphen HA. Operative treatment of spontaneous spinal epidural hematomas: a study of the factors determining postoperative outcome. Neurosurgery 1996;39:494.

Appendix 5.1
Localization of Spinal Cord Lesions at Different Levels*

Foramen Magnum Syndrome and Lesions of the Upper Cervical Cord

Suboccipital pain and neck stiffness, Lhermitte's sign, occipital and fingertip paresthesias.

Sensory dissociation may be present.

Sensory findings of posterior column dysfunction may be present.

High cervical compressive findings (spastic tetraparesis, long tract sensory findings, bladder disturbance).

Lower cranial nerve palsies (CN IX-XII) may occur from regional extension of the pathologic process.

Lesions at the foramen magnum may be associated with downbeat nystagmus, papilledema, and cerebellar ataxia.

Where the pyramidal tract decussates at the medullocervical junction with segregation of arm fibers (rostral) and leg fibers (caudal), a lesion can cause the unusual combination of contralateral upper extremity paresis and ipsilateral lower extremity paresis (hemiplegia cruciata).

Compression lesions at C1-C4 segments may compromise CN XI, which innervates the sternocleidomastoid muscle and the upper portion of the trapezius.

Possible diaphragmatic paralysis with lesions involving C3-C5 cord segments.

Lesions of the Fifth and Sixth Cervical Segments

Compression of the lower cervical cord causes lower motor neuron signs at the corresponding segmental levels and upper motor neuron signs below the lesion.

Lesions affecting the C5 segment may compromise the diaphragm.

With C5 segment lesions, biceps and brachioradialis reflexes are absent or diminished, whereas the triceps reflex and the finger flexor reflex are exaggerated (because of corticospinal tract compression at C5). The result is *inversion of the brachioradialis reflex*.

With C6 segment lesions, biceps, brachioradialis, and triceps reflexes are diminished or absent, but the finger flexor reflex (C8-T1) is exaggerated.

Lesions of the Seventh Cervical Segment

Paresis involves flexors and extensors of the wrists and fingers.

Biceps and brachioradialis reflexes are preserved, and the finger flexor reflex is exaggerated.

May result in *paradoxical triceps reflex* with flexion of the forearm following olecranon tap. (Weakness of the triceps prevents its contraction

*Data from Biller J, Brazis PW. The Localization of Lesions Affecting the Spinal Cord. In PW Brazis, JC Masdeu, J Biller (eds), Localization in Clinical Neurology. Boston: Little, Brown and Company, 1985.

and elbow extension, whereas muscles innervated by normal segments above the lesion are allowed to contract.)

Sensory loss at and below the third and fourth digits (including medial arm and forearm).

Lesions of the Eighth Cervical and First Thoracic Segments

Weakness that predominantly involves the small hand muscles, with associated spastic paraparesis.

With C8 lesions, the triceps reflex (C6-C8) and finger flexor reflex (C8-T1) are decreased.

With T1 lesions, the triceps reflex is preserved, but the finger flexor reflex is decreased.

Possible unilateral or bilateral Horner's syndrome with C8-T1 lesions.

Sensory loss involves the fifth digit, medial forearm and arm, and rest of the body below the lesion.

Lesions of the Thoracic Segments

Root pain or paresthesias that mimic intercostal neuralgia.

Segmental lower motor neuron involvement is difficult to detect clinically.

Paraplegia, sensory loss below a thoracic level, and bowel and bladder disturbances occur.

With lesions above T5, vasomotor control may be impaired.

With a cord lesion at the T10 level, upper abdominal musculature is preserved but lower abdominal muscles are weak. For example, when the head is flexed against resistance with the patient supine, the intact upper abdominal muscles pull the umbilicus upward (*Beevor's sign*).

If the lesion lies above T6, superficial abdominal reflexes are absent.

If the lesion is at or below T10, upper and middle abdominal reflexes are present.

If the lesion is below T12, all the abdominal reflexes are present.

Lesions of the First Lumbar Segment

Weakness in all muscles of the lower extremities, lower abdominal paresis.

Sensory loss includes both the lower extremities up to the level of the groin and the back to a level above the buttocks.

With long-standing lesions, the patellar and ankle jerks are brisk.

Lesions of the Second Lumbar Segment

Spastic paraparesis but no weakness of abdominal musculature.

Cremasteric reflex (L2) is not elicitable, and patellar jerk may be depressed.

Ankle jerks are hyperactive.

Lesions of the Third Lumbar Segment

Some preservation of hip flexion (iliopsoas and sartorius) and leg adduction (adductor longus, pectineus, and gracilis).

Patellar jerks are decreased or not elicitable.

Ankle jerks are hyperactive.

Lesions of the Fourth Lumbar Segment

Better hip flexion and leg adduction than is found in L1-L3 lesions.

Knee flexion and leg extension are better performed,and the patient is able to stand by stabilizing the knees.

Patellar jerks are absent, and ankle jerks are hyperactive.

Lesions of the Fifth Lumbar Segment

Normal hip flexion and adduction and leg extension.

Patient can extend legs against resistance when extremities are flexed at the hip and knee (normal quadriceps).

Patellar reflexes are present.
Ankle jerks are hyperactive.

Lesions of the First Sacral Segment

Achilles reflexes are absent, but patellar reflexes are preserved.
Complete sensory loss over the sole, heel, and outer aspect of the foot and ankle.
Anesthesia over medial calf, posterior thigh.

Conus Medullaris Lesions

Paralysis of the pelvic floor muscles and early sphincter dysfunction.
Disruption of the bladder reflex arc results in autonomous neurogenic bladder characterized by loss of voluntary initiation of micturition, increased residual urine, and absent bladder sensation.
Constipation and impaired erection and ejaculation common.
May have symmetrical saddle anesthesia.
Pain may involve thighs, buttocks, and perineum.
Pain uncommon.

Cauda Equina Lesions

Early radicular pain in the distribution of the lumbosacral roots due to compression below the L3 vertebral level.
Pain may be unilateral or asymmetrical and is increased by Valsalva's maneuver.
With extensive lesions, flaccid, hypotonic, areflexic paralysis develops that affects the glutei, posterior thigh muscles, and anterolateral muscles of the leg and foot, resulting in a true peripheral type of paraplegia.
Sensory testing reveals asymmetrical sensory loss in the saddle region, involving the anal, perineal, and genital regions and extending to the dorsal aspect of the thigh, anterolateral aspect of the leg, and outer aspect of the foot.
Achilles reflexes are absent, and the patellar reflexes are variable in response.
Sphincter changes are similar to those with a conus lesion, but occurrence tends to be late in the clinical course.
Although it can be concluded that lesions of the conus result in early sphincter compromise, late pain, and symmetrical sensory manifestations, whereas cauda lesions have early pain, late sphincter manifestations, and asymmetrical sensory findings, this distinction is difficult to establish and is of little practical value.

Appendix 5.2

British Medical Research Council Scale of Muscle Strength*

0 No muscular contraction
1 Muscular contraction without joint involvement
2 Muscular contraction moves joint but not against gravity
3 Muscular contraction moves joint, just overcoming gravity
4 Muscular contraction overcoming gravity and appreciable force
5 Muscular contraction not overcome by the examiner

*Modified from Aids to the Examination of the Peripheral Nervous System. London: Baillière Tindall, 1986. By permission of the Guarantors of Brain.

Part II

Catastrophic Neurologic Disorders Due to Specific Causes

Chapter 6

Aneurysmal Subarachnoid Hemorrhage

Contrary to common perception, patients with aneurysmal subarachnoid hemorrhage (SAH) come to the emergency department with headache only, alert or drowsy, and minimal neurologic findings.[1] The disastrous consequences for a patient with aneurysmal SAH thus may come later, and outcome may not be determined at the onset of the rupture. Although the time spent in the emergency room is short, these patients need frequent neurologic assessment and close cardiopulmonary monitoring.

The recognition of SAH (Capsule 6.1) may seem straightforward in many cases, but errors may arise in the evaluation of patients with presumed normal findings on computed tomography (CT) scans but typical onset of severe headache. The difficulties in assessment of patients with alleged SAH often can be traced back to misinterpretation of CT scans, failure to distinguish between bloody spinal fluid from needle trauma and true SAH, and, more simply but far more important, unreliable history-taking.

This chapter provides the necessary tools to appropriately assess these patients in the emergency department and transfer them to the intensive care unit.

Clinical Presentation

Fundamental in history-taking for a patient with acute headache is determination of the precise time of onset, quality of the headache, and whether the patient had similar earlier events. The type of headache in aneurysmal SAH is characteristic. A history of a severe "never experienced before," "in the middle of a sentence," "flashlike," "explosive," acute headache is very suggestive of SAH.[9] Many patients describe a brief sense of panic, because they are stunned by the unexpected presentation. The often-quoted "worst headache of my life" in textbooks may not necessarily indicate acute onset or precisely define the severity of the headache. (For example, patients with chronic headaches or migraine have episodes that they commonly first classify as "the worst headache ever.")

This headache must be differentiated from a rapidly worsening severe headache, brief volleys of stabbing pain, and a throbbing type of headache. It is useful to ask the patient whether the headache was acute by demonstrating it with a clap of the hands. The headache usually is persistent, but resolution with the use of medication, such as nonsteroidal anti-inflammatory agents, aspirin, or even narcotics, should not be mistakenly misinterpreted as an argument against SAH. The headache of acute SAH may have different levels of severity, but most of the time it is truly extremely severe. Less severe headaches have been confused with more common explanations, such as neck sprain or migraine, in patients visiting emergency departments.[10–14]

Vomiting may occur several minutes into the ictus as a result of further distribution of blood

Capsule 6.1. Aneurysmal Rupture

What causes aneurysms to rupture is puzzling. Risk factors have included recent documented enlargement (rupture of aneurysms less than 4 mm is very rare, most ruptured aneurysms are 7 to 8 mm, and risk of rupture increases significantly in aneurysms 10 mm or greater), hypertension, cigarette smoking, and family history of aneurysms and SAH.[2–4] Aneurysmal rupture has been reported to have occurred during weight lifting, sexual orgasm, and brawling, events that suggest acute hypertensive stress on a thin aneurysmal wall. However, at least 50% of patients have SAH at rest.[5,6]

Intracranial pressure rises dramatically to at least the level of the diastolic blood pressure but may briefly increase to the level of the systolic blood pressure, causing a cerebral perfusion standstill.[7] The increase in intracranial pressure decreases within 15 minutes but may persist if acute hydrocephalus or shift from intracerebral hematoma has occurred. Rupture stops within 3 to 6 minutes after ejection of up to 15 to 20 mL/minute into the basal cistern[8] (Color Plate 7).

throughout the subarachnoid space. It occurs in 50% of patients but is nonspecific. Profuse vomiting may override the headache and has been mistaken for a "gastric flu" by the patient or initially consulted physician. Clinical presentations have included acute paraplegia (anterior cerebral artery rupture) and severe thoracic and lumbar pain caused by meningeal irritation. These presentations obviously have resulted in a delay in cranial CT scan imaging, but fortunately they are extremely unusual as sole clinical manifestations.[1]

Acute severe headache, although less accurately defined in reported cases, is also seen in patients with viral meningoencephalitis,[15] cerebellar hematoma, pituitary apoplexy, acute bilateral carotid dissection, cerebral sinus thrombosis, and medical disorders such as acute sinusitis and pheochromocytoma. In more benign types of acute headache, the circumstances may provide a further clue to the cause, but they can be misleading. Examples are ingestion of ice cream (ice cream headache), exertion, including sexual activity (benign exertional head-ache), and a flurry of coughing (cough headache) (Table 6.1).

The clinical examination of patients with SAH should include grading of the severity of the SAH with use of the Glasgow coma scale and determining whether the patient has a motor deficit (World Federation of Neurological Surgeons [WFNS] scale; Table 6.2). However, stupor or coma in SAH (so-called poor-grade SAH) has many possible explanations. Impaired consciousness frequently is the result of a direct impact of the arterial jet and a massive increase in intracranial pressure, which significantly decrease cerebral perfusion pressure and thus result in global bihemispheric ischemia. Respiratory or cardiac arrest during the rupture followed by resuscitation may also result in an additional postanoxic-ischemic encephalopathy.[28] Other causes of poor-grade SAH are intracranial hematoma with brain shift and brain stem compression and acute hydrocephalus.

Neck stiffness from cervical meningeal irritation may take some time to develop and is absent in coma. Nuchal rigidity can be demonstrated by failure to flex the neck in the neutral position and failure to retroflex when both shoulders are lifted. Flat-topped retinal hemorrhages (subhyaloid hemorrhages) are characteristic of aneurysmal SAH and indicate profound SAH. Flat-topped retinal hemorrhages occur when outflow in the optic nerve venous system is suddenly obstructed by the intracranial pressure wave. Visual loss may be severe, with perception of light or hand motion only, if the hemorrhage expands and ruptures into the vitreous, becoming dome-shaped (Terson's syndrome; Figure 6.1; Color Plates 8, 9, and 10).[29,30]

Neuro-ophthalmologic signs can localize the site of the aneurysm. Rupture of a posterior communicating artery or carotid artery aneurysm can produce a third nerve palsy with total ptosis and a primary gaze abnormality, with the affected eye in a "down and out" position. The pupil is dilated and unreactive to light because of compression of the exteriorly

Table 6.1. Acute Headache Syndromes

Disorder	Location	Time profile	Quality	Pathognomonic features
Aneurysmal subarachnoid hemorrhage	Occipital, neck, bilateral	Acute, persistent, maximal at onset, split-second	Excruciating, may decrease to moderate intensity	Vomiting, brief loss of consciousness
Thunderclap headache	Occipital, bilateral	Maximal at onset, split-second	Excruciating	Exertion, sexual intercourse, normal CT and CSF, may have reversible cerebral vasospasm
Cluster headache	Oculofrontal, temporal	30 to 90 minutes	Severe, stabbing	Rocking, restless, Horner's syndrome, rhinorrhea
Chronic paroxysmal hemicrania	Unilateral	2 to 30 minutes	Severe	Conjunctival injection, female, not restless, lacrimation on symptomatic side
Acute migraine	Mostly unilateral	6 to 30 hours	Moderately severe	Nausea and photophobia in ~80%
Trigeminal neuralgia	Unilateral (face only)	Seconds	Severe, electrical	Chewing, cold wind, shaving
Carotid or vertebral artery dissection	Frontotemporal, unilateral, or occipital	Acute, minutes, median duration of 3 days	May be thunderclap, pulsating, or constant	May have carotid bruit, hemiparesis, aphasia, or dysarthria
CSF hypotension syndrome, ruptured arachnoid cyst	Bilateral	Acute, typically worse with standing	Dull	MRI shows additional marked meningeal enhancement from CSF hypotension
Acute sinusitis	Frontal, maxilla	Hours	Severe	Fever, pressure pain on maxillary or frontal sinus
Pheochromocytoma	Bilateral	Rapidly increasing in intensity	Severe when supine	Hypertension, sweating, pallor

(CSF = cerebrospinal fluid; CT = computed tomography; MRI = magnetic resonance imaging.)
See references 16–27.

located fibers that form the light reflex. However, up to 15% of posterior communicating artery aneurysms may occur with a pupil-sparing third nerve palsy.[31] Aneurysm of the basilar artery may produce unilateral or bilateral third or sixth nerve palsy. If the basilar artery aneurysm enlarges and progressively compresses oculomotor nuclei of the pons, horizontal gaze paralysis, skew deviation, internuclear ophthalmoplegia, and nystagmus occur, commonly in association with long tract signs such as hemiparesis and ataxia. Occlusion of the proximal posterior cerebral artery, often encased in a giant aneurysm, may occur, causing either a classic Weber syndrome due to mesencephalon infarction (third nerve palsy with opposite hemiparesis) or homonymous hemianopia due to occipital lobe infarction.

Table 6.2. World Federation of Neurological Surgeons (WFNS) Grading System for Subarachnoid Hemorrhage

WFNS grade	GCS	Motor deficit
I	15	Absent
II	14–13	Absent
III	14–13	Present
IV	12–7	Present or absent
V	6–3	Present or absent

(GCS = Glasgow coma score. [See Chapter 1 for full description.])

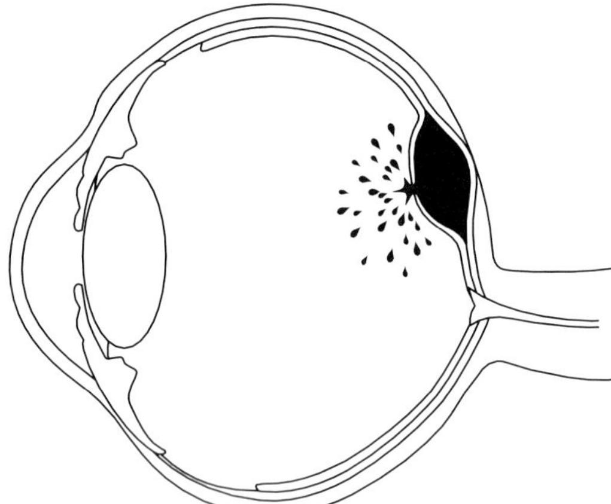

Figure 6.1. Terson's syndrome in aneurysmal subarachnoid hemorrhage. Drawing of rupture into the vitreous. (Modified from CE Swallow, JS Tsuruda, KB Digre, et al. Terson syndrome: CT evaluation in 12 patients. AJNR 1998;19:743. By permission of the American Society of Neuroradiology.) (See also Color Plates 8, 9, and 10.)

Hemiparesis that usually involves the face, arm, and leg in SAH should point to an intracranial hematoma. An anteriorly placed intracranial hematoma in the frontal lobe may not produce motor weakness but be associated with agitation and bizarre behavior. Many of the patients are confused, concoct bizarre stories, or ramble nonsensically (e.g., we cared for a physician with a ruptured anterior communicating aneurysm who repeatedly demanded to be signed up for a stroke prevention program). A Korsakoff syndrome with impaired recall and fabrications has been described in ruptured anterior communicating aneurysm. Abulia, a general sense of disinterest, and lackluster attention to daily living are also features, becoming apparent days later. Temporal lobe hematoma in the dominant hemisphere may produce aphasia, but often its associated brain shift decreases level of consciousness and word output.

Generalized tonic-clonic seizures are accompanied by aneurysmal rupture in 10% of patients or appear during rebleeding. Nonconvulsive status epilepticus or epilepsia partialis continua is very uncommon in aneurysmal SAH.

Systemic manifestations, besides vomiting, may include respiratory failure and oxygen desaturation from aspiration, pulmonary edema, or obstruction of the airways by a foreign object (e.g., pieces of teeth broken during clenching of the jaws at the time of a seizure). Cardiac arrhythmias may involve the entire gamut of supraventricular and ventricular arrhythmias. Most of the time they are associated with electrocardiographic changes, which may simulate anterior wall or subendocardial infarction. Thus, with an incomplete medical history and no inquiry about acute headache, patients may be wrongly transferred to a medical intensive care unit (cardiac resuscitation and pulmonary edema), gastrointestinal service (vomiting), or coronary care unit (cardiac arrhythmias with new electrocardiographic changes).

The clinical state of the patient may suddenly change in the emergency room. We have seen several patients who soon after presentation had acute worsening of the headache and became significantly more drowsy, with a drop of several points in the Glasgow coma score. Rebleeding could be demonstrated on CT scans in all instances. This sequence of events should be recognized, particularly because rebleeding is highly prevalent within the first 6 hours of initial rupture. Therefore, it can be expected to occur in the emergency department during the wait for results of neuroimaging studies and further disposition. Other causes of further worsening in the emergency room are acute obstructive hydrocephalus and herniation from swelling surrounding a hematoma.

Interpretation of Laboratory Tests

Computed Tomography Scanning

CT scanning has a very high sensitivity and specificity for SAH.[32,33] The sensitivity of a noncontrast CT scan for SAH alone is 93% for patients seen within the first day, 84% for those seen on the second day, 50% after day 5, and zero after day 10. The accumulation of subarachnoid blood on CT scans is characteristically diffuse, involving all basal cisterns, the interhemispheric and sylvian fissures, and the area along the convexity (Figure 6.2). Additional lobar hematomas point to more certain localization of an aneurysm[12,34–36] (Figures 6.3 and 6.4).

Hypodensity in both hemispheres and early loss of gray-white differentiation may develop in poor-grade SAH (Figure 6.5). They reflect periodic acute arrest of cerebral flow caused by a very large

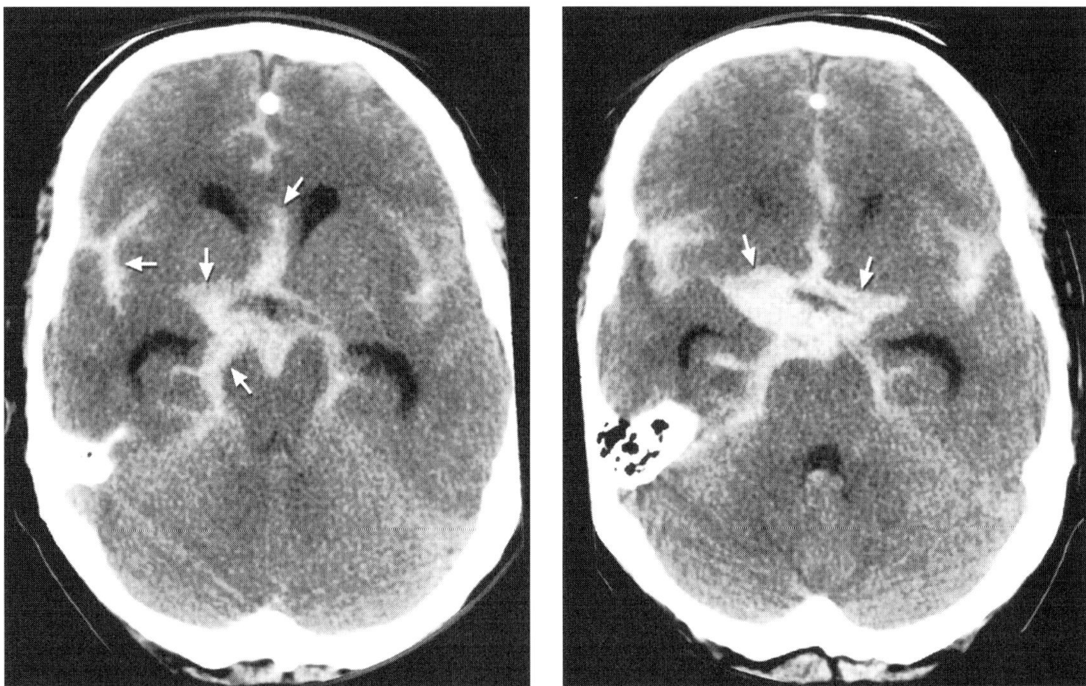

Figure 6.2. Computed tomography patterns of subarachnoid hemorrhage. Diffuse filling of basal cistern and fissures (*arrows*) produces a hyperdense cast.

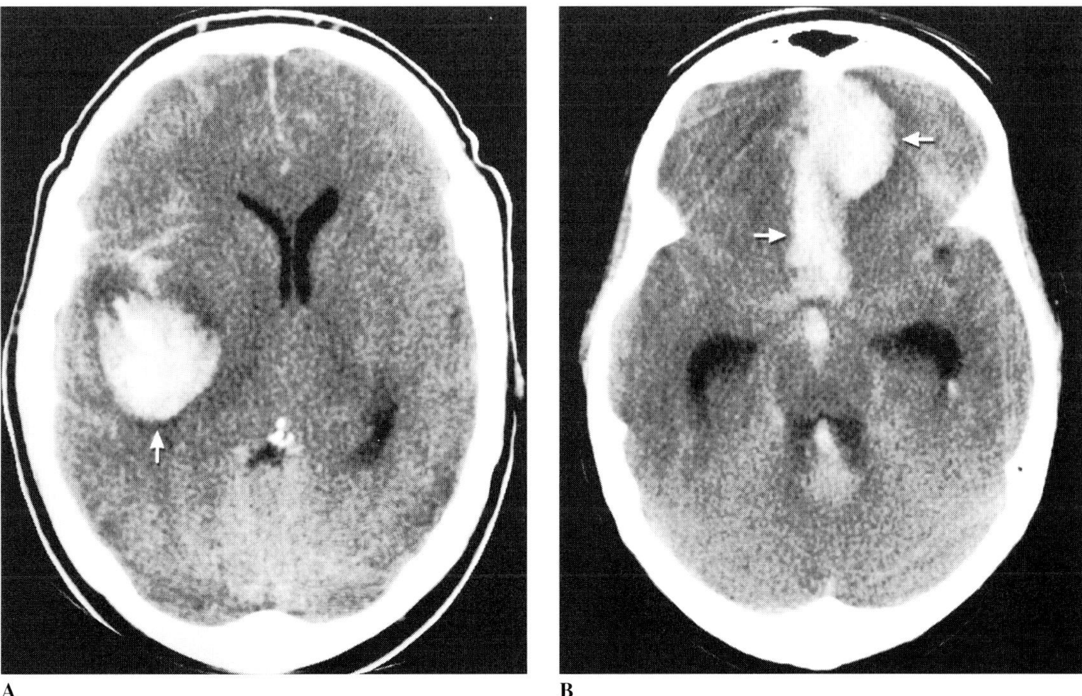

A B

Figure 6.3. Computed tomography patterns of subarachnoid hemorrhage with associated hematomas indirectly localizing ruptured aneurysms. **A.** Sylvian fissure (middle cerebral artery). **B.** Frontal hematoma (anterior cerebral artery).

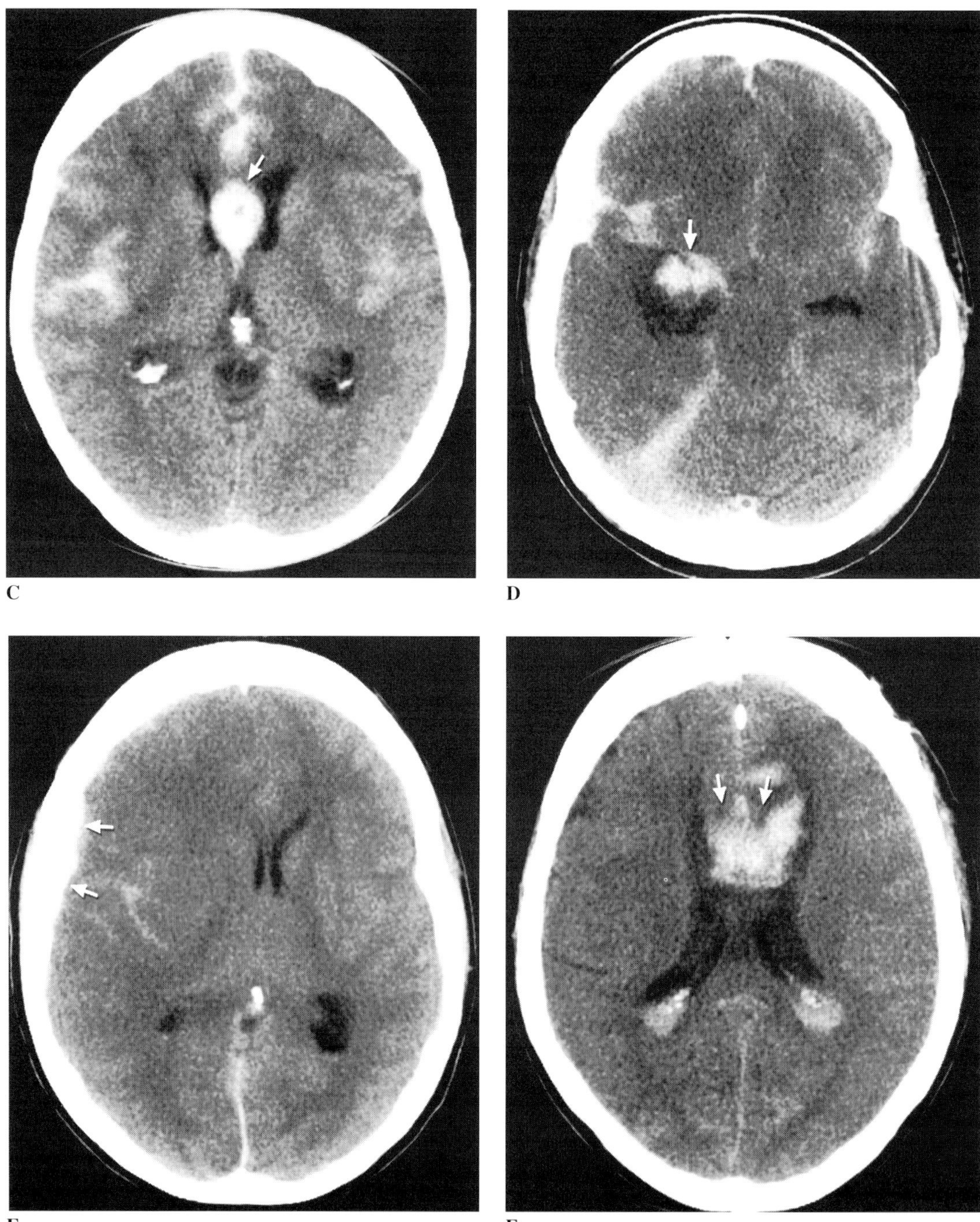

Figure 6.3. *Continued.* **C.** Hematoma in septum pellucidum. **D–E.** Medial temporal lobe with subdural hematoma (carotid artery). **F.** Corpus callosum (pericallosal artery).

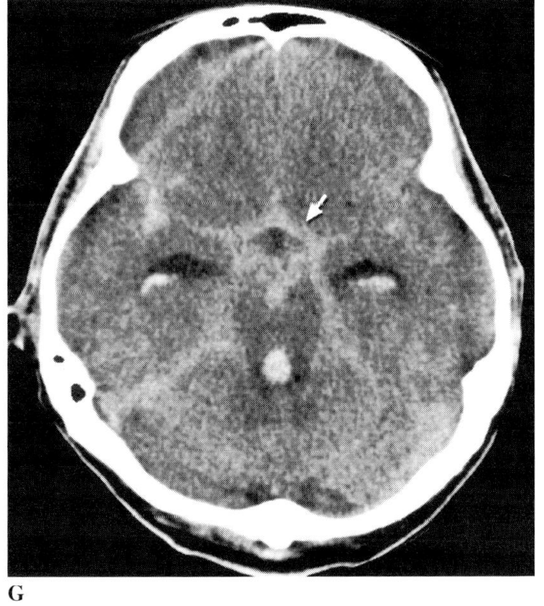

G

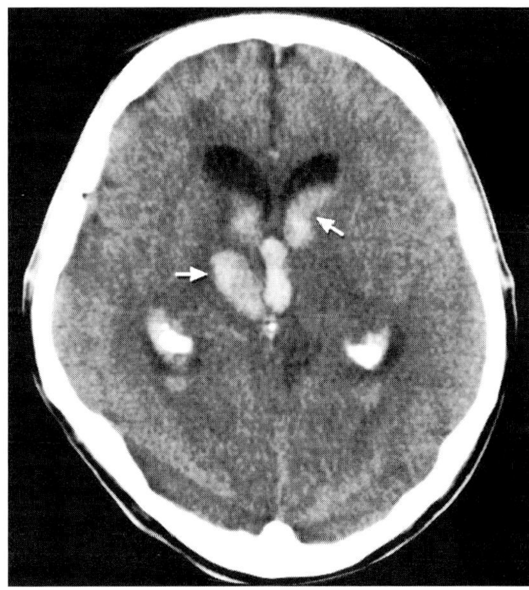

H

Figure 6.3. *Continued.* **G–I.** Thalamic hematoma with posterior cerebral artery (P1 segment) aneurysm identified on magnetic resonance imaging.

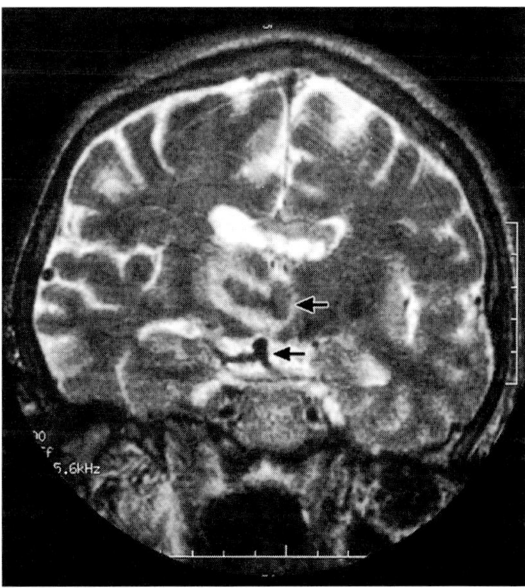

I

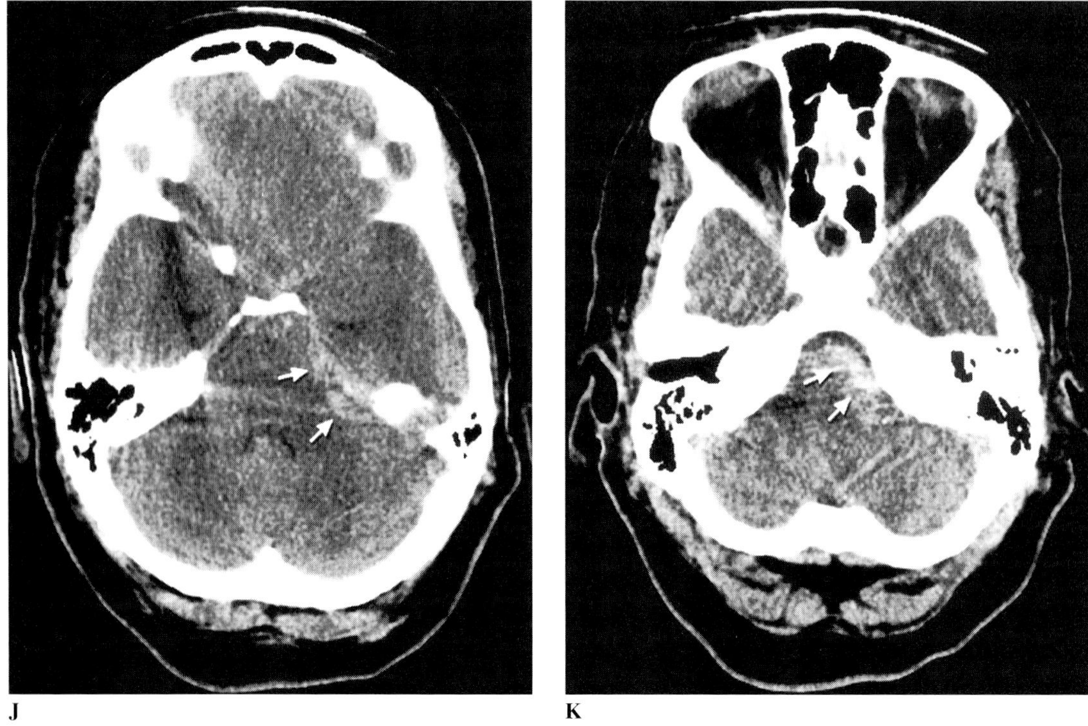

Figure 6.3. *Continued.* **J–K.** Premedullary hematoma with posterior inferior cerebellar artery aneurysm.

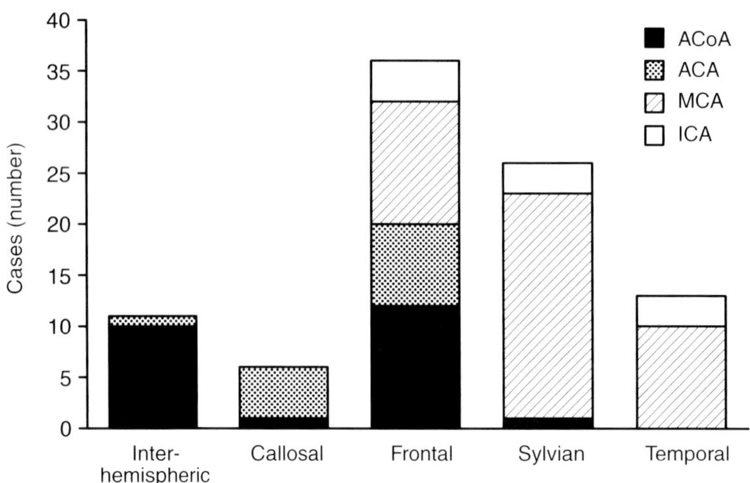

Figure 6.4. Prediction of hematoma. (Modified from Tokuda et al.[35] By permission of Elsevier Science.) (ACA = anterior cerebral artery; ACoA = anterior communicating artery; ICA = internal carotid artery; MCA = middle cerebral artery.)

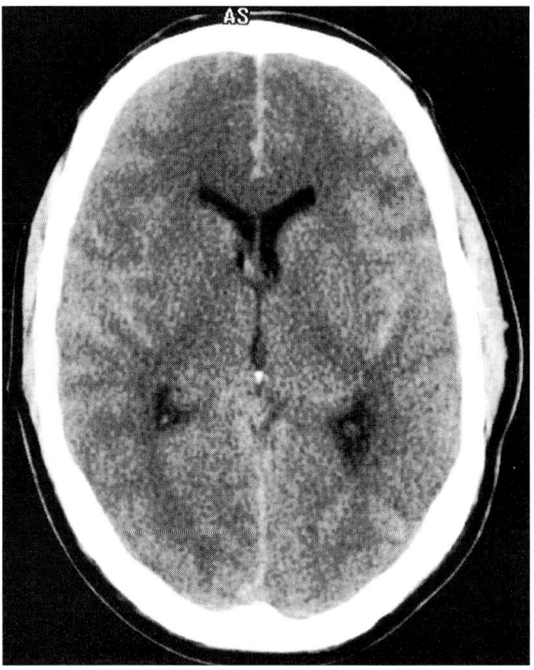

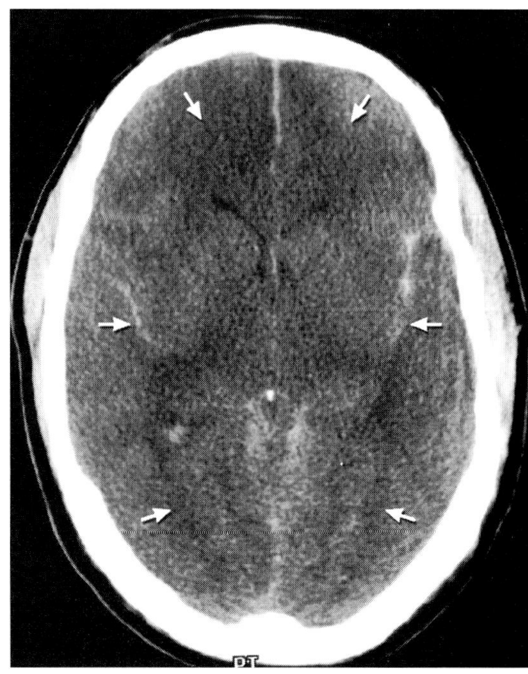

Figure 6.5. Development of bihemispheric ischemia (marked hypodensities; *arrows*) within 24 hours after subarachnoid hemorrhage.

increase in intracranial pressure at rupture. The CT scan findings are proof of early ischemic damage rather than cerebral vasospasm, which appears several days into the clinical course.

A clot in front of the brain stem with no extension beyond the suprasellar cisterns (so-called pretruncal SAH) highly predicts negative cerebral angiographic results,[37–39] but it has been estimated that in 10%, a posterior circulation aneurysm (most commonly, basilar tip) can be found on cerebral angiograms. The typical CT and MRI patterns of pretruncal SAH should be recognized (Capsule 6.2, Figures 6.6 and 6.7).

Blood can be difficult to detect on CT scans and may be very subtle, particularly in patients seen several days after the onset. The most commonly encountered false-negative CT scans are from patients with blood in the posterior horns of the ventricles (Figure 6.8A), sylvian fissure (Figure 6.8B), or prepontine region, in which hemorrhage may

Capsule 6.2. Pretruncal Nonaneurysmal Subarachnoid Hemorrhage

Pretruncal nonaneurysmal SAH (also called "perimesencephalic nonaneurysmal hemorrhage") is a benign variant of SAH. The entity is defined by blood before or surrounding the brain stem. Blood may extend to the middle of the basal part of the sylvian fissure but not in the interhemispheric fissure, convexity, or third ventricle and frontal horns of the ventricular system. In our experience, true perimesencephalic hemorrhage can also be due to trauma or SAH from a superior cerebellar artery or distal posterior cerebral artery or basilar tip aneurysm. Cerebral angiographic findings are normal, although cerebral vasospasm may occur and aneurysms may be found at far distant sites. Family members may harbor aneurysms as well. Patients do very well; rebleeding and cerebral infarction do not occur. The underlying pathologic lesion is not known, although occasionally pontine capillary telangectasias or focal dilatation of the basilar artery tip has been reported. It may represent a venous hemorrhage or intramural dissection.

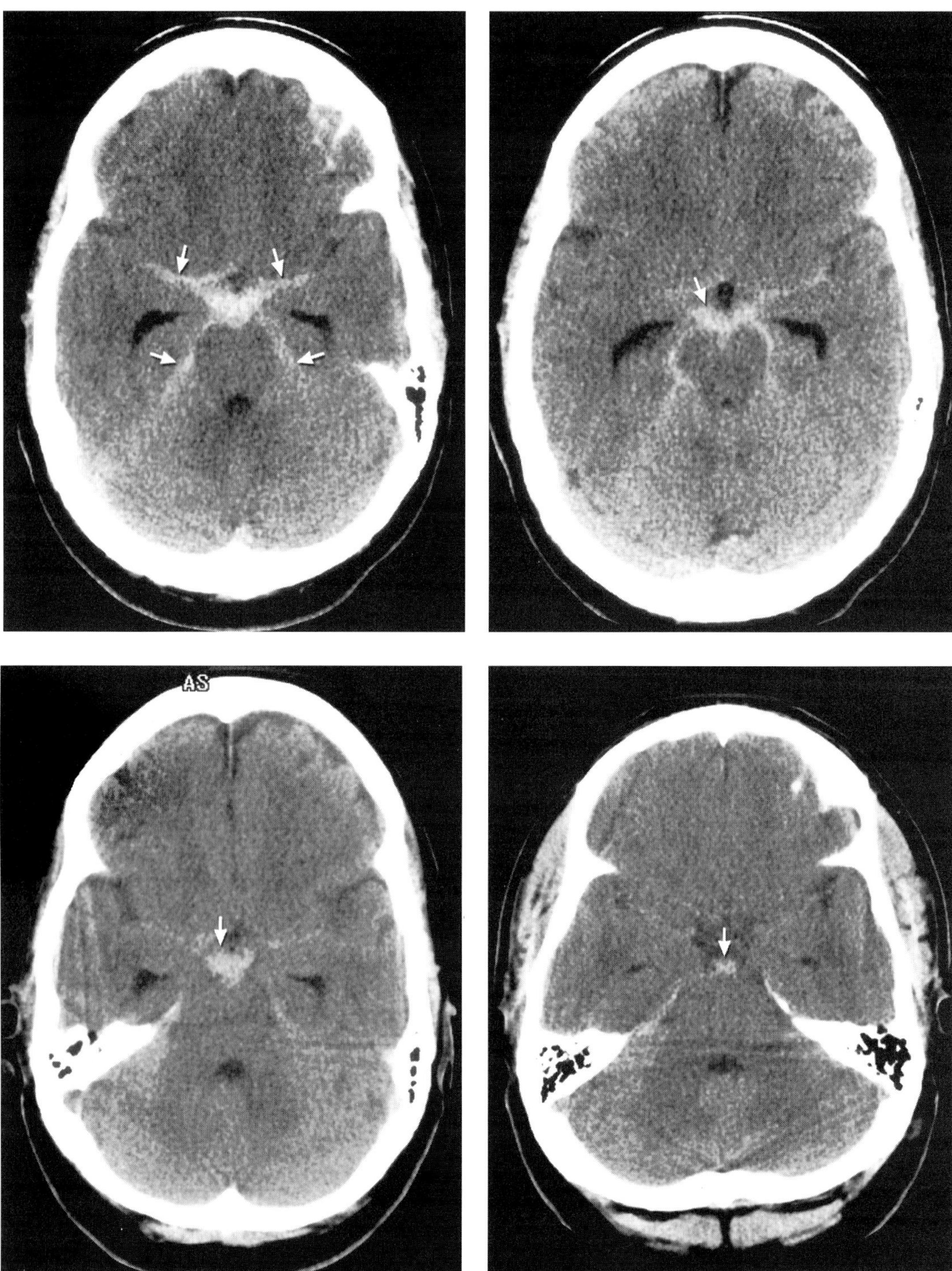

Figure 6.6. Computed tomography scan patterns of pretruncal nonaneurysmal subarachnoid hemorrhage in different patients. The spectrum includes complete filling of suprasellar cisterns and blood on the tentorium to more restricted clots and more subtle interpeduncular hematoma. The amount of blood is not critical in its recognition. The distribution of blood is limited and should not involve the entire lateral part of the sylvian fissure or the anterior hemisphere and ventricles.

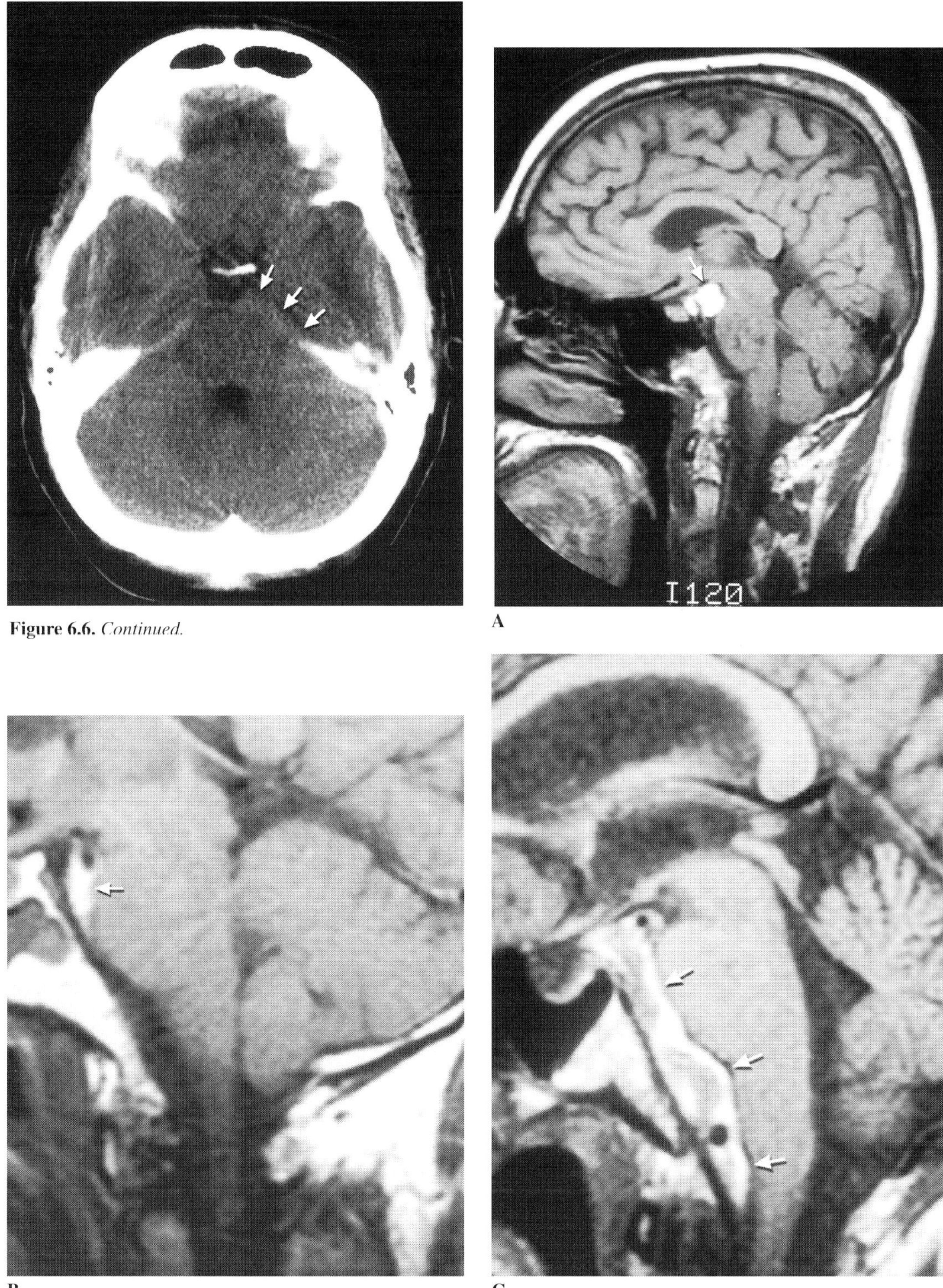

Figure 6.6. *Continued.*

A

B

C

Figure 6.7. A–C. Magnetic resonance imaging patterns of pretruncal nonaneurysmal subarachnoid hemorrhage. Blood may involve all or part of the cisterns in front of the brain stem.

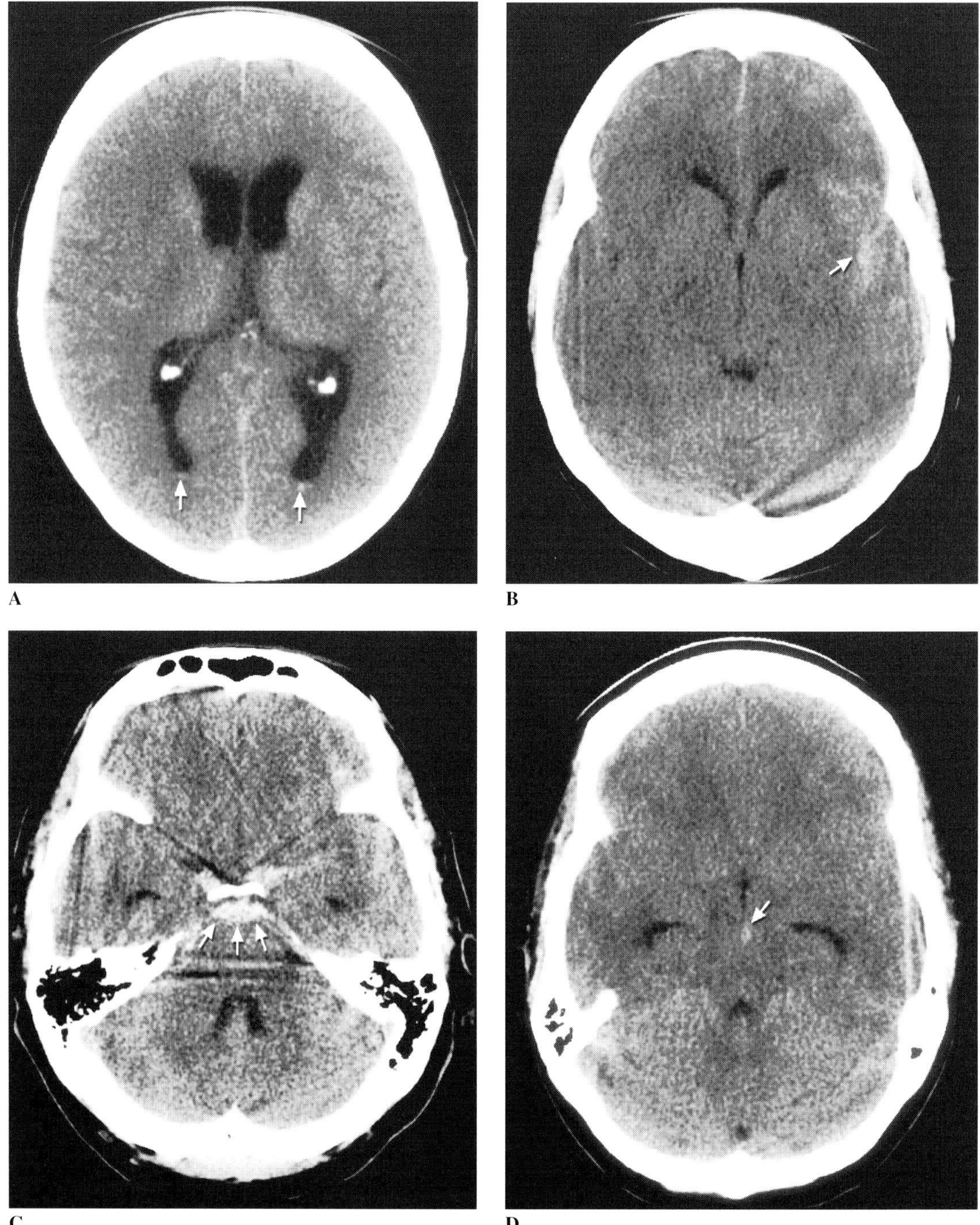

Figure 6.8. Subtle subarachnoid hemorrhage (false-negative computed tomography scans). **A.** Dependent blood in posterior horns. **B.** Blood in sylvian fissure. **C.** Prepontine layer of blood. **D.** Small area of interpeduncular blood.

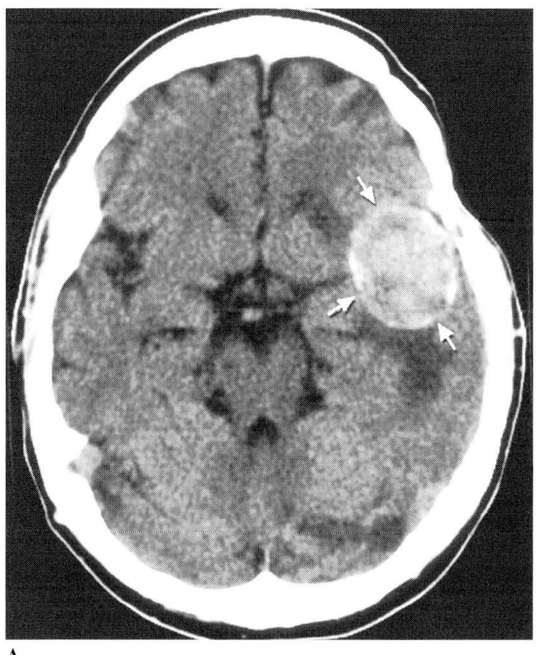

A

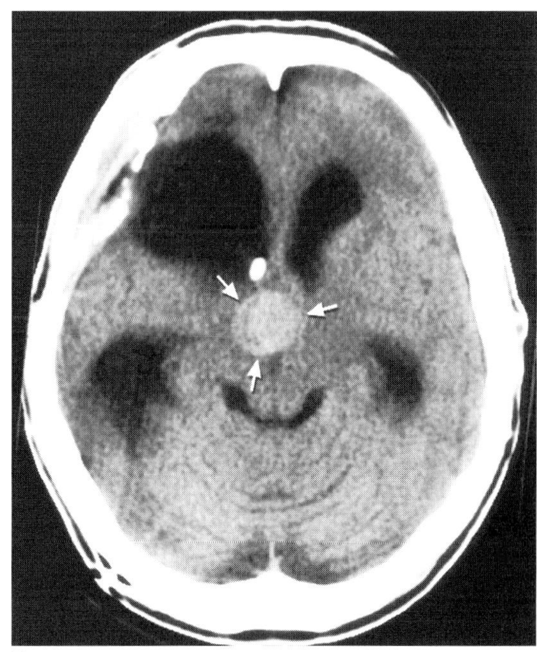

B

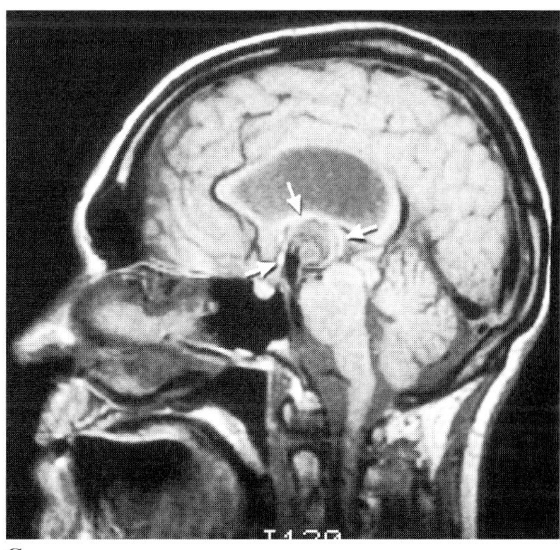

C

Figure 6.9. A. Computed tomography scan showing giant middle cerebral artery aneurysm. **B.** Giant basilar tip aneurysm. **C.** Magnetic resonance imaging further delineates compression of the third ventricle causing obstructive hydrocephalus.

affect only a small layer on the pons (Figure 6.8C). A tiny clot (involving a few pixels) may be localized in the interpeduncular cistern (Figure 6.8D). It is easily missed, particularly if the CT scan slices through the posterior fossa and basal cisterns are 10 mm.

CT detection of aneurysms has improved with a new generation of scanners, but contrast enhancement is needed to demonstrate an aneurysm, which is visualized only if larger than 5 mm. Larger aneurysms (more than 1 cm in diameter) or giant aneurysms (more than 2.5 cm) (Figures 6.9A and 6.9B) are disclosed on an unenhanced CT scan in most patients, although sometimes they are masked by an intracerebral hematoma. Magnetic resonance imaging (MRI) is most useful in further anatomical definition (Figure 6.9C).

SAH may also indicate a nonaneurysmal source and has been described in central nervous system vasculitis, trauma, coagulopathy, and subacute bacterial endocarditis with blood in sulci[40,41] (Figure 6.10). Typ-

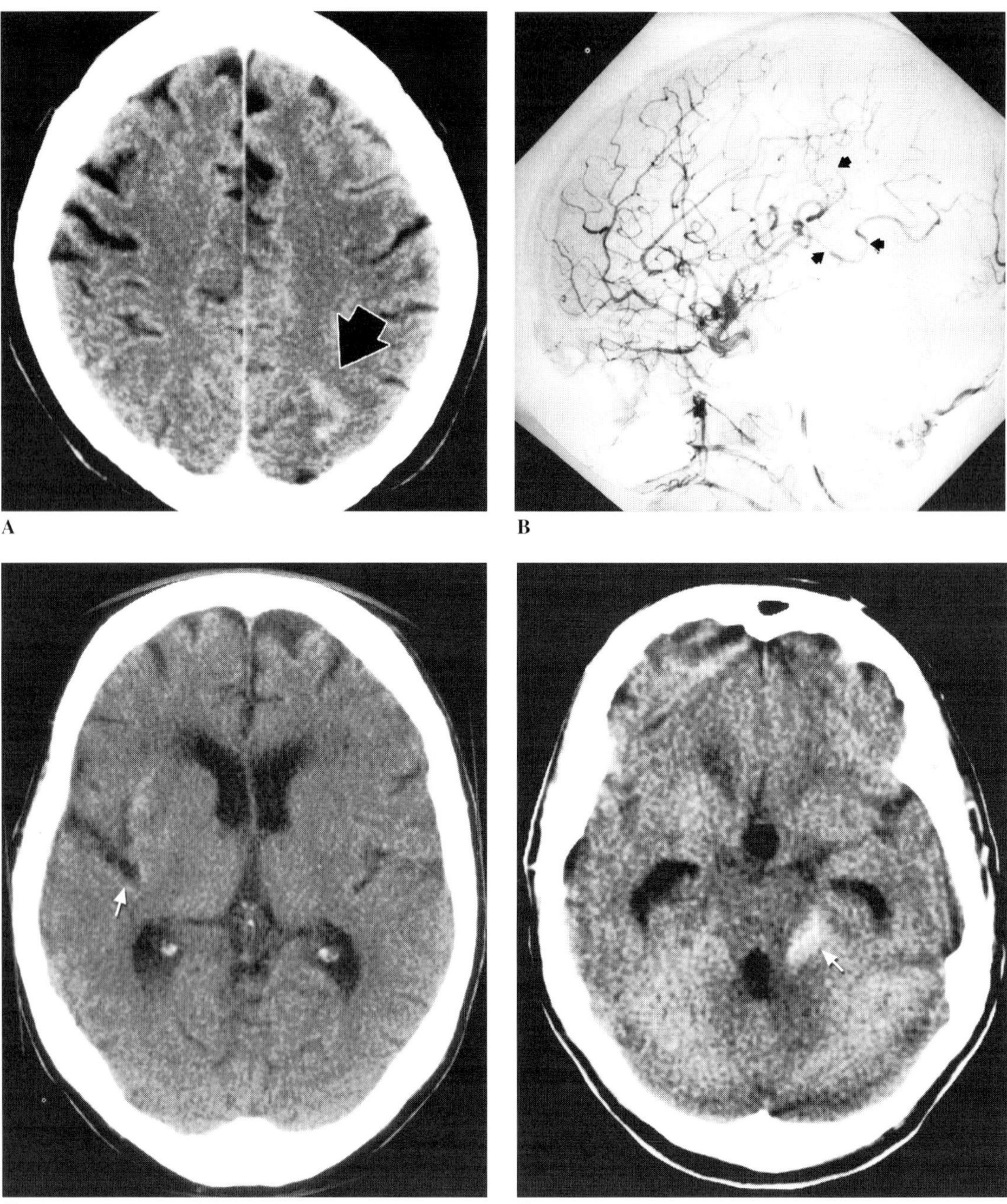

Figure 6.10. Typical nonaneurysmal locations of subarachnoid hemorrhage. **A–B.** Vasculitis. *Arrows* point to subarachnoid blood in a parietal sulcus and areas of segmental stenosis from vasculitis. **C–G.** Trauma (sulci and tentorium).

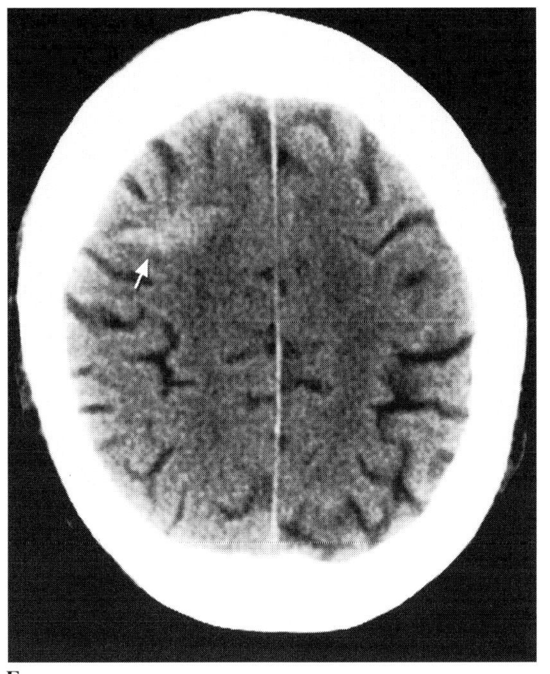

E

F

Figure 6.10. *Continued.*

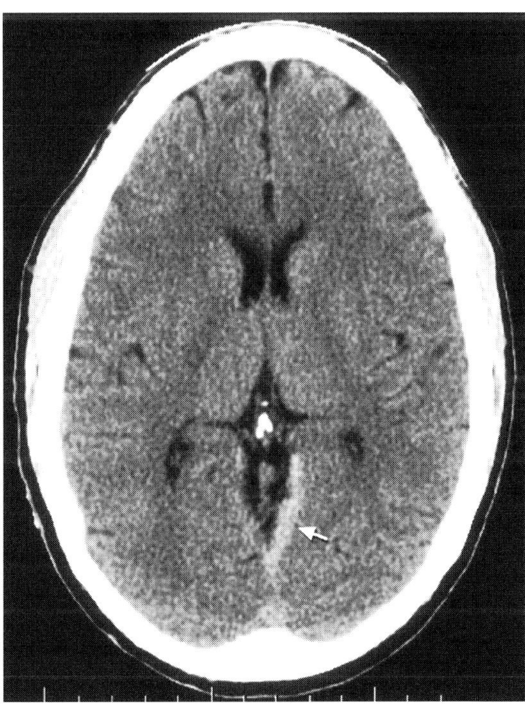

G

ical CT scan features of traumatic SAH are shown in Figures 6.10C through 6.10G. It is important to consider other causes of coma and false SAH, most commonly due to anoxia and contrast for evaluation of multitrauma. False SAH in massive anoxic cerebral edema in a resuscitated patient most likely represents stagnation of flow in the dura.[42,43] Anoxic brain swelling may emerge within 1 day after cardiac resuscitation, and CT may show hyperintensity in the basal cistern, falx, and tentorium. CT scan signs of edema are usually very obvious (Figures 6.11A and 6.11B). In addition, contrast enhancement may significantly mimic SAH. A contrast-enhanced study may have occurred before CT scanning, and contrast material may still be visualized in patients with poor renal function or shock or both (see Figures 6.11C and 6.11D).

Magnetic Resonance Imaging

MRI is usually not sensitive for SAH.[44,45] However, MRI may be able to show SAH when fluid attenuation inversion recovery (FLAIR) sequences are used. Recirculation of bloody cerebrospinal fluid (CSF) over the convexity is commonly seen as well[46] (Figure 6.12). MRI may be important in demonstrating an acute SAH in the posterior fossa, which, as mentioned previously, may be difficult to detect on CT scan because of beam-hardening artifacts.[47,48] Often in retrospect, CT scans showed a similar blood clot.[49] Sometimes a small deposit of blood in the sylvian fissure not visualized on CT scans can be demonstrated on MRI.

Magnetic resonance angiography (MRA) is useful in demonstrating the aneurysm,[50] and with three-dimensional time-of-flight MRA, aneurysms 3 mm in diameter and larger can be demonstrated[51,52] (Figure 6.13). At this time, however, MRA is not a substitute for conventional cerebral angiography.

Whether to perform MRI or MRA in a patient seen within 1 week of onset of a thunderclap headache who has entirely normal findings on neurologic examination, CSF study, and CT scan is a complex decision.[53] MRA may indeed demonstrate an aneurysm, a finding that can in fact a priori be expected in 4% of the general population. There has not been a published report of a patient with a typical thunderclap headache, normal neurologic CT and CSF findings, aneurysm after cerebral angiography, and hemorrhage in the close proximity of an aneurysm when explored with craniotomy. We have been able to diagnose pituitary apoplexy and bilateral carotid dissections with MRI (Chapter 8) as causes of thunderclap headache, but we remain reluctant about the routine use of MRA in these patients.

Cerebrospinal Fluid

Patients with normal CT scan findings and consistent history of thunderclap onset of headache should have a CSF examination in all instances. The fluid should be centrifuged, and the supernatant should be examined for xanthochromia. Xanthochromia is evaluated by comparing CSF with a tube of water in bright light, preferably daylight. If xanthochromia is found, absorption spectrophotometry is recommended to confirm oxyhemoglobin or bilirubin. This can be done hours later in stored, centrifuged CSF samples. CSF xanthochromia is detected by spectroscopy in specimens from all patients 12 hours before and up to 2 weeks after the onset of headache. Other tests that differentiate traumatic SAH from true SAH, such as measurements of D-dimer and the sequential tube test that demonstrates the clearing of tubes tinged with blood, are all very unreliable.

Finding only CSF evidence of SAH in patients with acute headache seen early after the ictus is uncommon, and a traumatic puncture is thus more probable. In a recent consecutive series of 175 patients with acute headache who had initial CT scans within 12 hours, only 2 patients had normal CT scan findings and positive results of spectrophotometric analysis of the CSF.[54] Finally, it is important also to measure the CSF pressure. Increased pressure in a patient with acute headache may suggest sagittal sinus thrombosis associated with sudden headache (Chapter 8), and MRI and magnetic resonance venography should be done for confirmation.

First Priority in Management

Stabilization of a patient with aneurysmal SAH also includes early institution of pain medication (codeine, 30 to 60 mg every 4 hours, or morphine, 10 mg every 4 hours). Management of increased blood pressure in the emergency room is a delicate balancing act. Many of the earlier studies suggesting an increased risk of rerupture with sustained hyper-

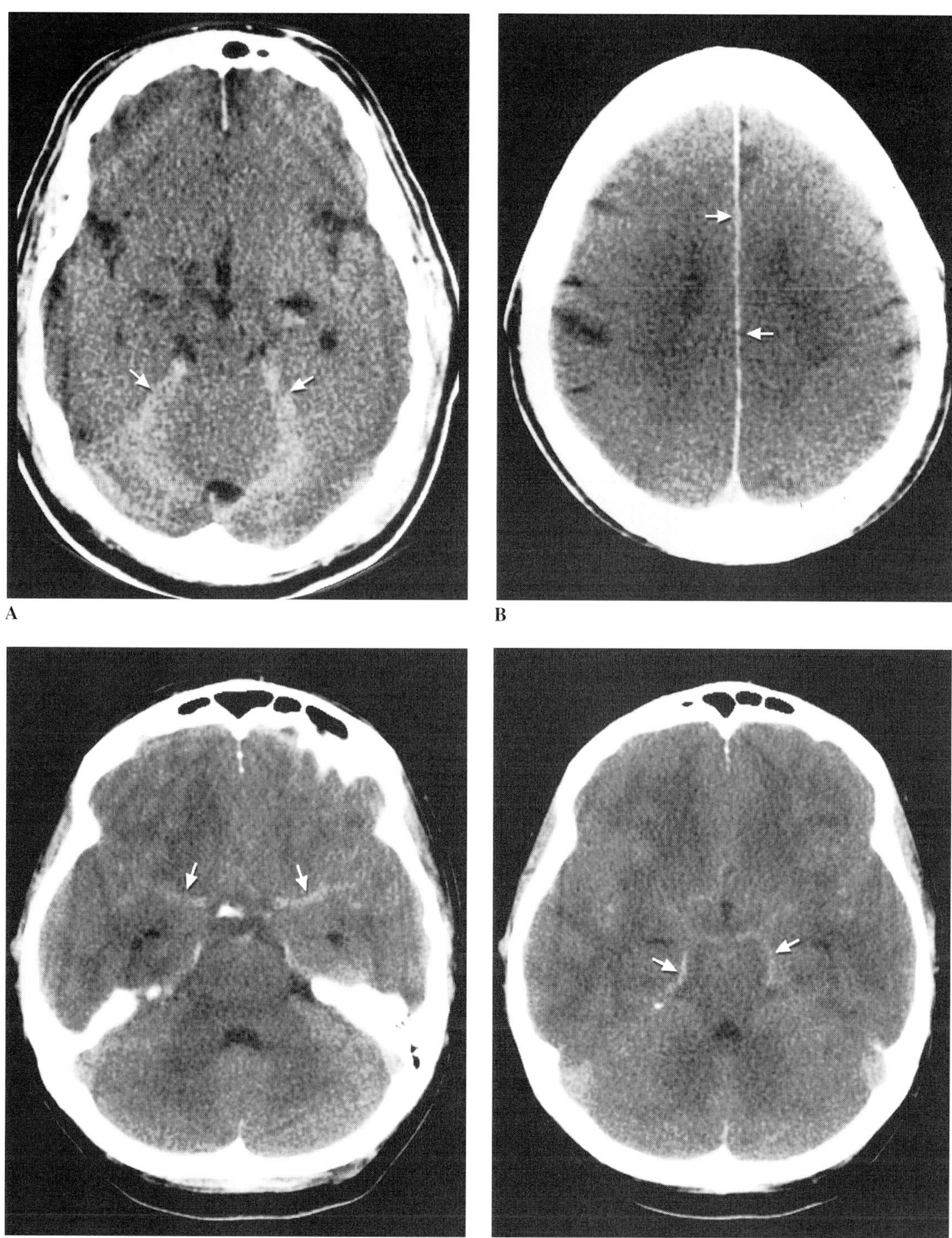

Figure 6.11. Pseudo–subarachnoid hemorrhage (SAH) (false-positive computed tomography [CT] scan). **A–B.** Cerebral edema and pseudo-SAH. **C–D.** Intravascular contrast, 150 mL, from prior abdominal CT. Contrast may remain in vessels when the patient is in shock, which is often the reason for contrast CT scanning of the abdomen.

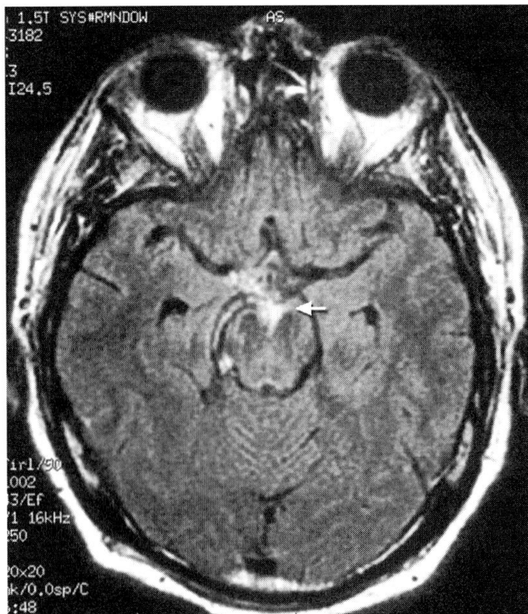

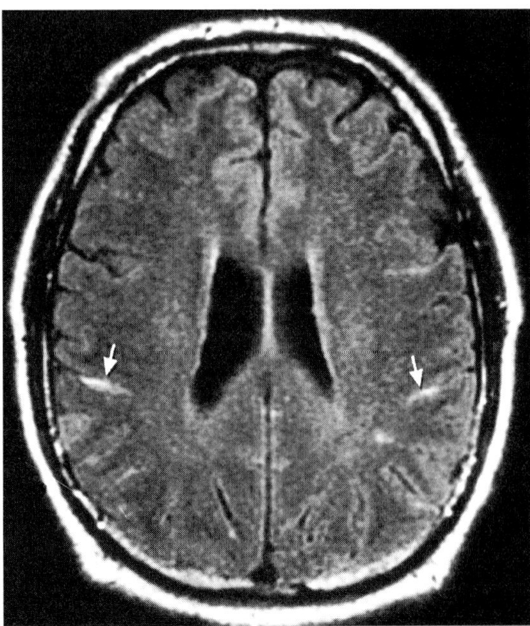

Figure 6.12. Magnetic resonance imaging with fluid attenuation inversion recovery (FLAIR) sequence: interpeduncular hemorrhage with subarachnoid blood over convexity. From Wijdicks, et al.[47] By permission of the American Heart Association.

tension should be devalued by lack of strict criteria for the diagnosis of rebleeding. Conversely, marked reduction of postrupture hypertension may precipitate a further reduction of cerebral perfusion pressure and possibly induce more ischemia. The initial management of aneurysmal SAH is shown in Table 6.3.

Surgical management is indicated in a patient with an acute temporal lobe hematoma and early mass effect. Craniotomy with immediate clipping of the ruptured middle cerebral artery aneurysm is warranted, with deferral of cerebral angiography in most instances. Immediate surgical management of a frontal hematoma is not indicated, because mass effect is lacking, and neurosurgical management of most anterior cerebral artery aneurysms is more complex, requiring better definition by cerebral angiography.

Figure 6.13. Magnetic resonance angiographic view of 6-mm aneurysm of the internal carotid artery (posterior communicating artery aneurysm).

Early surgical or endovascular management is also indicated if subarachnoid hemorrhage is caused by a dissecting vertebral aneurysm (Figure 6.14). Rebleeding is very common, often during a wait for emergency angiography or a coiling procedure. However, management remains uncertain because the natural history is not known. Aggressive treatment seems justified, with proximal balloon occlusion or coiling or proximal clipping or trapping to prevent early rebleeding.[55–58]

Acute hydrocephalus should be treated with a ventriculostomy but only when clinical deterioration can be attributed to CSF obstruction (see Chapter 4 for further discussion).

Sudden deterioration in the emergency department often is due to rebleeding (Figure 6.15), and emergency cerebral angiography is indicated.[3] Placement of a platinum coil should be considered (Figure 6.16) if the aneurysm is of sufficient size (4 to 10 mm). Neck size of the aneurysm should be less than 4 mm, because anything larger may permit free herniation of

Table 6.3. Initial Management of Aneurysmal Subarachnoid Hemorrhage in the Emergency Department

Endotracheal intubation in patients with GCS <10, pulmonary edema, or hypoxemia
Maintenance fluid intake of 2 L of 0.9% NaCl
Accept mean arterial blood pressure ≤130 mm Hg
Nimodipine, 60 mg 6 times a day
Fosphenytoin, 20 mg/kg intravenously (only with documented seizures)
Ventriculostomy in patients with acute hydrocephalus and GCS ≤10
Emergency neurosurgical evacuation in patients with progressive drowsiness and temporal lobe hematoma

(GCS = Glasgow coma score.)

the coil into the parent vessel, or the ratio of the largest diameter of the aneurysm to the size of its neck should be favorable, and patients should be poor surgical risks. However, the coil may become compacted after placement, increasing the risk of future rupture, and therefore repeat cerebral angiography is needed in 6 weeks. Whether platinum coil placement equals aneurysmal clipping in future risk of rupture remains to be investigated. One- to 2-year follow-up data are encouraging. However, rupture of a completely coil-occluded middle cerebral artery aneurysm after an 18-month interval was recently reported.[59] Recurrent filling of the aneurysm occurred in 15% of 259 aneurysms treated by coil embolization. Annual rebleeding rates were 0.8% in the first year, 0.6% in the second year, and 2.4% in the third year after coil placement, with no rebleeding in 2 subsequent years.[60]

Outcome Predictors

Favorable clinical and CT scan features in aneurysmal SAH are absence of syncope at the onset, full awareness at presentation,[60,61] lack of localizing neurologic signs, and subsequent early clipping of the aneurysm. Unfavorable signs are coma at ictus, older age, major comorbidity,[62] rebleeding, large amounts of blood on CT scan, and intraventricular hemorrhage.[61] The presence of intracerebral hematoma and retinal hemorrhage does not influence outcome. Basilar artery aneurysmal rupture has a worse outcome than rupture in other locations.[63] Visual loss from vitreous hemorrhage has a good outcome, but recovery may take up to 3 years (median, 9

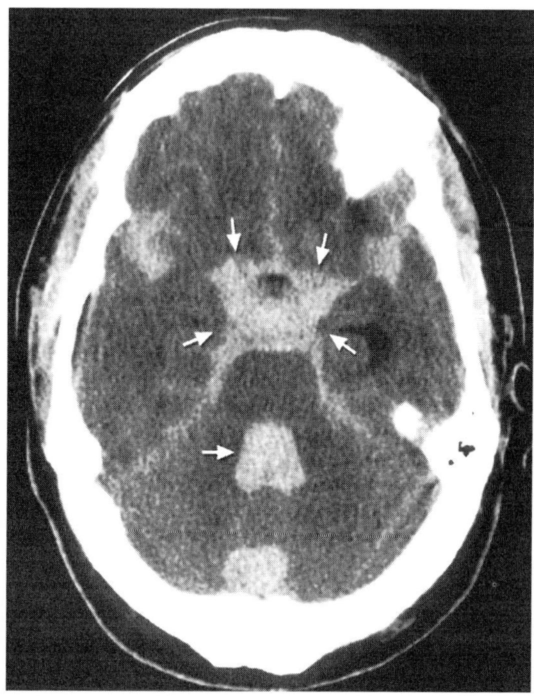

A

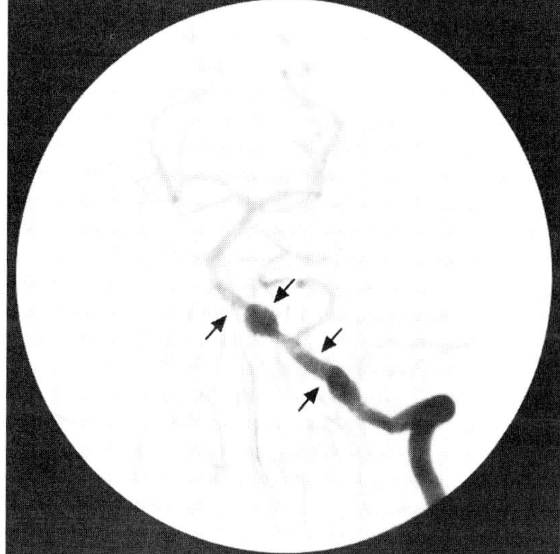

B

Figure 6.14. Massive subarachnoid hemorrhage with acute hydrocephalus and hemoventricle from dissecting vertebral aneurysm with fusiform dilatation. **A.** Computed tomography scan. **B.** Cerebral angiogram.

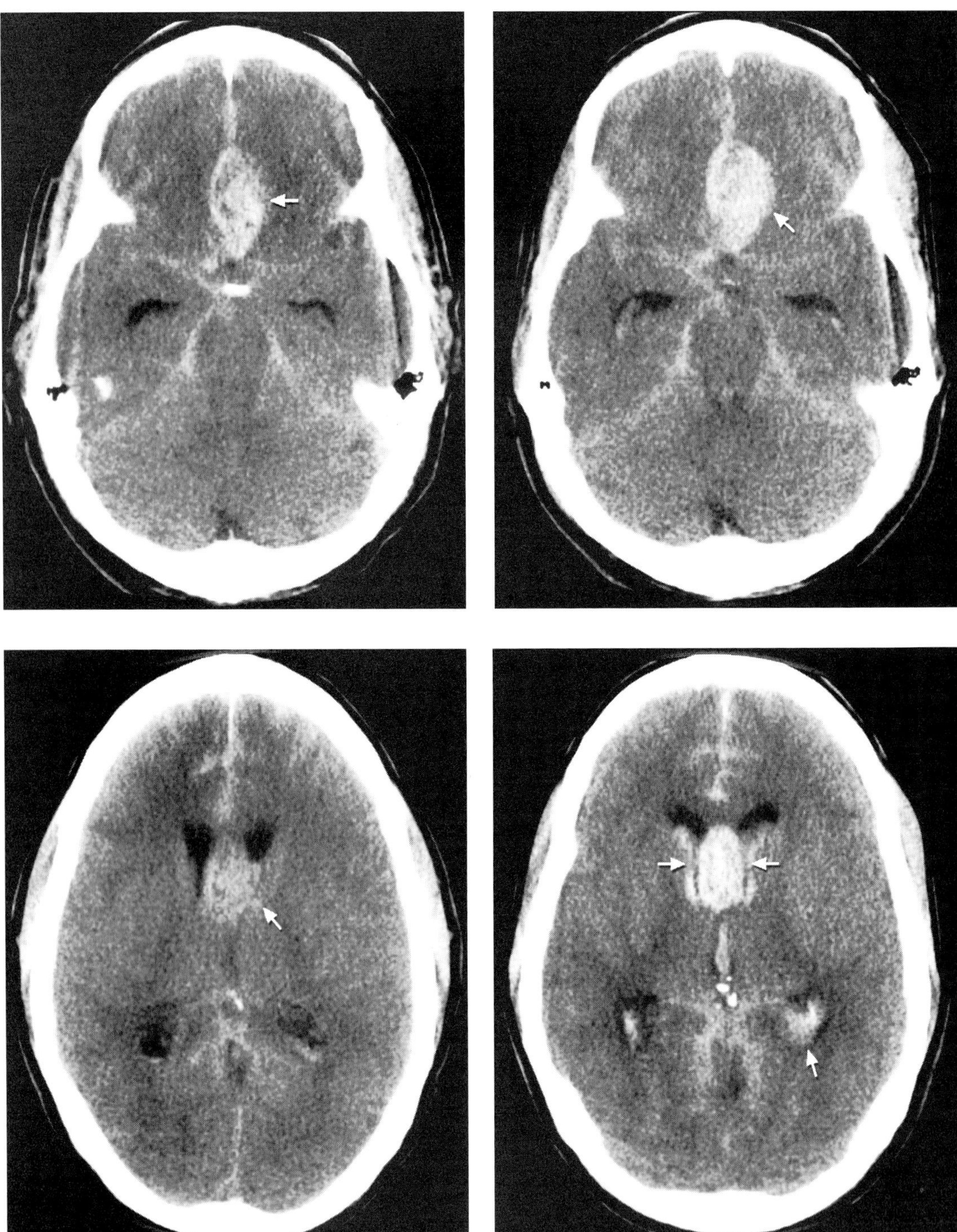

Figure 6.15. Rebleeding in the emergency department. Computed tomography scans at 2-hour intervals in a patient with new headache and drowsiness.

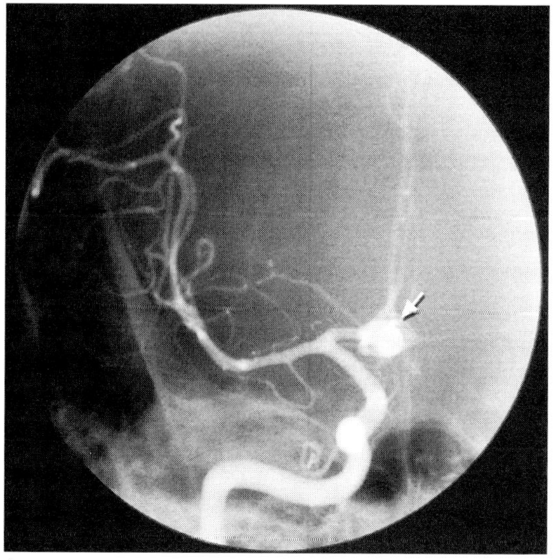
A

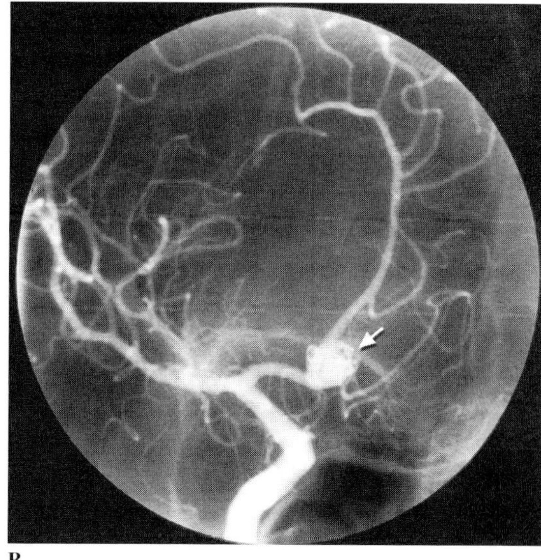
B

Figure 6.16. Successful endovascular coil placement in the patient in Figure 6.15. **A.** Before coiling. **B.** After coil placement.

months).[30] Vitrectomy, at least in one eye, to remove the clot should be considered after 6 to 12 months.

Triage

- In appropriate patients, placement of a platinum coil should have a place in treatment of poor-grade SAH to prevent rebleeding[64] and to safely increase cerebral perfusion pressure by volume replacement and pressure augmentation.
- Admission to a neurologic-neurosurgical intensive care unit, further observation for deterioration, and careful planning for cerebral angiography are followed by clipping of the aneurysm or endovascular occlusion with platinum coils.
- Early surgical intervention in patients with temporal lobe hematoma, documented rebleeding, and dissecting vertebral aneurysms if coiling is not possible.

References

1. Weir B. Subarachnoid Hemorrhage: Causes and Cures. New York: Oxford University Press, 1998.
2. Teunissen LL, Rinkel GJ, Algra A, van Gijn J. Risk factors for subarachnoid hemorrhage: a systematic review. Stroke 1996;27:544.
3. Lynch P. Ruptured cerebral aneurysm and brawling. BMJ 1979;1:1793.
4. International Study of Unruptured Intracranial Aneurysms Investigators. Unruptured intracranial aneurysms—risk of rupture and risks of surgical intervention. N Engl J Med 1998;339:1725.
5. Schievink WI, Karemaker JM, Hageman LM, van der Werf DJ. Circumstances surrounding aneurysmal subarachnoid hemorrhage. Surg Neurol 1989;32:266.
6. van der Jagt M, Hasan D, Bijvoet HW, et al. Validity of prediction of the site of ruptured intracranial aneurysms with CT. Neurology 1999;52:34.
7. Grote E, Hassler W. The critical first minutes after subarachnoid hemorrhage. Neurosurgery 1988;22:654.
8. McCormick PW, McCormick J, Zabramski JM, Spetzler RF. Hemodynamics of subarachnoid hemorrhage arrest. J Neurosurg 1994;80:710.
9. Lledo A, Calandre L, Martinez-Menendez B, et al. Acute headache of recent onset and subarachnoid hemorrhage: a prospective study. Headache 1994;34:172.
10. Duffy GP. The "warning leak" in spontaneous subarachnoid haemorrhage. Med J Aust 1983;1:514.
11. Leblanc R. The minor leak preceding subarachnoid hemorrhage. J Neurosurg 1987;66:35.
12. Leblanc R, Winfield JA. The warning leak in subarachnoid hemorrhage and the importance of its early diagnosis. CMAJ 1984;131:1235.
13. Okawara SH. Warning signs prior to rupture of an intracranial aneurysm. J Neurosurg 1973;38:575.

14. Waga S, Otsubo K, Handa H. Warning signs in intracranial aneurysms. Surg Neurol 1975;3:15.
15. Linn FH, Wijdicks EFM, van der Graaf Y, et al. Prospective study of sentinel headache in aneurysmal subarachnoid haemorrhage. Lancet 1994;344:590.
16. Biousse V, D'Anglejan-Chatillon J, Massiou H, Bousser MG. Head pain in non-traumatic carotid artery dissection: a series of 65 patients. Cephalalgia 1994;14:33.
17. Blau JN. Behaviour during a cluster headache. Lancet 1993;342:723.
18. Call GK, Fleming MC, Sealfon S, et al. Reversible cerebral segmental vasoconstriction. Stroke 1988;19:1159.
19. Clarke CE, Shepherd DI, Chishti K, Victoratos G. Thunderclap headache (letter to the editor). Lancet 1988;2:625.
20. Day JW, Raskin NH. Thunderclap headache: symptom of unruptured cerebral aneurysm. Lancet 1986;2:1247.
21. Dodick DW, Wijdicks EFM. Pituitary apoplexy presenting as a thunderclap headache. Neurology 1998;50:1510.
22. Fisher CM. Painful states: a neurological commentary. Clin Neurosurg 1984;31:32.
23. Kudrow L. Cluster Headache, Mechanisms and Management. Oxford: Oxford University Press, 1980.
24. Silbert PL, Mokri B, Schievink WI. Headache and neck pain in spontaneous internal carotid and vertebral artery dissections. Neurology 1995;45:1517.
25. Harling DW, Peatfield RC, Van Hille PT, Abbott RJ. Thunderclap headache: is it migraine? Cephalalgia 1989;9:87.
26. Slivka A, Philbrook B. Clinical and angiographic features of thunderclap headache. Headache 1995;35:1.
27. Wijdicks EFM, Kerkhoff H, van Gijn J. Long-term follow-up of 71 patients with thunderclap headache mimicking subarachnoid haemorrhage. Lancet 1988;2:68.
28. Shapiro S. Management of subarachnoid hemorrhage patients who presented with respiratory arrest resuscitated with bystander CPR. Stroke 1996;27:1780.
29. Lawn ND, Wijdicks EFM, Younge B. Blinding headache and two black eyes. J Neurol Neurosurg Psychiatry (in press).
30. Schultz PN, Sobol WM, Weingeist TA. Long-term visual outcome in Terson syndrome. Ophthalmology 1991;98:1814.
31. Nadeau SE, Trobe JD. Pupil sparing in oculomotor palsy: a brief review. Ann Neurol 1983;13:143.
32. Berlit P, Buhler B, Tornow K. CT findings in subarachnoidal haemorrhage (SAH). A retrospective study of 138 patients. Neurochirurgia (Stuttg) 1988;31:123.
33. Sames TA, Storrow AB, Finkelstein JA, Magoon MR. Sensitivity of new-generation computed tomography in subarachnoid hemorrhage. Acad Emerg Med 1996;3:16.
34. Jackson A, Fitzgerald JB, Hartley RW, et al. CT appearances of haematomas in the corpus callosum in patients with subarachnoid haemorrhage. Neuroradiology 1993;35:420.
35. Tokuda Y, Inagawa T, Katoh Y, et al. Intracerebral hematoma in patients with ruptured cerebral aneurysms. Surg Neurol 1995;43:272.
36. Kallmes DF, Lanzino G, Dix JE, et al. Patterns of hemorrhage with ruptured posterior inferior cerebellar artery aneurysms: CT findings in 44 cases. AJR Am J Roentgenol 1997;169:1169.
37. Duong H, Melancon D, Tampieri D, Ethier R. The negative angiogram in subarachnoid haemorrhage. Neuroradiology 1996;38:15.
38. Farrés MT, Ferraz-Leite H, Schindler E, Mühlbauer M. Spontaneous subarachnoid hemorrhage with negative angiography: CT findings. J Comput Assist Tomogr 1992;16:534.
39. Wijdicks EFM, Schievink WI, Miller GM. Pretruncal nonaneurysmal subarachnoid hemorrhage. Mayo Clin Proc 1998;73:745.
40. Kakarieka A. Review on traumatic subarachnoid hemorrhage. Neurol Res 1997;19:230.
41. Chukwudelunzu FE, Brown RB, Wijdicks EFM, et al. Nonaneurysmal subarachnoid hemorrhage associated with bacterial endocarditis (submitted for publication).
42. Spiegel SM, Fox AJ, Vinuela F, Pelz DM. Increased density of tentorium and falx: a false positive CT sign of subarachnoid hemorrhage. Can Assoc Radiol J 1986; 37:243.
43. Phan T, Wijdicks EFM, Worrel G, et al. False subarachnoid hemorrhage in anoxic brain swelling: an overlooked CT scan sign (submitted for publication).
44. Atlas SW. MR imaging is highly sensitive for acute subarachnoid hemorrhage … not! Radiology 1993;186:319.
45. Jenkins A, Hadley DM, Teasdale GM, et al. Magnetic resonance imaging of acute subarachnoid hemorrhage. J Neurosurg 1988;68:731.
46. Noguchi K, Ogawa T, Inugami A, et al. Acute subarachnoid hemorrhage: MR imaging with fluid-attenuated inversion recovery pulse sequences. Radiology 1995;196:773.
47. Wijdicks EFM, Schievink WI, Miller GM. MR imaging in pretruncal nonaneurysmal subarachnoid hemorrhage: is it worthwhile? Stroke 1998;29:2514.
48. Yoon HC, Lufkin RB, Vinuela F, et al. MR of acute subarachnoid hemorrhage. AJNR Am J Neuroradiol 1988;9:404.
49. Schievink WI, Wijdicks EFM, Spetzler RH. Severe diffuse vasospasm in pretruncal subarachnoid hemorrhage (submitted for publication).
50. Curnes JT, Shogry ME, Clark DC, Elsner HJ. MR angiographic demonstration of an intracranial aneurysm not seen on conventional angiography. AJNR Am J Neuroradiol 1993;14:971.
51. Ida M, Kurisu Y, Yamashita M. MR angiography of ruptured aneurysms in acute subarachnoid hemorrhage. AJNR Am J Neuroradiol 1997;18:1025.
52. Vieco PT, Shuman WP, Alsofrom GF, Gross CE. Detection of circle of Willis aneurysms in patients with acute subarachnoid hemorrhage: a comparison of CT angiography and digital subtraction angiography. AJR Am J Roentgenol 1995; 165:425.

53. Raps EC, Galetta SL, Rogers J, et al. Unruptured aneurysms and headache (letter to the editor). Arch Neurol 1994;51:447.
54. van der Wee N, Rinkel GJ, Hasan D, van Gijn J. Detection of subarachnoid haemorrhage on early CT: is lumbar puncture still needed after a negative scan? J Neurol Neurosurg Psychiatry 1995;58:357.
55. Tsukahara T, Wada H, Satake K, et al. Proximal balloon occlusion for dissecting vertebral aneurysms accompanied by subarachnoid hemorrhage. Neurosurgery 1995;36:914.
56. Lylyk P, Ceratto R, Hurvitz D, Basso A. Treatment of a vertebral dissecting aneurysm with stents and coils: technical case report. Neurosurgery 1998;43:385.
57. Yamaura A, Watanabe Y, Saeki N. Dissecting aneurysms of the intracranial vertebral artery. J Neurosurg 1990;72:183.
58. Halbach VV, Higashida RT, Dowd CF, et al. Endovascular treatment of vertebral artery dissections and pseudoaneurysms. J Neurosurg 1993;79:183.
59. Hodgson TJ, Carroll T, Jellinek DA. Subarachnoid hemorrhage due to late recurrence of a previously unruptured aneurysm after complete endovascular occlusion. AJNR Am J Neuroradiol 1998;19:1939.
60. Byrne JV, Sohn MJ, Molyneux AJ, Chir B. Five-year experience in using coil embolization for ruptured intracranial aneurysms: outcomes and incidence of late rebleeding. J Neurosurg 1999;90:656.
61. Kassell NF, Torner JC, Jane JA, et al. The International Cooperative Study on the Timing of Aneurysm Surgery. I. Overall management results. II. Surgical results. J Neurosurg 1990;73:18,37.
62. Solenski NJ, Haley EC Jr, Kassell NF, et al. Medical complications of aneurysmal subarachnoid hemorrhage: a report of the Multicenter Cooperative Aneurysm Study. Participants of the Multicenter Cooperative Aneurysm Study. Crit Care Med 1995;23:1007.
63. Schievink WI, Wijdicks EF, Piepgras DG, et al. The poor prognosis of ruptured intracranial aneurysms of the posterior circulation. J Neurosurg 1995;82:791.
64. Wijdicks EFM. Worst-case scenario: management in poor grade aneurysmal subarachnoid hemorrhage. Cerebrovasc Dis 1995;5:163.

Chapter 7
Intracerebral Hematomas

By and large, intracerebral hematomas are caused by a ruptured penetrating arterial branch damaged by the effects of long-standing hypertension. Hypertension or, in certain circumstances, an acute hypertensive crisis produces hemorrhages in the caudate nucleus, putamen, thalamus, cerebellum, or pons. Hematomas involving the subcortical white matter and cortex may have different causes, including vascular malformations. This fundamental distinction is important, because cerebral angiography may be urgently indicated in a lobar hematoma.

Intraparenchymal hemorrhage, in one form or another, poses significant management and triage problems in the first hours.[1] Some types of intracerebral hematomas are surgically accessible, and early recognition of clinical and computed tomography (CT) scan predictors of deterioration may lead to surgical evacuation. Thus, it is important to separate lobar hematoma from ganglionic hemorrhage and cerebellar hematoma from pontine hemorrhage. Another task is to determine at an early stage whether survival is remote or whether salvage with a reasonable opportunity for rehabilitation is possible.

Interpretation of different aspects of neuroimaging, management, stabilization, and indications for neurosurgical treatment of spontaneous intracerebral hematomas are discussed. Traumatic intracerebral hematoma is discussed in Chapter 12.

Ganglionic Hemorrhages

Location of the hemorrhage typically is in the putamen or caudate nucleus. The cause is a ruptured lateral branch of the lenticulostriate artery. Equally common are hematomas in the thalamus from ruptured thalamoperforating arteries. Many of these hemorrhages are apoplectic, creating large destructive volumes with extension into the ventricular system.

Clinical Presentation

Supratentorial intracerebral hemorrhage may be manifested in many ways. Coma or any impaired level of consciousness can be explained by the space-occupying effect of the hematoma, causing significant shift of the brain stem; extension of the hemorrhage of the putamen into the thalamus, compressing the opposite thalamic nuclei; and rupture into the ventricular system, resulting in an acutely pronounced hydrocephalus.

A hemorrhage in the putamen may produce global aphasia, hemianopia, conjugate deviation of the eyes, flaccid hemiplegia, loss of sensation, or neglect of the left side of the body. A cataclysmic progression to loss of many brain stem functions is not unusual. The clinical syndromes in patients with hemorrhages into the putamen have been further divided on the basis of whether the lesion affects

Capsule 7.1. Growth of Parenchymal Hematoma

The volume of a hematoma may increase from continued bleeding, edema formation, and rebleeding. Continued bleeding occurs from a cascade effect. The mass exerts pressure and stretch on surrounding arteries, which subsequently rupture and build a mass in consecutive layers of fibrin. Edema in intracerebral hematoma is due to both cytotoxic and vasogenic mechanisms. It is maximal 1 to 3 days after the initial hemorrhage and resolves by day 5. The perilesional edematous regions contain significant clot-derived protein and expand the extracellular space, increasing the distance of white matter axons and cells from their blood supply and creating hypoxia. This may be further enhanced by systemic hypoxemia.[3] Thrombin is important in perilesional edema[4,5] because it causes inflammation, reactive gliosis, and retraction of axons and dendrites. In one experimental study, the effects of thrombin could be blocked by hirudin, which is a specific thrombin inhibitor, and edema could not be produced by other blood products.[4] Single-photon emission computed tomography suggested that edema is a form of reperfusion injury due to early ischemia after the hematoma, with flow improving significantly over time.[6] A recent study of regional cerebral blood flow that used radiolabeled microspheres failed to detect an ischemic penumbra in nonhypertensive animals with large-volume clots.[7]

only the anterior part of the putamen close to the anterior limb of the internal capsule, the middle part of the putamen, or the posterior part. Hemorrhage localized to the anterior part of the putamen may produce purely motor hemiparesis, eye deviation to the site of the lesion, and abulia. Extension into the middle part of the putamen may additionally involve spatial neglect and decreased sensation evidenced by diminished awareness of pinprick, touch, and position. Extension of the clot into the posterior putamen leads to a more prominent left-sided neglect in right-sided lesions and fluent aphasia in left-sided lesions. Large hemorrhages in the putamen may dissect along the white matter tracts into the temporal lobe, causing a Wernicke-type aphasia, but surrounding edema may also impair the function of the temporal lobe.

The neurologic deficit in a putaminal hemorrhage is commonly stable when the patient is admitted to the emergency department. Neurologic deficits may become more pronounced, signaled by stupor instead of drowsiness or by new development of a gaze preference. Progression of neurologic symptoms, indicating enlargement of the hematoma with more mass effect, is commonly noted clinically within the first 6 hours after presentation.

Clinical features of a thalamic hematoma are excessive sleepiness and abulia. Stupor may ensue if the hematoma causes pressure effects on the opposite thalamus or causes acute hydrocephalus due to extension into the third ventricle. A thalamic hematoma with dissection into a mesencephalon causes a fluctuating level of consciousness, and episodes of stupor alternate with slow responses (see Chapter 1). Left-sided thalamic hemorrhages are associated with fluent aphasia, with nonexistent phrases and poor naming but conspicuously good comprehension of spoken language. When the hematoma affects the internal capsule, hemiplegia occurs. Right-sided thalamic hematomas produce left visual neglect and hemiplegia.

Caudate hemorrhage is the least common of the classic hypertensive hemorrhages, and its clinical manifestations often can be inferred mainly from an extension to the ventricular system. More commonly, agitation, confusion, and thrashing around occur at the onset without localizing neurologic findings.[2] When the hematoma enlarges and extends from the caudate nucleus into the white matter, involving the internal capsule or putamen, level of consciousness decreases because of brain shift. Extension of the hemorrhage into the hypothalamus and diencephalon might produce complete Horner's syndrome on one side, a diagnostic clue to a large extending caudate hematoma (Capsule 7.1). The clinical features are summarized in Table 7.1.

Table 7.1. Hypertension-Associated Intracerebral Supratentorial Hemorrhages

Primary site	Extension	Telltale signs
Caudate nucleus	Localized intraventricular hemorrhage	Headache, confusion, drowsiness-stupor, abulia
	Capsule, putamen, diencephalon	Hemiparesis, eye deviation, Horner's syndrome
Putamen	Localized	Hemiparesis, eye deviation, global aphasia
	Posterior extension	Fluent aphasia
Thalamus	Localized	Paresthesia, hemineglect, nonfluent aphasia (often preserved repetition), disorientation to place
	Mesencephalon	Slow syndrome

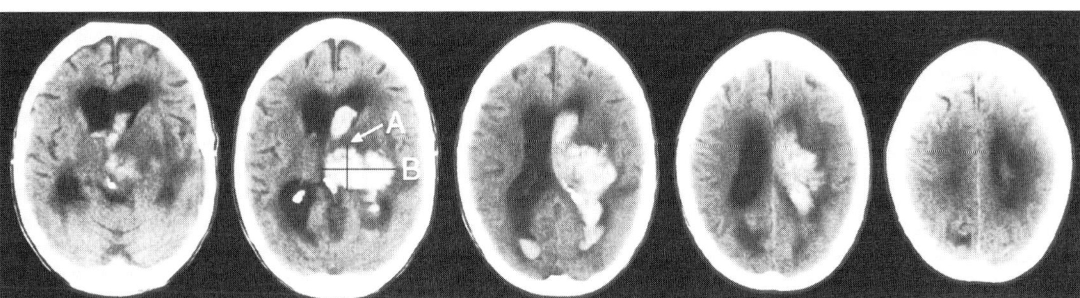

Figure 7.1. Volume of a thalamic hemorrhage as measured by the ABC method (ABC ÷ 2). In this example, A is 3 cm, B is 5 cm, and the number of slices (C) is 4 (hemorrhage is visible on four computed tomography slices at 10-mm intervals). The total volume is calculated as 60 ÷ 2, or 30 cm^3.

Interpretation of Diagnostic Tests

The volume in cubic centimeters can be measured on CT scan by the ellipsoid method: $(A \times B \times C)/2$ (Figure 7.1). (A is the maximum diameter, B is the diameter perpendicular to A, and C is the number of slices on which the hematoma is seen, assuming 10-mm cuts.[8]) The projected grid on CT scan films is 1 cm per single step. This approximation of hemorrhagic volume assumes that every hematoma is ellipsoidal. Nonetheless, the value obtained correlates well with a direct CT scan measurement, and thus the method is a simple, practical means of ad hoc volume analysis in the emergency department. In 25% of patients, enlargement of the ganglionic hematoma may appear on CT scans obtained within the first 3 hours of presentation. In contrast, patients with CT scans obtained more than 6 hours after the ictus and a volume of less than 25 cm^3 are unlikely to have deterioration from further growth of the hematoma.

Putaminal hemorrhages are most prevalent and usually massive. The volume on CT scan commonly approaches 60 cm^3, but smaller hematomas may occur without further enlargement on serial CT scans. Common types of putaminal hemorrhage are shown in Figure 7.2.

Thalamic hematomas are usually small, but because of close proximity to the ventricles, intraventricular hemorrhage may occur. Hydrocephalus may develop from obstruction of the cerebrospinal fluid (CSF) at the level of the foramen of Monro, more commonly with medially located thalamic hemorrhages (Figure 7.3). Enlargement of the hematoma has been observed in thalamic hemorrhages, typically in conjunction with progression to coma, and markedly reduces the outlook for independent recovery[9] (Figure 7.4). The CT scan and MRI features producing coma in patients with thalamic hematomas are shown in Figure 7.5. Caudate hemorrhage (Figure 7.6) may be difficult to separate from intraventricular hemorrhage on CT scans, and often magnetic resonance imaging (MRI) is needed to locate the source in the caudate nucleus.

Finally, CT scan interpretation of spontaneous intracerebral hematoma may be deceiving. Possibly,

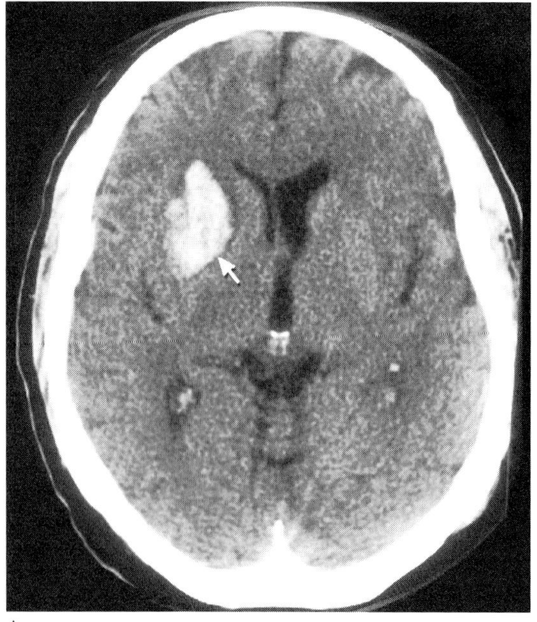
A

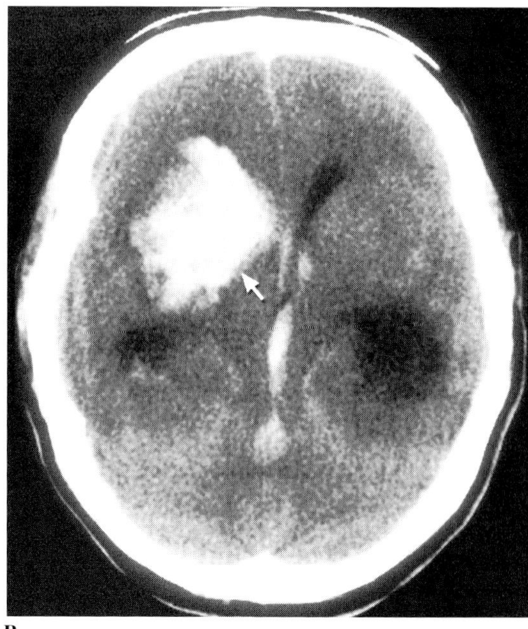
B

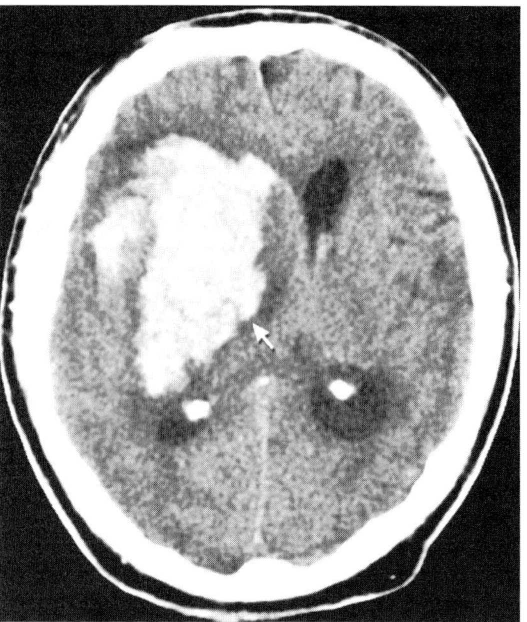
C

Figure 7.2. Computed tomography scan examples of putaminal hemorrhage: **(A)** localized, **(B)** extensions to capsule and frontal lobe and intraventricular extension, and **(C)** extension into the thalamus.

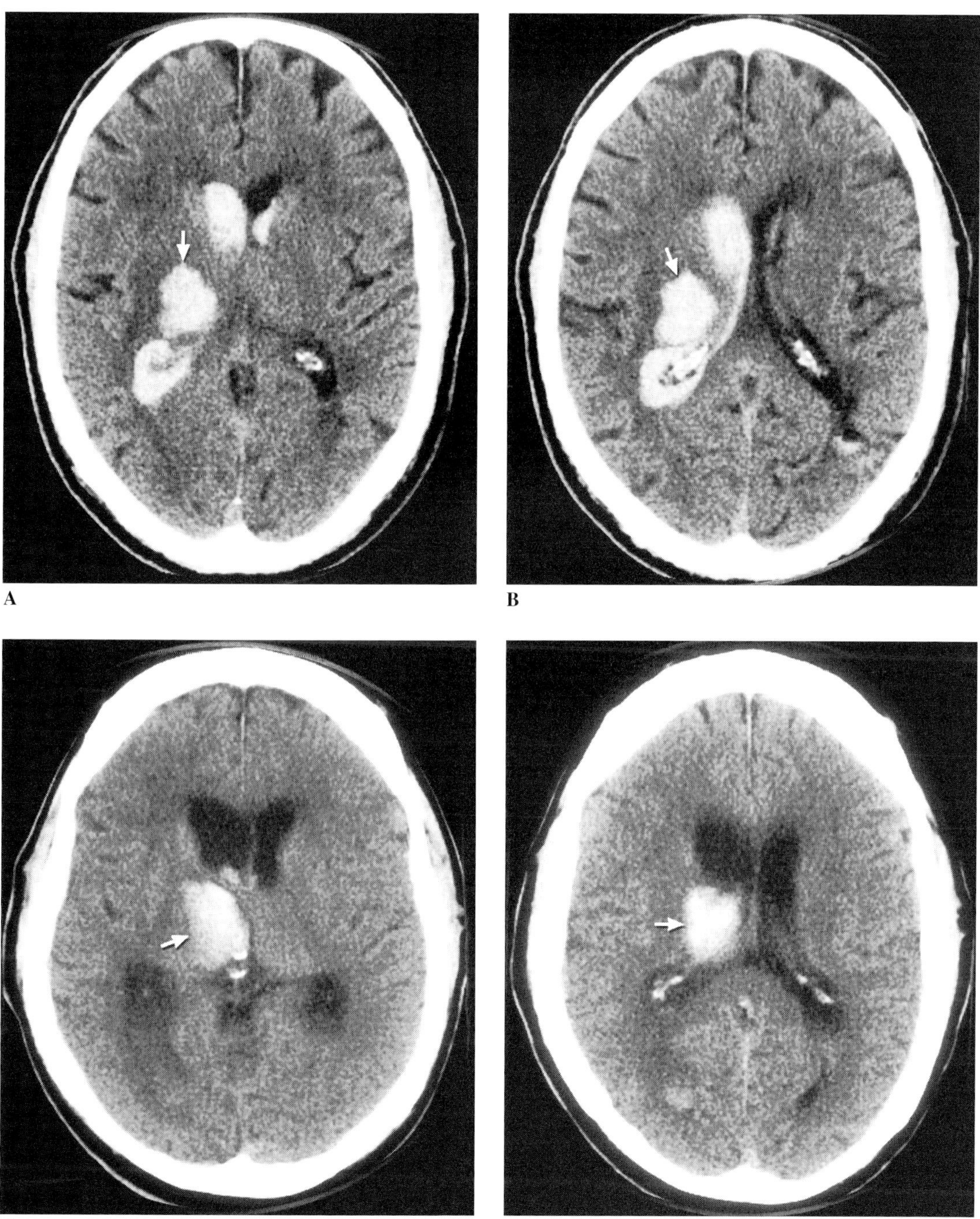

Figure 7.3. Computed tomography scans of thalamic hemorrhage (*arrows*). **A–B.** Lateral. **C–D.** Medial.

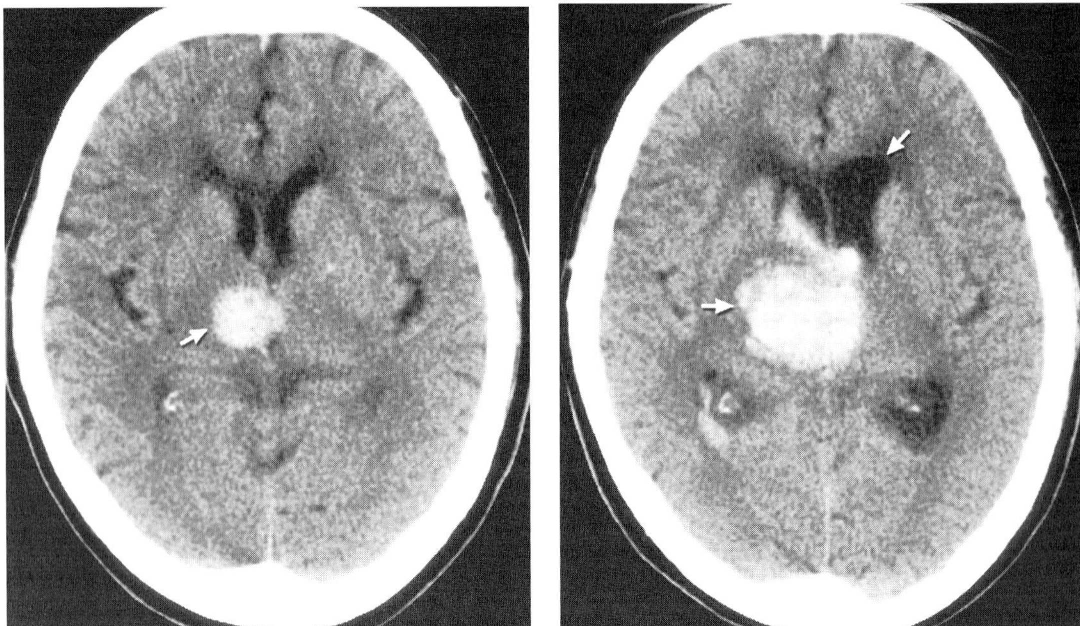

Figure 7.4. Computed tomography images of enlargement of thalamic hemorrhage, intraventricular extension, and hydrocephalus.

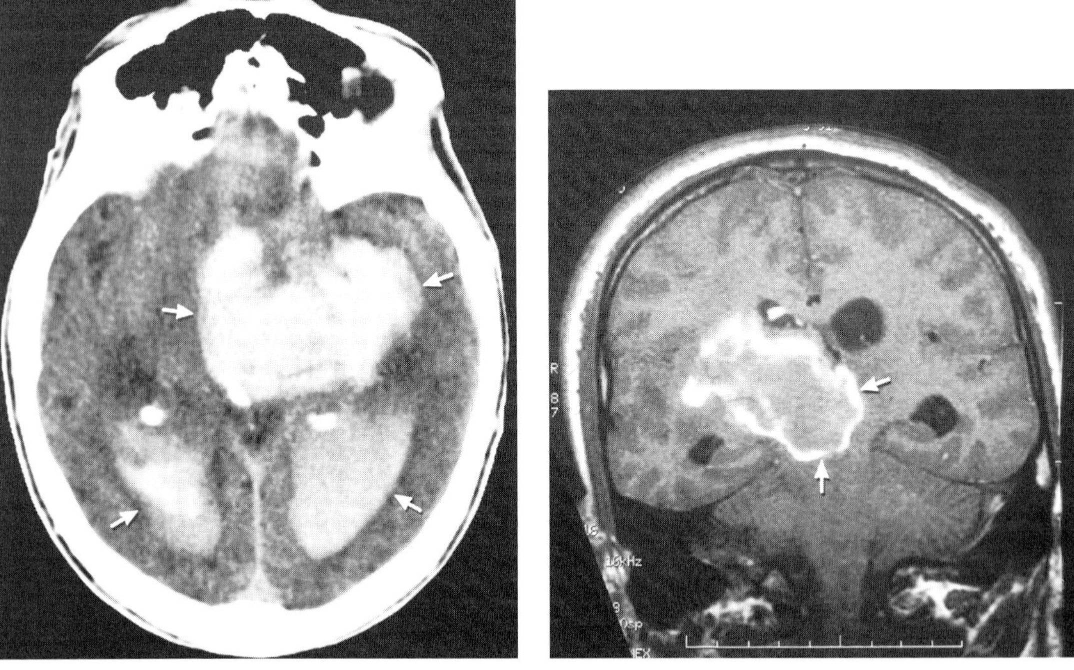

Figure 7.5. Coma caused by thalamic hemorrhage. *Left*, Massive extension and enlargement of ventricles. *Right*, Magnetic resonance image of the thalamic hemorrhage with extension into the midbrain.

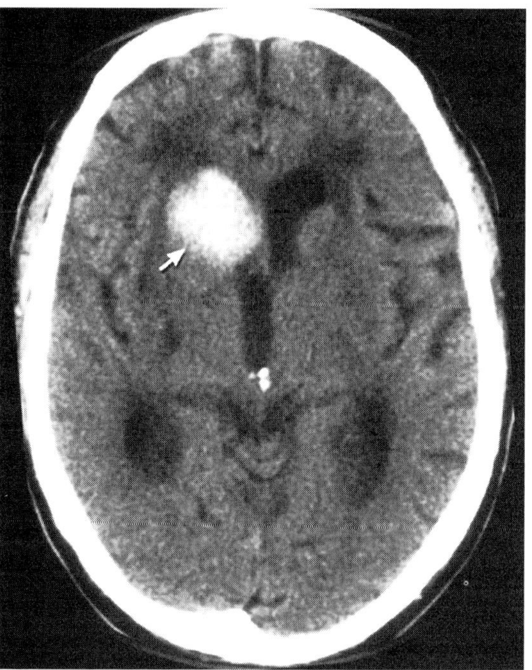
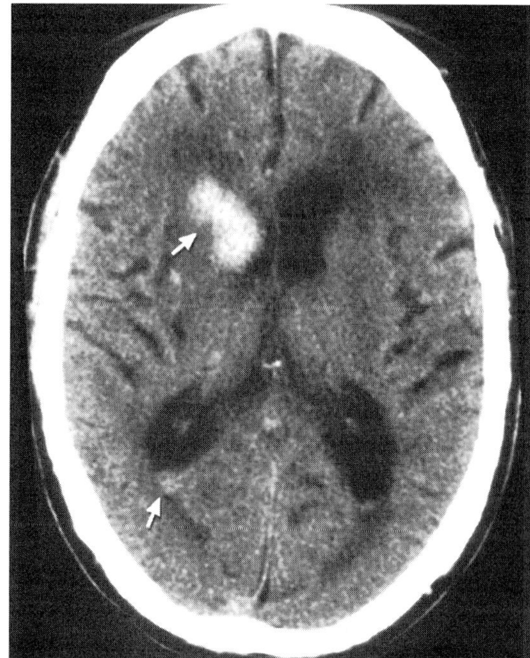

Figure 7.6. Computed tomography images of caudate hemorrhage and intraventricular extension (*arrows*).

some represent hemorrhagic infarcts rather than primary intracerebral hematomas. This possibility should be particularly considered in patients who have had transient ischemic attacks, who have a potential cardioembolic source for emboli, such as atrial fibrillation or left ventricle hypokinesis, and who have silent infarcts revealed on CT scans[10] (Figure 7.7). Later, a localized putaminal hemorrhage may mimic an infarct by leaving a slit-like lesion (Figure 7.8).

First Priority in Management

Most academic institutions in the United States and Europe manage patients with ganglionic hemorrhages medically.[11] This policy implies supportive care and monitoring of further deterioration from enlargement in volume caused by development of surrounding edema or continuous bleeding. Reversal of anticoagulation is essential, and fresh frozen plasma (and vitamin K) or, if appropriate, platelets should be infused in the emergency department.[12] In patients with a metallic heart valve or otherwise high cardioembolic risk, for example, marked ventricular hypokinesis or atrial fibrillation and echocardiographic evidence of atrial thrombus, there is an increased risk of thromboembolization or valve thrombosis, but it appears that discontinuation of anticoagulation for less than a week in these patients rarely leads to systemic embolization.[13]

Hypertensive crisis is very common but seldom produces congestive heart failure or brief ventricular arrhythmias from a catecholamine surge. Only when blood pressure remains high (mean arterial pressure >140 mm Hg) and electrocardiographic changes or cardiac arrhythmias appear is reduction with β-blockers indicated.[14] No evidence suggests that persistent acute hypertension provokes a recurrence of bleeding in patients with a spontaneous intracranial hematoma.[15] However, vasogenic edema may develop and persistent hypertension may possibly contribute to an increase in intracranial pressure.[16] Aggressive treatment of hypertension might theoretically reduce cerebral edema in these patients, but it may increase the risk of producing further perilesional ischemia in patients with prior hypertension. It is generally accepted that when the mean arterial blood pressure reaches 145 to 150 mm Hg, the risk of enlargement of the hematoma from continuous leakage or cerebral

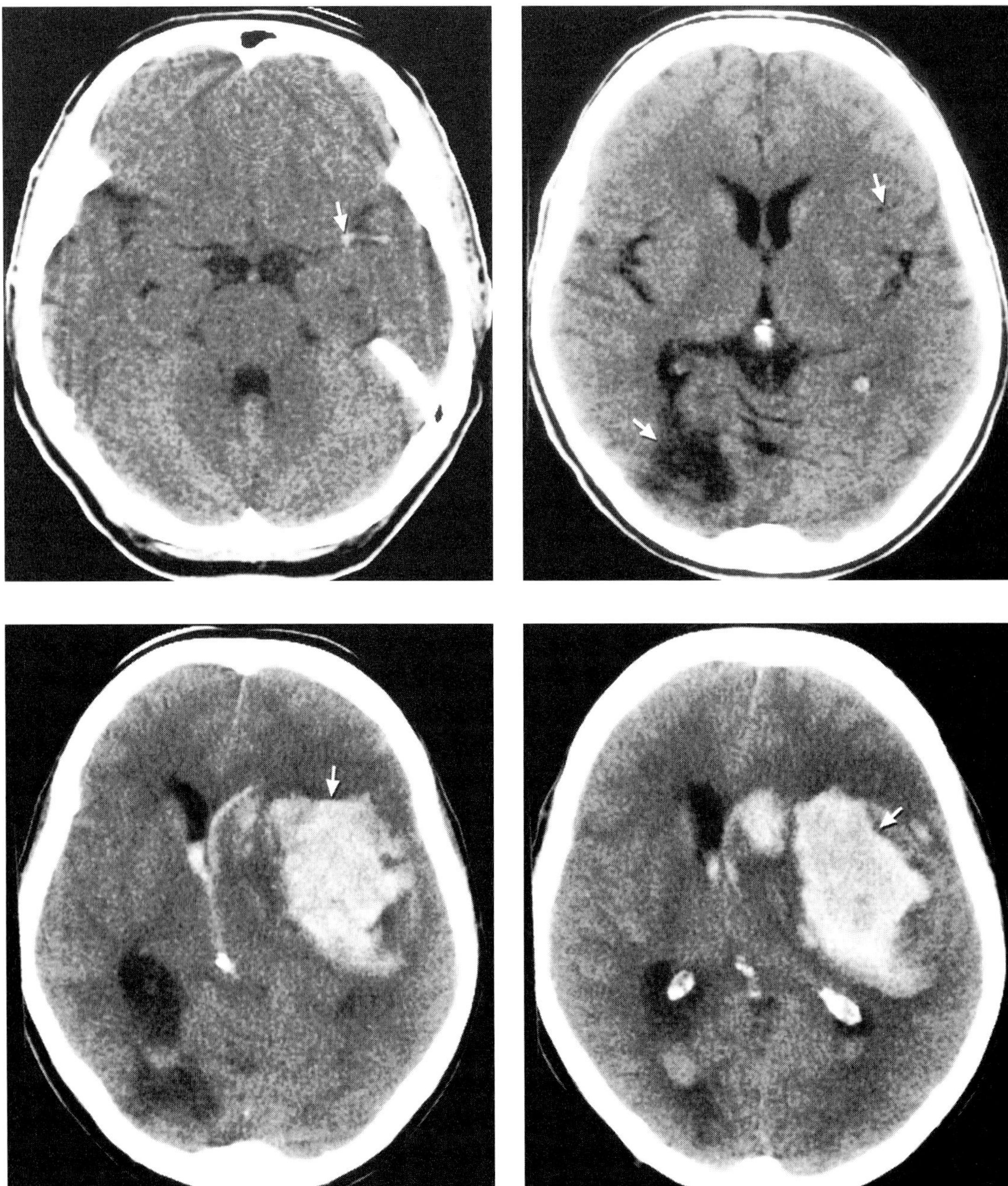

Figure 7.7. Series of computed tomography scans in a patient with rapidly progressing neurologic deficit. *Top row*, There is a hyperdense middle cerebral artery sign, but, except for a dubious difference in sylvian fissure width (*arrow*) and an old infarct in the posterior cerebral artery territory (*arrow*), there is no evidence of a recent ischemic stroke by computed tomography. *Bottom row*, Several hours later, a large putaminal hemorrhage represents a hemorrhagic infarct rather than a primary putaminal hemorrhage.

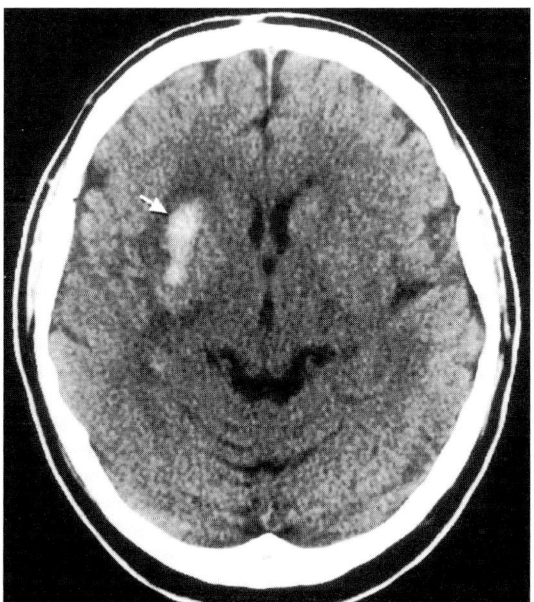
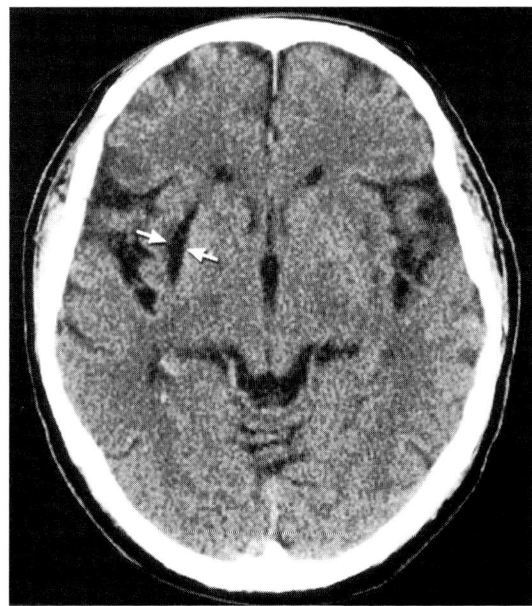

Figure 7.8. Putaminal hemorrhage (localized type) recognized 3 years later on subsequent computed tomography scan as a slit-like lesion (*right*; *arrows*).

edema is too high. Blood pressure should be reduced gradually to a mean arterial pressure around 130 mm Hg. The recommended antihypertensive medication is labetalol, 10 to 40 mg intravenously every 10 minutes up to 300 mg. In patients with asthma, sodium nitroprusside (0.5 to 10 μg/kg per minute) can be considered.[1,14]

There is no benefit from corticosteroids,[17] and in susceptible patients, they may increase the risk of severe hyperglycemia or enhance pulmonary infection triggered by aspiration. The benefit of mannitol in deep ganglionic hemorrhage is not known. It is unlikely to result in improvement in outcome unless its effect on intracranial pressure and cerebral perfusion pressure is documented, nor is it known whether it may assist in the bridging period before surgical evacuation. More likely, the direct destructive effect in this type of hematoma rather than brain shift determines outcome.

Enlargement may have occurred during transport, and any further deterioration should be evaluated with a new CT scan. Enlargement 24 hours after onset is rare. Several systemic factors have been identified that increase the probability of enlargement, such as liver disease and poorly controlled diabetes with high systolic blood pressure (>200 mm Hg).[9]

Surgery in large ganglionic hemorrhages is only lifesaving, and awakening from coma rarely occurs without devastating morbidity (Capsule 7.2).

Predictors of Outcome

A large volume of putaminal blood (>60 cm^3 by ellipsoid volume measurement) associated with coma is likely to result in death.[22] Extension of the hematoma into the middle putamen most likely results in persistent hemiplegia. The prognosis in thalamic hemorrhage is determined by diameter and extension to the mesencephalon. If a thalamic hematoma exceeds 2.5 cm in greatest diameter, outcome is worse. Unilateral hydrocephalus in ganglionic hemorrhage caused by trapping of the ventricular system is a CT scan sign that indicates poor outcome despite surgical evacuation.

Triage

- Observation for at least 24 hours in a neurologic-neurosurgical intensive care unit.
- Evacuation of hematoma if enlargement causes brain herniation syndromes.

Capsule 7.2. Surgical Management of Ganglionic Supratentorial Hemorrhage

Most neurosurgeons prefer surgical evacuation in a deteriorating patient. Randomized surgical trials of supratentorial hemorrhage have been hampered by selection and marginal statistical power. Surgical evacuation of a ganglionic hematoma through open craniectomy did not improve outcome. Endoscopic aspiration reduced mortality, with no improvement in morbidity in large hematomas (>50 mL) but a trend in improved outcome in smaller hematomas. Very early removal of intracerebral hematoma is currently under investigation.[18–20]

A recent small randomized pilot trial (STICH study)[21] documented reduced mortality at 1 month but not at 6 months in patients treated with surgery (median Glasgow coma score = 11; median volume = 49 mL) compared with those given medical management (median Glasgow coma score = 11; median volume = 44 mL). Future trials should analyze lobar hematomas separately from ganglionic hemorrhage and study patients at high risk of deterioration to demonstrate a possible surgical benefit. Ventriculostomy may be performed in patients with intraventricular rupture, but its effect on outcome is marginal, if any.

Lobar Hemorrhages

Intracranial hematomas can be found dissecting throughout the subcortical white matter and often involving the cortex. The clinical features are related to topography. The source of lobar hematomas is unclear in many instances. Mechanisms include a ruptured vascular malformation, cerebral amyloid angiopathy,[23] hemorrhage inside an existing brain tumor, metastatic lesion or infectious lesion (e.g., aspergillosis, toxoplasmosis), coagulation disorders, and use of sympathomimetic drugs or fibrinolytic agents.

A temporal lobe hematoma may be caused by a ruptured middle cerebral artery aneurysm.[24] Any patient with a temporal lobe hematoma, transient loss of consciousness, and a much lower level of consciousness than expected on the basis of size or brain shift should be considered to have a ruptured aneurysm of the middle cerebral artery. A temporal lobe hematoma may indicate a hemorrhagic necrotic mass due to herpes simplex encephalitis, and febrile agitation may be the only manifestation (see Chapter 10). Multiple hematomas should point to a possible devastating sagittal sinus thrombosis with multiple hemorrhagic infarcts (see Chapter 8).

Use of thrombolytic agents has increased the frequency of intracerebral hematomas associated with thrombolysis.[25] The frequency of symptomatic intracerebral hematomas after intravenous administration of tissue-type plasminogen activator (tPA) for ischemic stroke has increased to 6%. These hemorrhages occur within 36 hours after the infusion. Decrease in level of consciousness is most prevalent, but increased weakness, headaches, and increased blood pressure have also been noted.[25] A major neurologic deficit (defined as a score of more than 20 on the National Institutes of Health Stroke Scale; see Chapter 8, Table 8.1) and early hypodensity or edema on CT scans increase the odds of later development of symptomatic intracerebral hematoma after tPA use. The risk of intracerebral hematoma after tPA for myocardial infarction is very low, but old age, dose, and history of stroke are major predisposing factors.[26]

Clinical Presentation

Frontal hematomas cause abulia, contralateral arm weakness, and gaze preference toward the side of the hematoma, but when the hemorrhages are located superiorly above the frontal horn, leg weakness may be more apparent.[27] Headache is frequently present and associated with vomiting. Approximately one-third of the patients have seizures within the first hours of presentation. Temporal lobe hematomas may cause Wernicke's aphasia and right-sided homonymous hemianopia. Temporal lobe hematomas in the nondominant hemisphere may produce only confusional episodes without any localizing neurologic symptoms. Parietal lobe hematoma produces prominent hemisensory symptoms, but if it extends into the posterior parietal lobe, constructional apraxia or dressing apraxia may be found if specifically tested for. Patients with an occipital lobe hematoma have a sudden visual field defect, most commonly an easily identifiable homonymous hemianopia with only transient motor or sensory abnormalities. Multiple hematomas commonly immediately involve the level of consciousness unless they are localized within one hemisphere or are small. Clinical features are determined by the largest hematoma.

Interpretation of Diagnostic Tests

Several CT scan characteristics of hematoma suggesting its origin should be recognized,[28] and they are summarized in Table 7.2. Shift of midline structures on the initial CT scan in patients with lobar hematoma admitted to the emergency department is highly predictive of further clinical deterioration. The specific features are shift of the septum pellucidum, obliteration of the opposite ambient cistern, and early trapping of the temporal horn[29] (Figure 7.9). Some of the CT scan changes may be subtle and involve effacement of the supracerebellar cistern from edema (Figure 7.10).

Lobar hematoma may indicate an underlying metastatic lesion or primary brain tumor, and it is evident by marked fingerlike white matter edema notably out of proportion to the size of the hematoma and seldom causing brain shift (Figure 7.11).

Superficially located hematomas commonly are a result of amyloid angiopathy, and MRI may show earlier hemorrhages (Figure 7.12). Coagulation-associated hematomas are commonly multiple, involving multiple compartments (Figure 7.13).

Intracerebral hematomas after intravenous tPA for myocardial infarction characteristically are hemorrhages in multiple compartments, and fluid levels from continuing anticoagulation are evident (Figure 7.14).

MRI is a crucial study in lobar hematoma because it may identify an underlying structural lesion. In young adults, an arteriovenous malformation is common; in older adults, earlier amyloid hemorrhages may be found, although MRI may be unrewarding.

Cerebral angiography is warranted in patients with a lobar hematoma and MRI evidence of arteriovenous malformation (Figure 7.15). Its yield in a patient with normal findings on MRI is very low.

Table 7.2. Computed Tomography Scan Characteristics of Lobar Hematoma That Suggest the Cause

Coagulopathy	Multiple locations and compartments Fluid level from poor clot formation
Amyloid angiopathy	Superficially located Irregular border Recurrent hematomas White matter hypodensities
Tumoral hemorrhage	Central or eccentric location of hemorrhage Tumor mass visible Proportionally more white matter edema
Arteriovenous malformation	Calcification in hemorrhage mass Enhancement with contrast medium

First Priority in Management

The approach to lobar hematoma is similar to that in ganglionic hemorrhages.

Multiple intracranial lobar hematomas are often found in patients who have recently received tPA for acute myocardial infarction.[30] Fresh-frozen plasma (2 units) should be used initially. It is important to repeat a CT scan, preferably 1 to 3 hours after the onset, to assess the true extension and dimension of the hematomas.[25]

The decision to proceed with surgery is determined by clinical presentation. Craniotomy with evacuation of a lobar hematoma should be strongly considered in patients with evidence of brain shift on CT scan and a decrease in the Glasgow coma score, because there is a high probability of further deterioration in the next hours. Early surgical management is also indicated if an intracerebral hematoma is associated with a ruptured middle cerebral artery aneurysm or arteriovenous malformation, but mostly after further definition by cerebral angiography.[31]

Predictors of Outcome

Poor outcome can be expected in patients with deterioration from hematoma enlargement who need emergency surgical evacuation. Poor outcome is more common in patients with a decreased Glas-

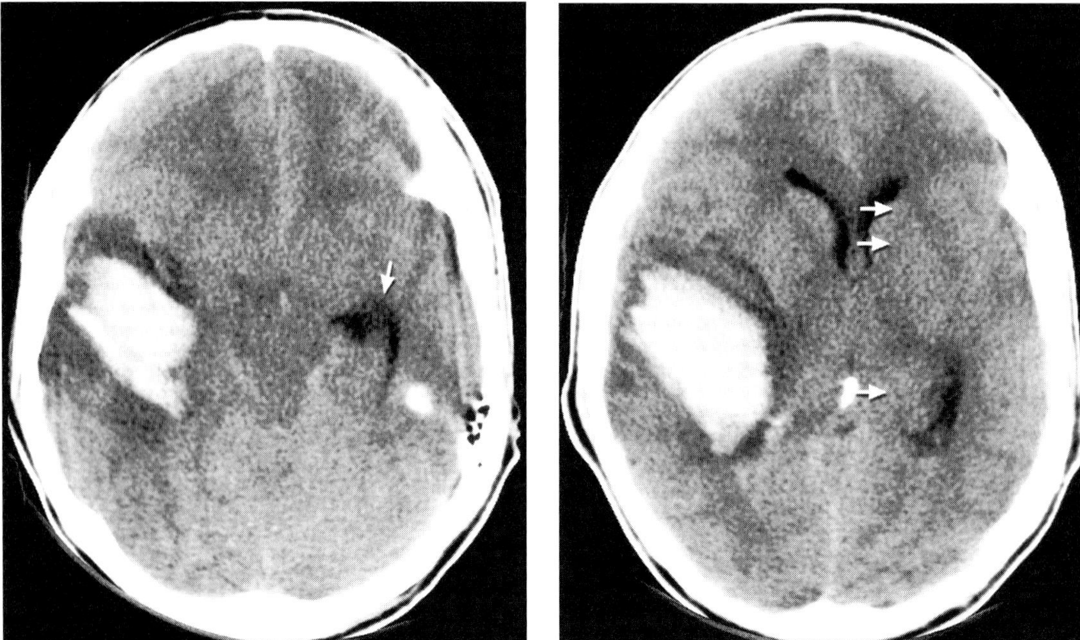

Figure 7.9. Computed tomography scan signs predictive of deterioration in lobar hematoma (*arrows*). Note shift of septum pellucidum, effacement of ambient cistern, and early temporal horn entrapment.[32]

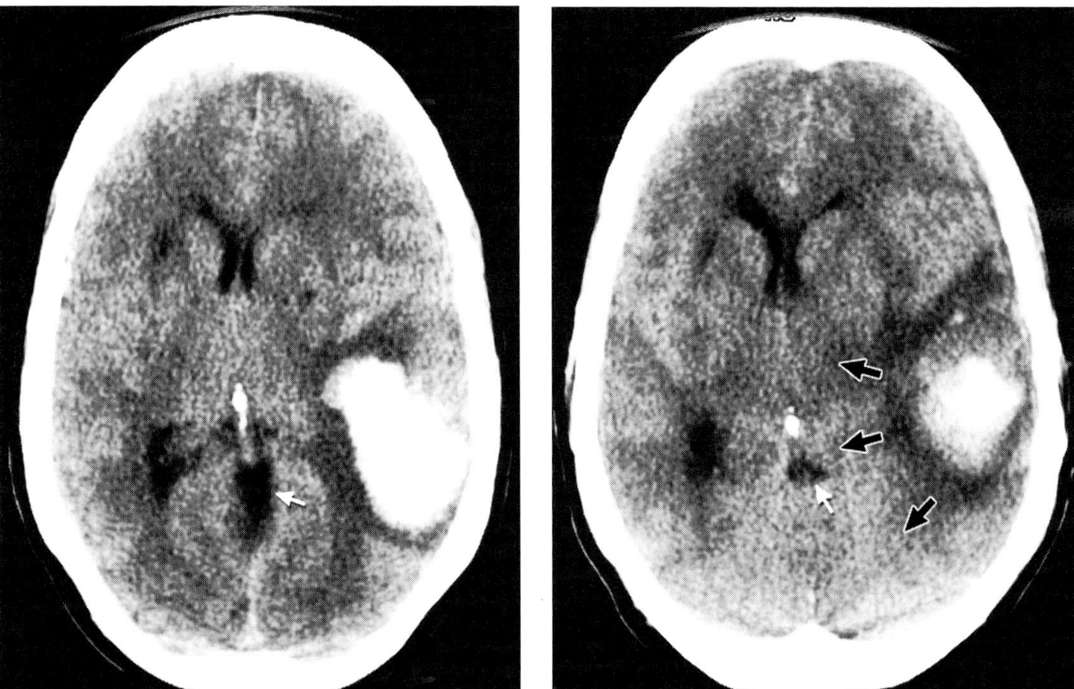

Figure 7.10. Computed tomography scans showing lobar hematoma with some mass effect and bowing of the midline structures. *Right*, Two days later, the hematoma has resolved but edema is more pronounced, with progressive obliteration of the supracerebellar cistern without appreciable shift of the pineal gland from edema.

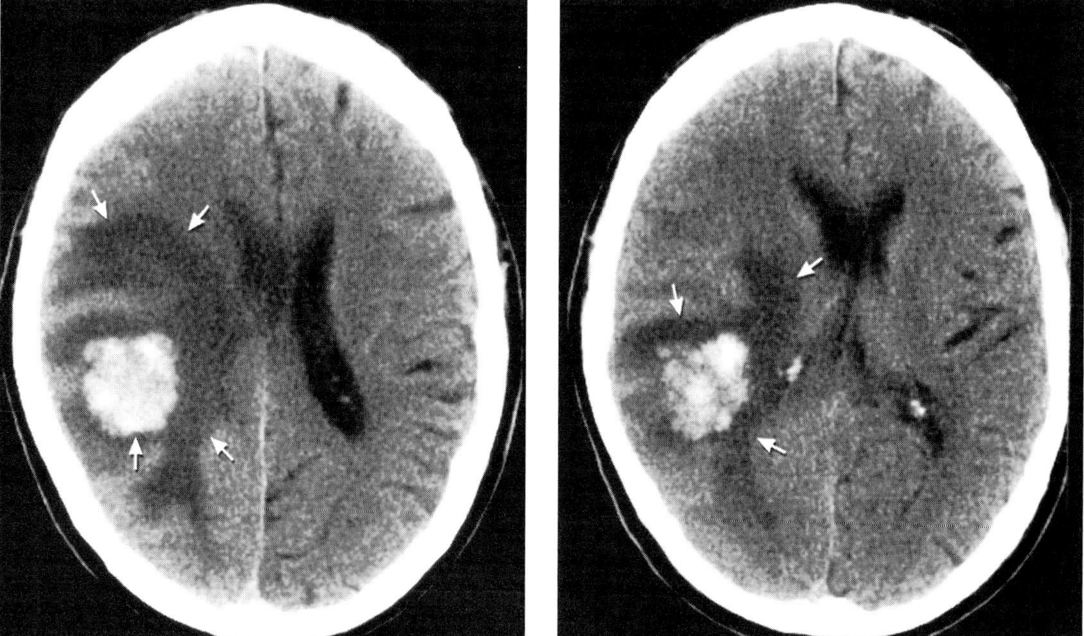

Figure 7.11. Hemorrhage in metastasis. Note the comparatively large fingerlike edema in the white matter out of proportion to the size of the hematoma. Computed tomography scans mask underlying metastasis, which may be more evident by magnetic resonance imaging.

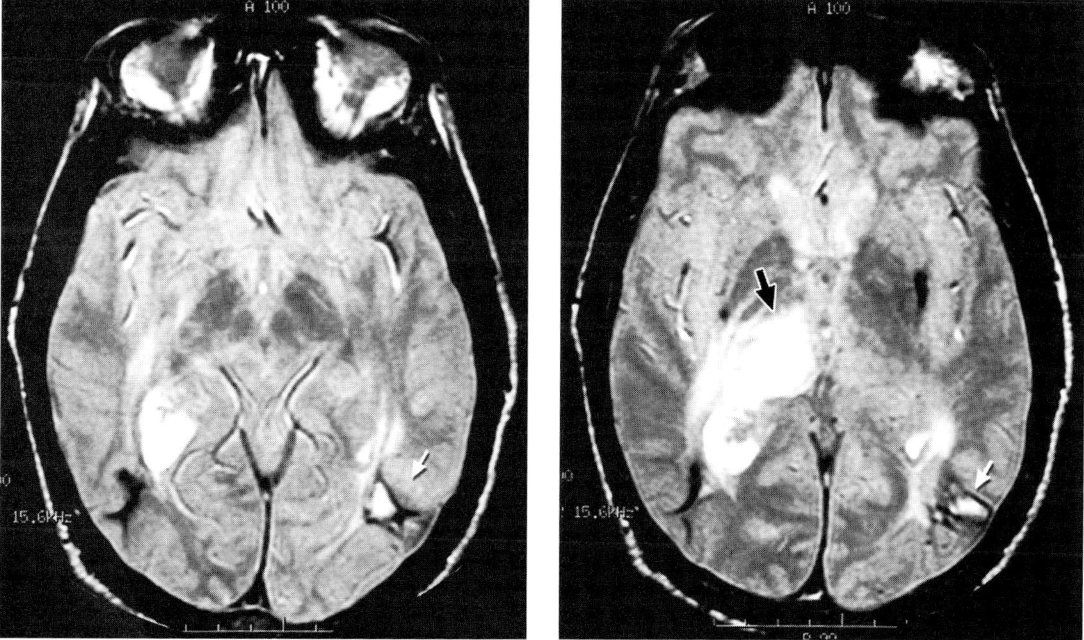

Figure 7.12. Amyloid angiopathy-associated hematoma. Magnetic resonance images show a thalamic hemorrhage and multiple areas of hemosiderin (*white arrows*), which are clues to earlier hemorrhages.

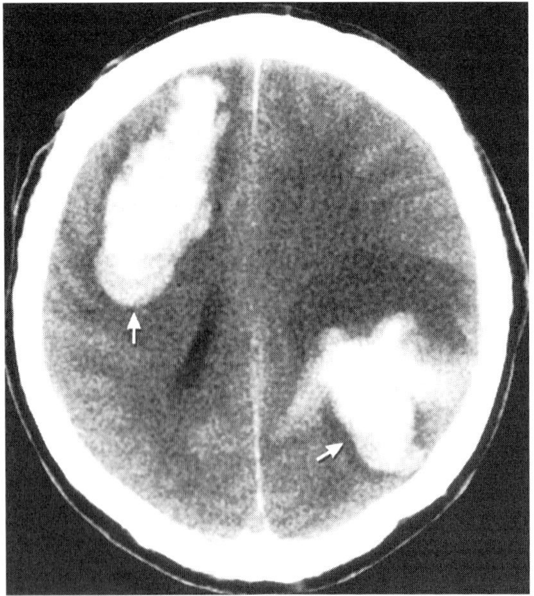

Figure 7.13. Computed tomography scan shows multiple hemorrhages in coagulopathy.

gow coma score and a septum pellucidum shift of more than 6 mm.[32] Lobar hematomas associated with tPA administration are commonly fatal. Outcome is good after rehabilitation if the lobar hematoma is less than 40 cm^3 on CT scan and there is no shift on CT scan in a patient seen several hours after ictus.[32]

Triage

- ♦ Neurologic intensive care unit if level of consciousness is decreased and mass effect appears on CT scan.
- ♦ Smaller-sized hematomas (<30 cm^3) in alert patients can be observed in the ward if the time of ictus and presentation is beyond 6 hours.
- ♦ Surgical evacuation in patients with CT scan evidence of mass effect and documented deterioration.

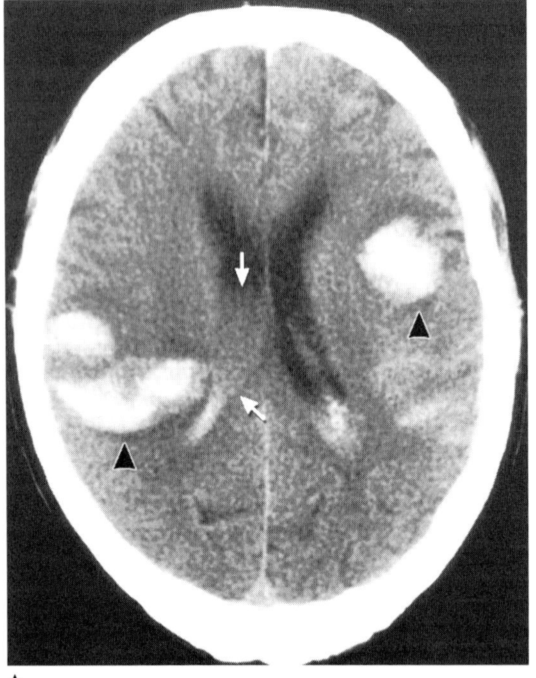

A

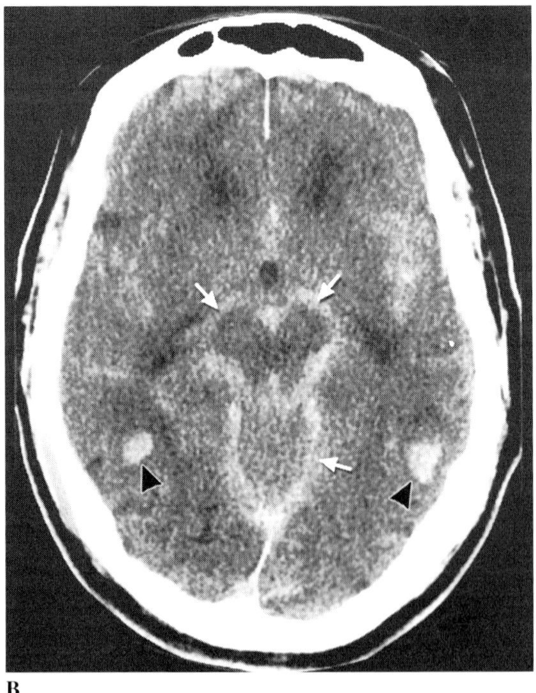

B

Figure 7.14. Examples of hemorrhage associated with tissue-type plasminogen activator. **A.** *Arrows* point to different compartments, convexity subarachnoid hemorrhage, and lobar and intraventricular hemorrhages with fluid level. **B.** Massive subarachnoid hemorrhage and lobar hematomas.

Intraventricular Hemorrhage

It may be difficult clinically and by CT scan criteria to differentiate spontaneous intraventricular hemorrhage from a small thalamic or caudate nucleus hemorrhage with overwhelming filling of the lateral portion of the ventricles. In many situations, intraventricular hemorrhage is caused by a rupture of the anterior communicating aneurysm, which can dissect through the lamina terminalis to enter the third ventricle and connecting ventricles (see Chapter 6). Primary intraventricular hemorrhage may be caused by arteriovenous malformations in the proximity of the ventricular system, intraventricular tumors, and, more recently, use of thrombolytic agents. Uncommon causes are coagulopathy in patients with severe thrombocytopenia associated with a hematologic malignancy and moyamoya disease from rupture of the dilated periventricular arteries.

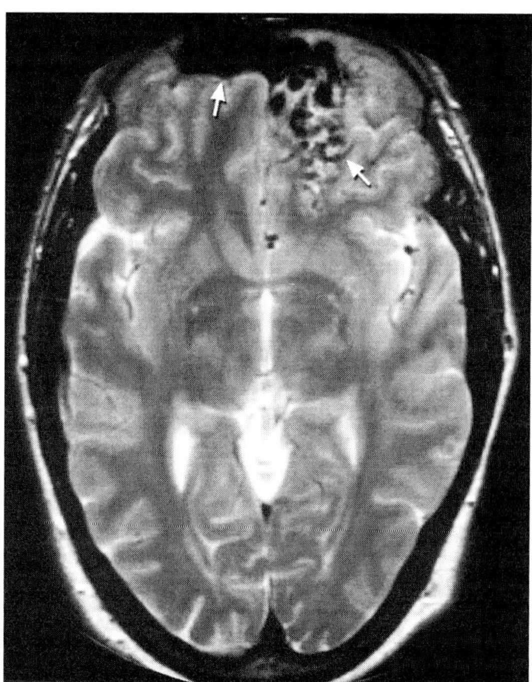

Figure 7.15. Magnetic resonance features of large arteriovenous malformation in right frontal lobe with large vein draining to the sagittal sinus.

Clinical Presentation

Primary intraventricular hemorrhage has a clinical presentation similar to that of poor-grade aneurysmal subarachnoid hemorrhage.[33–35] Onset is acute, with immediate loss of consciousness but with extensor posturing that occurs spontaneously or with any manipulation of the patient. Nonspecific shivering, myoclonic jerks, and well-characterized generalized tonic-clonic seizures are common. Many patients have rapid breathing with periods of apnea or barely audible air displacement and need to be immediately placed on a mechanical ventilator. Increased blood pressure most likely is a consequence of transmitted intracranial pressure affecting the brain stem, particularly at the flush of arterial blood through the ventricular system. Pupil reflexes may become sluggish and pupil size smaller if acute hydrocephalus develops rapidly. Any change in this direction should prompt a repeat CT scan to evaluate progression of ventricular enlargement and need for ventriculostomy.

Interpretation of Diagnostic Tests

Entire filling of all components of the ventricular system is characteristic, with acute ballooning out of the ventricular system (Figure 7.16). The CT scan is notoriously unreliable in demonstrating a potential cause of intraventricular hemorrhage. Thus, some patients with a thalamic or caudate hemorrhage have only a hint of parenchymal bleeding on CT scanning, and this is markedly overshadowed by the massive intraventricular hemorrhage, often filling only one ventricle. The anatomical location may provide additional clues to the origin of the hemorrhage[36,37] (Table 7.3).

MRI can demonstrate hemorrhage into the thalamus or caudate nucleus and is also more sensitive to visualization of arteriovenous malformations and cavernous angiomas. Cavernous angiomas may be found at other locations inside the parenchyma, providing further clues to cavernous angioma as the main culprit in the ventricular hemorrhage. Magnetic resonance angiography should also be performed to exclude the possibility of a large anterior communicating aneurysm or to document a much less common moyamoya vascular pattern. This pattern is the consequence of bilateral internal carotid artery occlusion causing dilatation to develop in the lenticulostriate, thalamoperforating, and thalamogeniculate arteries.

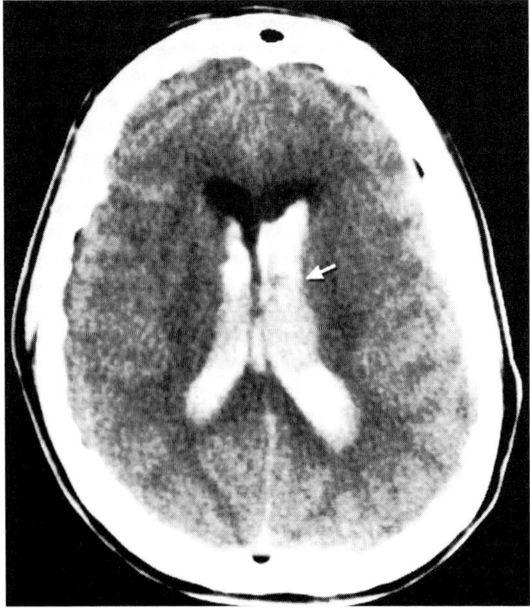

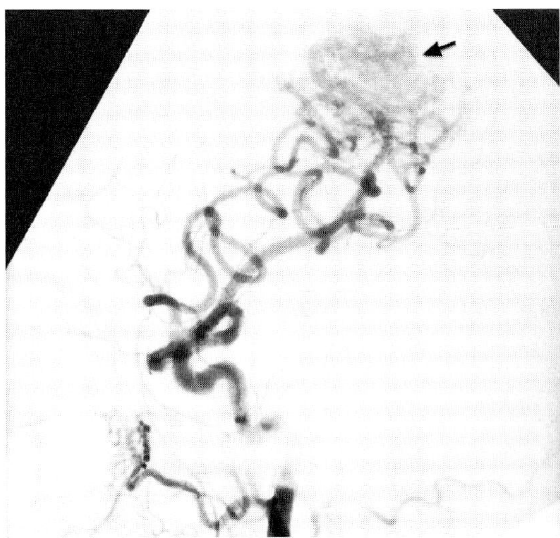

Figure 7.16. Primary intraventricular hemorrhage. *Right*, Cerebral angiography disclosed an arteriovenous malformation.

Microaneurysms are often formed in these arteries, and they may rupture into the ventricular system.

Not only is cerebral angiography imperative to exclude an anterior communicating aneurysm, but the posterior circulation should also be visualized bilaterally with multiple projections, because blood in the fourth ventricle might have an origin in the ruptured aneurysm of the distal posteroinferior cerebellar artery. One study claimed an arteriovenous malformation or an aneurysm in 50% to 70% of the patients, with a higher yield in patients younger than 45 years.[38]

First Priority in Management

The management of primary ventricular hemorrhage is immediate ventriculostomy in patients with a Glasgow coma score of less than 8 and marked ventricular dilatation on CT scan (Chapter 3). Experimental studies are under way to use intraventricular thrombolysis when no cause is found by cerebral angiography (which should then be performed immediately). Dramatic resolution of the obstructing clot has been described, but experience with this potentially dangerous therapy is very limited. It should not be used in intraparenchymal hemorrhages with intraventricular extension, even if the intraventricular compartment produces most of the clot volume.[39,40]

Predictors of Outcome

Outcome remains poor (severe disability or vegetative state) in patients with primary intraventricular hemorrhage associated with acute hydrocephalus. Survival is common but with a severe amnesic state.[34]

Table 7.3. Intraventricular Hemorrhage

Intraventricular	
Unilateral ventricle	Caudate hemorrhage Thalamic hemorrhage
Biventricular	Arteriovenous malformation of ependymal lining or choroid plexus Ependymoma Cocaine or amphetamine
Cavum septum pellucidum	Anterior artery complex aneurysm
Fourth ventricle only	Posterior inferior cerebellar artery aneurysm

Data from Terayama et al.[15]

Triage

- Consider immediate cerebral angiography after ventriculostomy.
- Neurologic-neurosurgical intensive care unit for monitoring of development of acute hydrocephalus, intracranial pressure, or drainage of a ventriculostomy.

Cerebellar Hemorrhages

Cerebellar hemorrhages are commonly caused by rupture of a branch of the superior cerebellar artery afflicted by fibroid necrosis from long-standing hypertension. Much less frequent causes are hemorrhages associated with anticoagulation, arteriovenous malformation, and a metastatic lesion. Patients arriving in the emergency department often are initially alert but may have rapid deterioration to a lower level of consciousness and development of new brain stem signs. Features that predict clinical deterioration have recently been identified, as have clinical and CT scan features associated with such a poor prospect that even suboccipital craniotomy for clot evacuation may be discouraged.[41,42]

Clinical Presentation

Acute severe headache associated with vertigo and vomiting and acute gait imbalance are presenting findings. At onset, patients are unable to take a single step if standing and cry out for immediate assistance; some fall, are unable to stand up, and have to roll themselves to a telephone. Speech is slurred, and clumsiness may become apparent in one limb. A cerebellum hematoma can be further suspected if a clinical triad of ipsilateral limb ataxia, horizontal gaze palsy, and peripheral facial palsy is demonstrated, although two or fewer of these signs may be present. Other common neurologic findings are skew deviation, horizontal nystagmus, and decreased corneal reflex. In this condition, pinprick-sized pupils indicate significant pontine compression and imply a high risk of further deterioration. Unilateral ataxia and dysarthria point to a cerebellar hemispheric hematoma. Dysautonomic features are frequent in large-sized cerebellar hematomas, and they include episodic bradycardia and hypertension, not necessarily coupled together.

Interpretation of Diagnostic Tests

Two major types of cerebellar hemorrhage have been described. Cerebellar hemispheric hemorrhages are most common (Figures 7.17A, 7.17B, and 7.17C). Vermis hematomas are more frequently seen in hemorrhages associated with acquired coagulopathy (Figure 7.17D). Both may involve extension into the ventricle and compression of the brain stem. The typical features of brain stem compression often involve effacement of the quadrigeminal cistern, and when cerebellar tissue is herniated upward, the supracerebellar cisterns are effaced as well (so-called tight posterior fossa). These CT findings should be regarded as an urgent indication for evacuation of the hematoma. CT scan features highly predictive of further deterioration are extension to the vermis and acute hydrocephalus.[39]

An arteriovenous malformation should be considered in a young patient with no history of hypertension. Cerebellar hemispheric arteriovenous malformations have a characteristic bleeding pattern on CT scans and blood tracts in the direction of the cerebellar folia, particularly in the primary cerebellar fissure. The malformation may extend, rather symmetrically, into the midline as well. Blood in the quadrigeminal cisterns and tracts on the tentorium are characteristic (Figure 7.17E). These cerebellar hemispheric arteriovenous malformations are unmasked by MRI and should be further defined by cerebral angiography.

First Priority in Management

Attending physicians should be primed for surgical evacuation in many patients. At our institution, clinicians usually wait for clinical deterioration before operating. Another commonly accepted precept is to remove a clot when it is 3 cm or larger in axial diameter on CT scans.[43] In patients with significant swelling, a bolus of mannitol, 1 g/kg, should be administered to bridge the time to the operating room. Administration of a corticosteroid can be considered as well, but valid data about its efficacy are not available.

Bradycardia may be frequently observed but should be left alone. Runs of bradycardia, however, should be treated with atropine, 0.5 mg intravenously, if hypotension occurs.

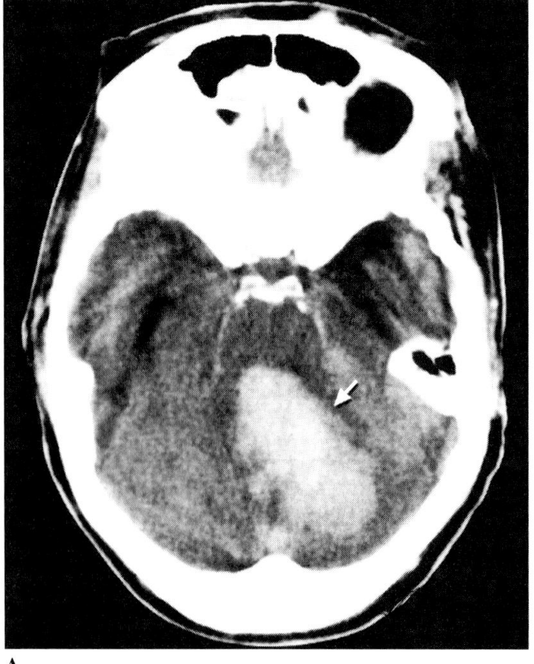

A

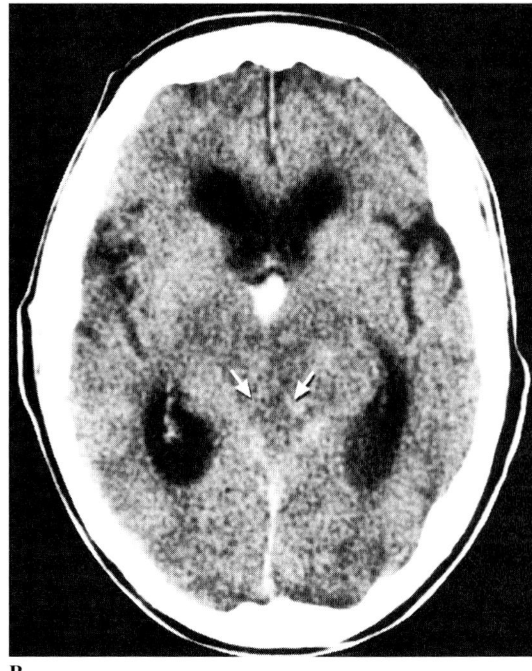

B

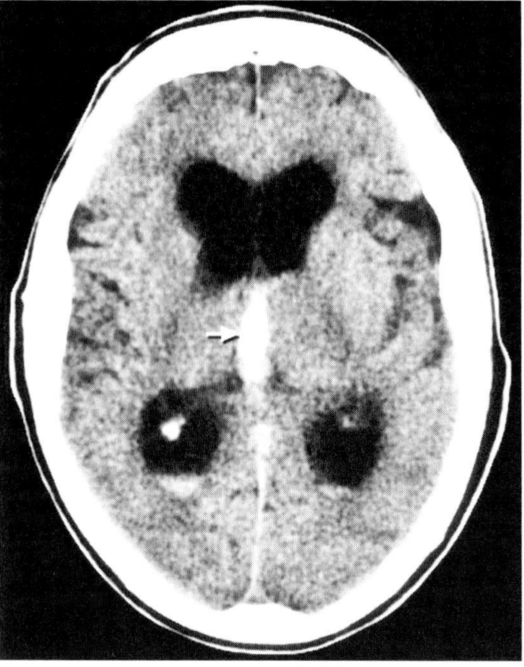

C

Figure 7.17. Types of cerebellar hematomas on computed tomography. **A–C.** Cerebellar hemisphere. Note effacement of the quadrigeminal cisterns, intraventricular extension, and hydrocephalus.

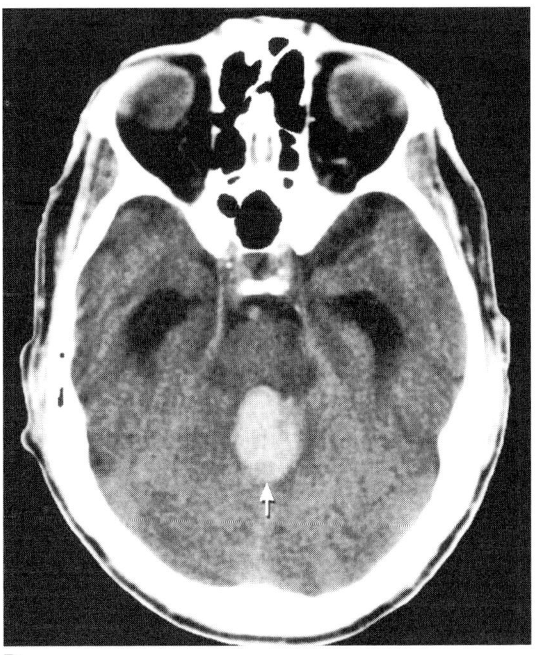

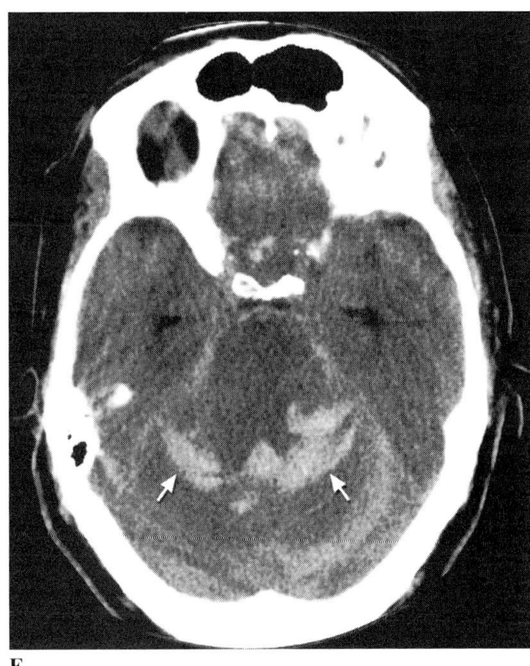

Figure 7.17. *Continued.* **D.** Vermis hemisphere. **E.** Cerebellar hemorrhage from arteriovenous malformation.

Predictors of Outcome

Alert or minimally drowsy patients are at high risk of further deterioration when they have a midline extension of the hematoma or acute hydrocephalus. Poor outcome after surgery is very likely when acute hydrocephalus is present and corneal and doll's eye reflexes are absent. Good outcome after surgery can be expected in younger patients with intact brain stem reflexes.[41,44]

Triage

- Surgical evacuation if CT scan shows signs of "tight posterior fossa."
- Observation in a ward if the hematoma is small (<3 cm) and not localized in the vermis, no deterioration has occurred, and the patient does not have a coagulation disorder.

Pontine Hemorrhage

A pontine hemorrhage is associated with high rates of death and neurologic morbidity. Hypertension is the usual cause, and arteriovenous malformation or rupture of a cavernous angioma is less common. At presentation, most patients are in a cataclysmic state and are comatose with small pupils (diameter, 2 to 3 mm), loss of horizontal gaze, and apneic spells requiring mechanical ventilation. Quadriplegia with extreme rigidity is frequent, but if the hematoma is unilaterally localized in the pons, hemiplegia may occur. Extension to the mesencephalon may cause significant anisocoria that can be clinically misinterpreted as an uncal herniation syndrome (see Chapter 1). Abnormalities of eye movement have been described, such as ocular bobbing (sudden downward jerking with slow return to midcentral position), skew deviation, and abnormal horizontal conjugate gaze that is more apparent after caloric stimulation with ice water. Complete destruction of the mid pons is common, and the tegmentum is seldom spared; thus, a locked-in syndrome is rarely found in this condition. Dysautonomic features with marked hypertension, tachycardia, and hyperthermia (>39.5°C) may be profound. In contrast, pontine hemorrhages in cavernous hemangioma are not catastrophic and are manifested by acute oculomotor abnormalities or ataxia only.

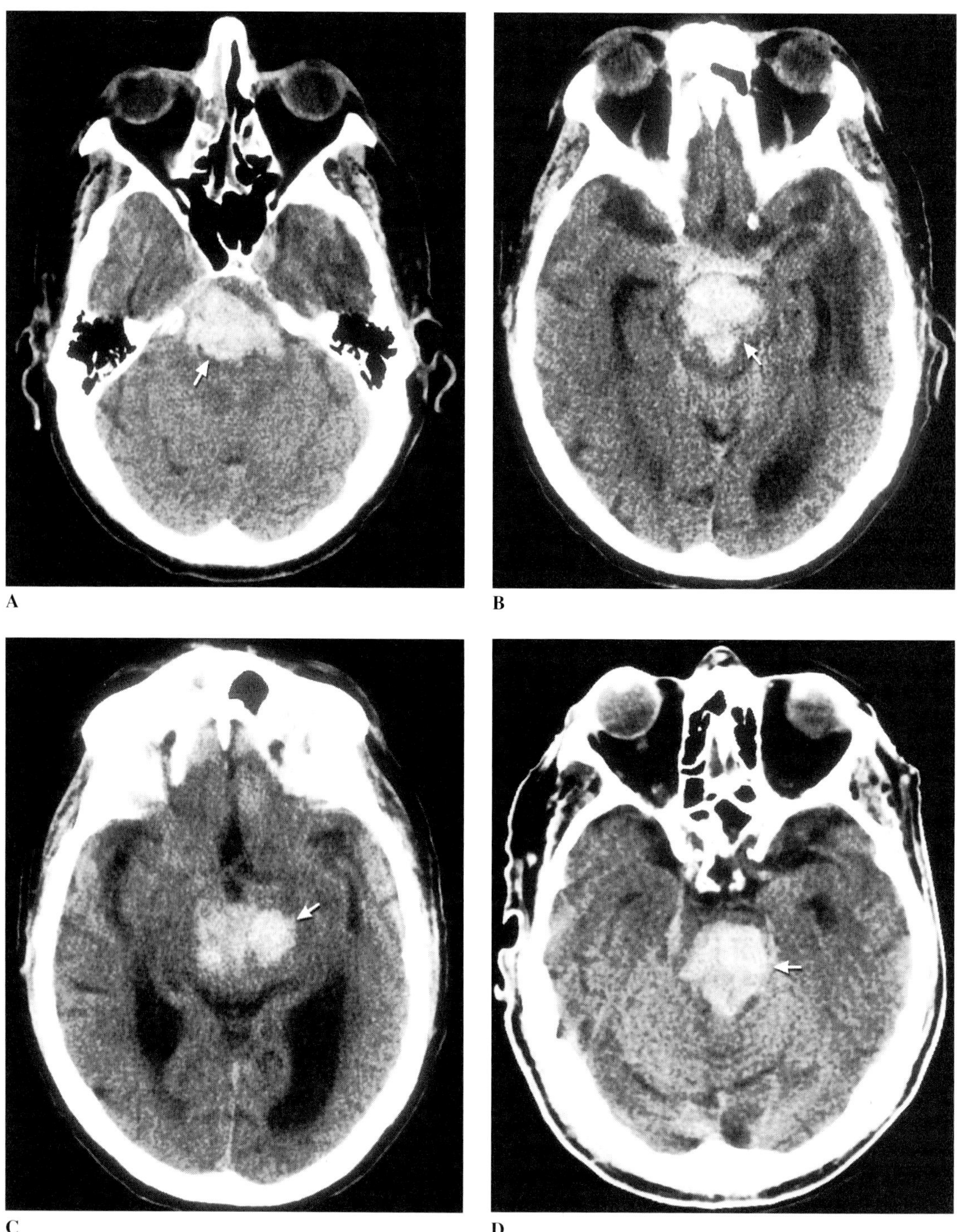

Figure 7.18. Types of pontine hemorrhages on computed tomography images. **A–C.** Extension to midbrain and thalamus. **D.** Massive destructive hemorrhage limited to pons.

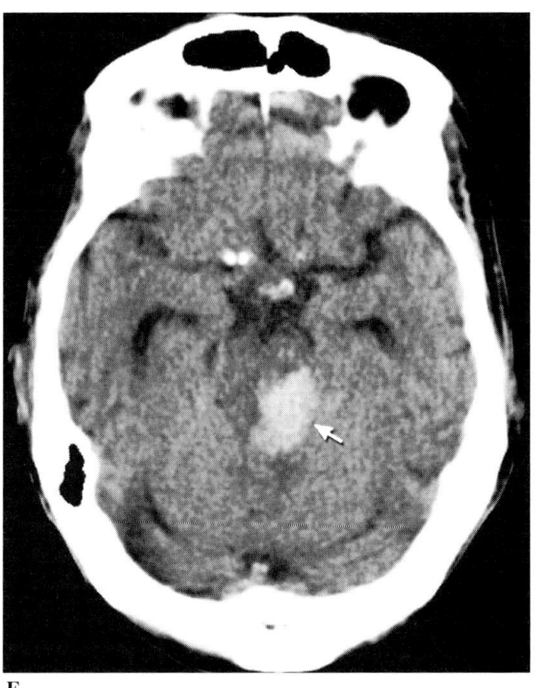

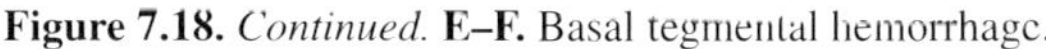

E

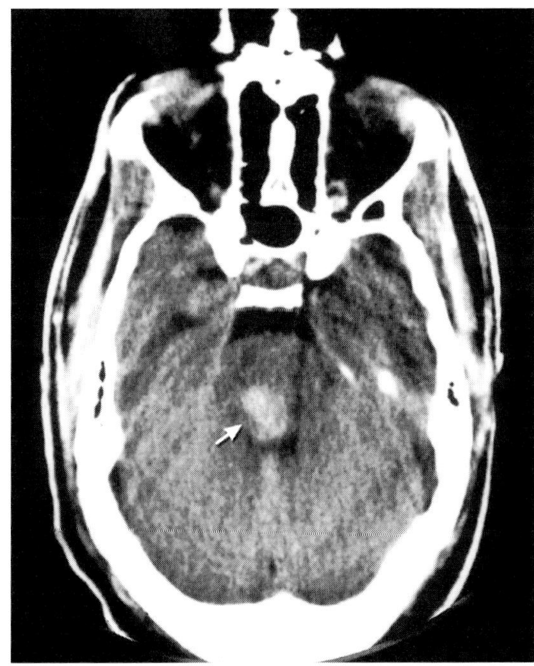

F

Figure 7.18. *Continued.* **E–F.** Basal tegmental hemorrhage.

Interpretation of Diagnostic Tests

The CT scan patterns are shown in Figure 7.18. Pontine hemorrhages can be divided into massive pontine hemorrhage with extension to the midbrain and thalamus, pontine hemorrhage with unilateral extension to the midbrain, and basal tegmental pontine hemorrhage. The lesion should be differentiated from a large fusiform aneurysm, which may produce identical clinical features due to basilar artery thrombosis (Figure 7.19). Rarely, a unilateral tegmental hemorrhage is found; it is usually very circumscribed and barely involves the pontine structures. It may be caused by a cavernous hemangioma (Figure 7.20).

First Priority in Management

Endotracheal intubation is needed in virtually all patients. Blood pressures are markedly increased, but aggressive management does not appear to have much effect on size. Blood pressure may become very high, with diastolic pressure in the range of 140 to 150 mm Hg. Labetalol or a vasodilator, such as nitroprusside, may be needed to reduce the pressure to a more acceptable level. Ventriculostomy is not indicated, because deterioration is related to evolving swelling surrounding the hematoma. Stereotactic surgical evacuation has not been shown to improve outcome, and morbidity remains substantial. The effect of corticosteroids is unknown.

Predictors of Outcome

Good recovery occurs only in patients who are alert on admission and have small unilateral pontine hemorrhages. Cavernous malformations of the brain stem may continue to cause repeated hemorrhages. In one selected population of treated patients, the rate was up to 30% per person per year. Whether stereotactic radiosurgery improves outcome is uncertain, and resection should be strongly considered to prevent devastating future morbidity.[45] Clinical or CT scan features observed only in patients with a fatal outcome are a core temperature in excess of 39.8°C, tachycardia defined as more than 110 beats/minute, CT evidence of extension to the midbrain and thalamus, and acute hydrocephalus on the initial CT scans.[46]

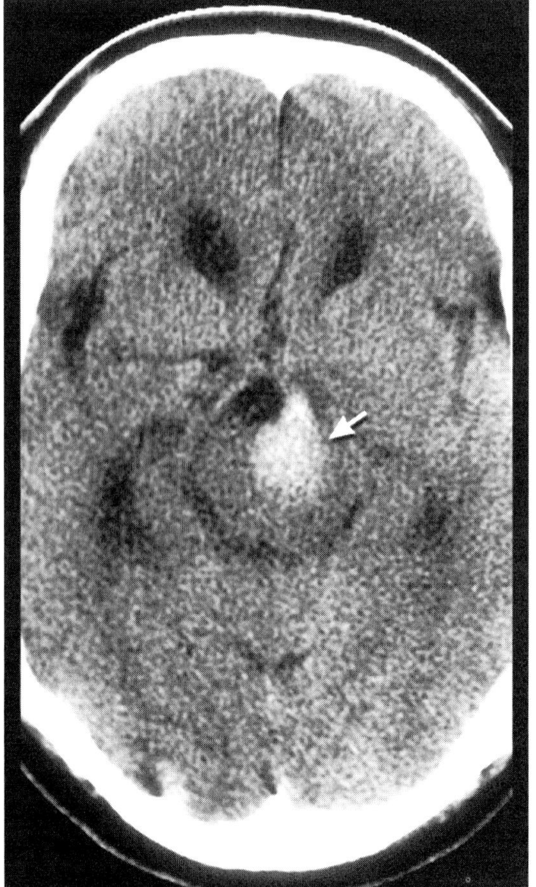

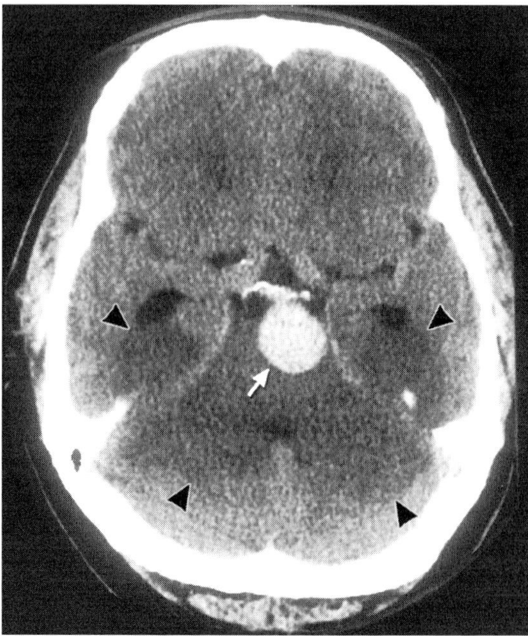

Figure 7.19. Pseudopontine hemorrhage. Fusiform basilar aneurysm associated with acute basilar artery occlusion mimics pontine bleeding. Note development of hypodensities on follow-up computed tomography scan and better delineation of the aneurysm.

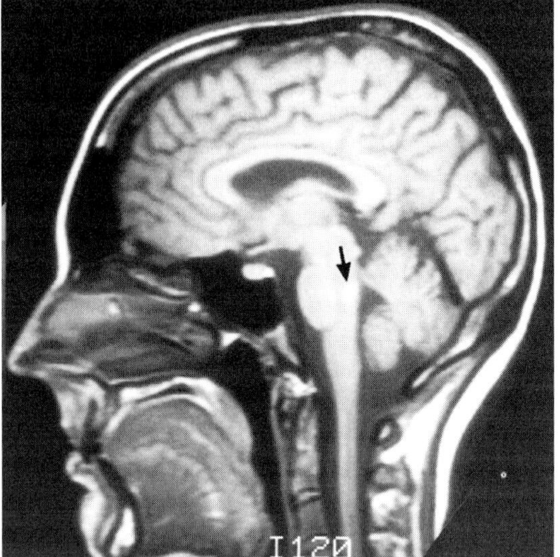

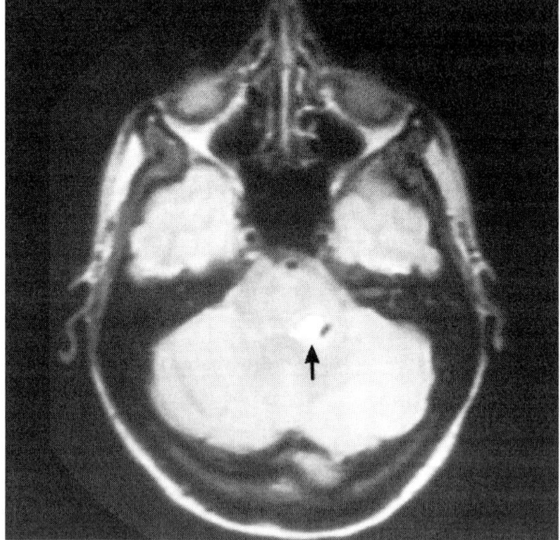

Figure 7.20. Magnetic resonance images showing limited pontine hemorrhage from cavernous hemangioma.

Triage

- Neurologic intensive care unit for observation. Brain stem death may occur, and organ harvesting should be anticipated.
- Patients with small pontine hemorrhages from cavernous hemangioma may be transferred to a ward for elective MRI, cerebral angiography, and surgical evacuation.

References

1. Diringer MN. Intracerebral hemorrhage: pathophysiology and management. Crit Care Med 1993;21:1591.
2. Stein RW, Kase CS, Hier DB, et al. Caudate hemorrhage. Neurology 1984;34:1549.
3. Sutton LN, Barranco D, Greenberg J, et al. Cerebral blood flow and glucose metabolism in experimental brain edema. J Neurosurg 1989;71:868.
4. Lee KR, Colon GP, Betz AL, et al. Edema from intracerebral hemorrhage: the role of thrombin. J Neurosurg 1996;84:91.
5. Xi G, Wagner KR, Keep RF, et al. Role of blood clot formation on early edema development after experimental intracerebral hemorrhage. Stroke 1998;29:2580.
6. Mayer SA, Lignelli A, Fink ME, et al. Perilesional blood flow and edema formation in acute intracerebral hemorrhage: a SPECT study. Stroke 1998;29:1791.
7. Qureshi AI, Wilson DA, Hanley DF, Traystman RJ. No evidence for an ischemic penumbra in massive experimental intracerebral hemorrhage. Neurology 1999;52:266.
8. Kothari RU, Brott T, Broderick JP, et al. The ABCs of measuring intracerebral hemorrhage volumes. Stroke 1996;27:1304.
9. Kazui S, Naritomi H, Yamamoto H, et al. Enlargement of spontaneous intracerebral hemorrhage. Incidence and time course. Stroke 1996;27:1783.
10. Bogousslavsky J, Regli F, Uske A, Maeder P. Early spontaneous hematoma in cerebral infarct: is primary cerebral hemorrhage overdiagnosed? Neurology 1991;41:837.
11. Weir B. The clinical problem of intracerebral hematoma. Stroke 1993;24(Suppl 12):I93.
12. Radberg JA, Olsson JE, Radberg CT. Prognostic parameters in spontaneous intracerebral hematomas with special reference to anticoagulant treatment. Stroke 1991;22:571.
13. Wijdicks EFM, Schievink WI, Brown RD, Mullany CJ. The dilemma of discontinuation of anticoagulation therapy for patients with intracranial hemorrhage and mechanical heart valves. Neurosurgery 1998;42:769.
14. Tietjen CS, Hurn PD, Ulatowski JA, Kirsch JR. Treatment modalities for hypertensive patients with intracranial pathology: options and risks. Crit Care Med 1996;24:311.
15. Terayama Y, Tanahashi N, Fukuuchi Y, Gotoh F. Prognostic value of admission blood pressure in patients with intracerebral hemorrhage. Keio Cooperative Stroke Study. Stroke 1997;28:1185.
16. Powers WJ. Acute hypertension after stroke: the scientific basis for treatment decisions (editorial). Neurology 1993;43:461.
17. Poungvarin N, Bhoopat W, Viriyavejakul A, et al. Effects of dexamethasone in primary supratentorial intracerebral hemorrhage. N Engl J Med 1987;316:1229.
18. Hankey GJ, Hon C. Surgery for primary intracerebral hemorrhage: is it safe and effective? A systematic review of case series and randomized trials. Stroke 1997;28:2126.
19. Prasad K, Browman G, Srivastava A, Menon G. Surgery in primary supratentorial intracerebral hematoma: a meta-analysis of randomized trials. Acta Neurol Scand 1997;95:103.
20. Schaller C, Rohde V, Meyer B, Hassler W. Stereotactic puncture and lysis of spontaneous intracerebral hemorrhage using recombinant tissue-plasminogen activator. Neurosurgery 1995;36:328.
21. Morgenstern LB, Frankowski RF, Shedden P, et al. Surgical treatment for intracerebral hemorrhage (STICH): a single-center, randomized clinical trial. Neurology 1998;51:1359.
22. Lampl Y, Gilad R, Eshel Y, Sarova-Pinhas I. Neurological and functional outcome in patients with supratentorial hemorrhages. A prospective study. Stroke 1995;26:2249.
23. Wakai S, Kumakura N, Nagai M. Lobar intracerebral hemorrhage. A clinical, radiographic, and pathological study of 29 consecutive operated cases with negative angiography. J Neurosurg 1992;76:231.
24. Tokuda Y, Inagawa T, Katoh Y, et al. Intracerebral hematoma in patients with ruptured cerebral aneurysms. Surg Neurol 1995;43:272.
25. Hart RG, Boop BS, Anderson DC. Oral anticoagulants and intracranial hemorrhage. Facts and hypotheses. Stroke 1995;26:1471.
26. Gurwitz JH, Gore JM, Goldberg RJ, et al. Risk for intracranial hemorrhage after tissue plasminogen activator treatment for acute myocardial infarction. Ann Intern Med 1998;129:597.
27. Ropper AH, Davis KR. Lobar cerebral hemorrhages: acute clinical syndromes in 26 cases. Ann Neurol 1980;8:141.
28. Weisberg LA. Subcortical lobar intracerebral haemorrhage: clinical-computed tomographic correlations. J Neurol Neurosurg Psychiatry 1985;48:1078.
29. Flemming KD, Wijdicks EFM, St Louis EK, Li H. Predicting deterioration in patients with lobar haemorrhages. J Neurol Neurosurg Psychiatry 1999;66:600.
30. Kaufman HH, McAllister P, Taylor H, Schmidt S. Intracerebral hematoma related to thrombolysis for myocardial infarction. Neurosurgery 1993;33:898.

31. Griffiths PD, Beveridge CJ, Gholkar A. Angiography in non-traumatic brain haematoma. An analysis of 100 cases. Acta Radiol 1997;38:797.
32. Flemming K, Wijdicks EFM, Li H. Prognosis in lobar hematoma. (Submitted for publication.)
33. Gates PC, Barnett HJ, Vinters HV, et al. Primary intraventricular hemorrhage in adults. Stroke 1986;17:872.
34. Darby DG, Donnan GA, Saling MA, et al. Primary intraventricular hemorrhage: clinical and neuropsychological findings in a prospective stroke series. Neurology 1988;38:68.
35. Findlay JM, Grace MG, Weir BK. Treatment of intraventricular hemorrhage with tissue plasminogen activator. Neurosurgery 1993;32:941.
36. Naff NJ, Tuhrim S. Intraventricular hemorrhage in adults: complications and treatment. New Horizons 1997;5:359.
37. Yeh HS, Tomsick TA, Tew JM Jr. Intraventricular hemorrhage due to aneurysms of the distal posterior inferior cerebellar artery. Report of three cases. J Neurosurg 1985;62:772.
38. Chang DS, Lin CL, Howng SL. Primary intraventricular hemorrhage in adult—an analysis of 24 cases. Kao Hsiung I Hsueh Ko Hsueh Tsa Chih 1998;14:633.
39. Schwarz S, Schwab S, Steiner HH, Hacke W. Secondary hemorrhage after intraventricular fibrinolysis: a cautionary note: a report of two cases. Neurosurgery 1998;42:659.
40. Coplin WM, Vinas FC, Agris JM, et al. A cohort study of the safety and feasibility of intraventricular urokinase for nonaneurysmal spontaneous intraventricular hemorrhage. Stroke 1998;29:1573.
41. St Louis EK, Wijdicks EFM, Li H. Prognostic features of spontaneous cerebellar hematomas (submitted for publication).
42. St Louis EK, Wijdicks EFM, Li H. Predicting neurologic deterioration in patients with cerebellar hematomas. Neurology 1998;51:1364.
43. Wijdicks EFM, St Louis EK, Atkinson JD, et al. Clinicians' biases toward surgery in cerebellar hematomas. Cerebrovasc Dis 1999 (in press).
44. Donauer E, Loew F, Faubert C, et al. Prognostic factors in the treatment of cerebellar haemorrhage. Acta Neurochir (Wien) 1994;131:59.
45. Porter RW, Detwiler PW, Spetzler RF, et al. Cavernous malformations of the brainstem: experience with 100 patients. J Neurosurg 1999;90:50.
46. Wijdicks EFM, St Louis E. Clinical profiles predictive of outcome in pontine hemorrhage. Neurology 1997;49:1342.

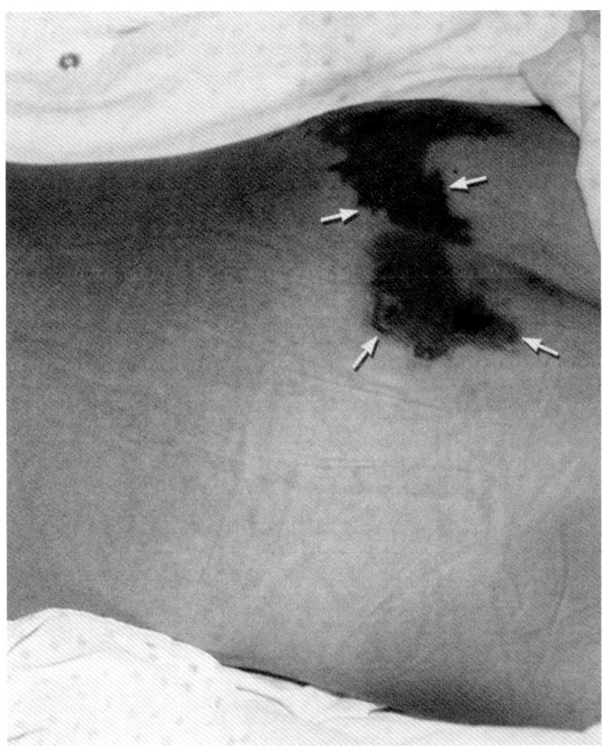

Color Plate 1. Excoriated blisters (*arrows*) at typical pressure in a patient found in coma from an overdose of a barbiturate.

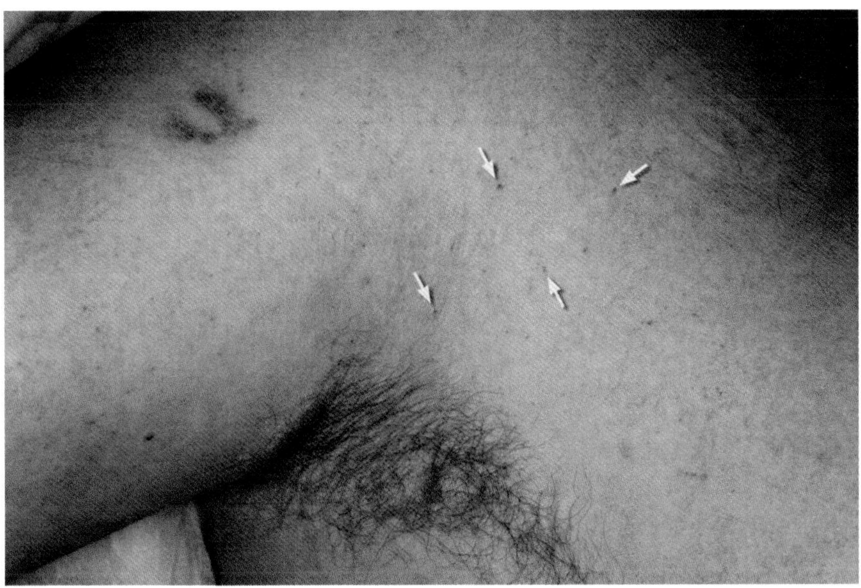

Color Plate 2. Typical axillary petechiae in a multitraumatized patient with fat emboli.

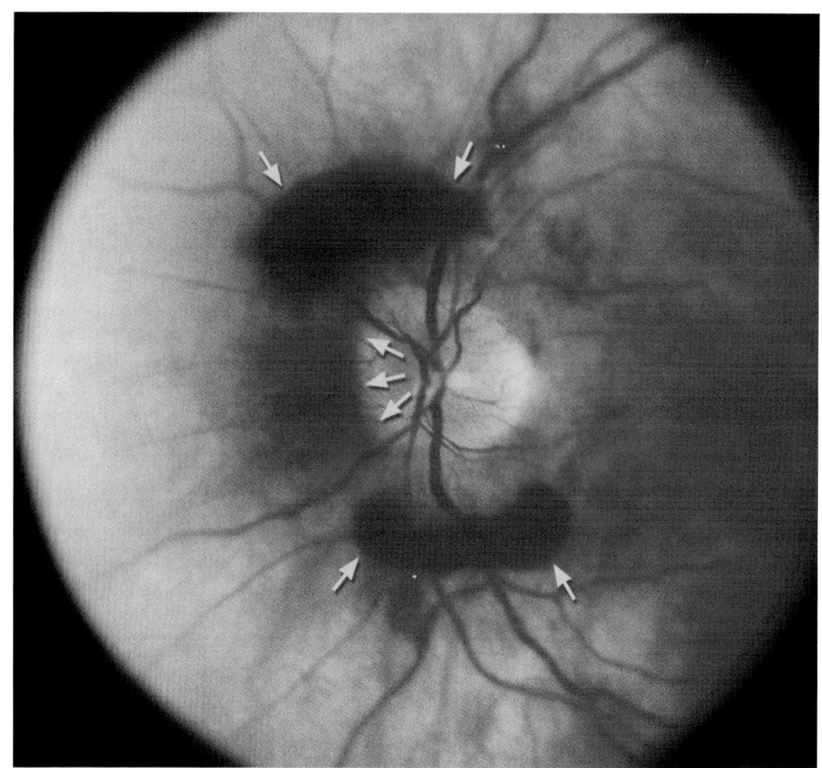

Color Plate 3. Subhyaloid hemorrhage (*arrows*) in subarachnoid hemorrhage.

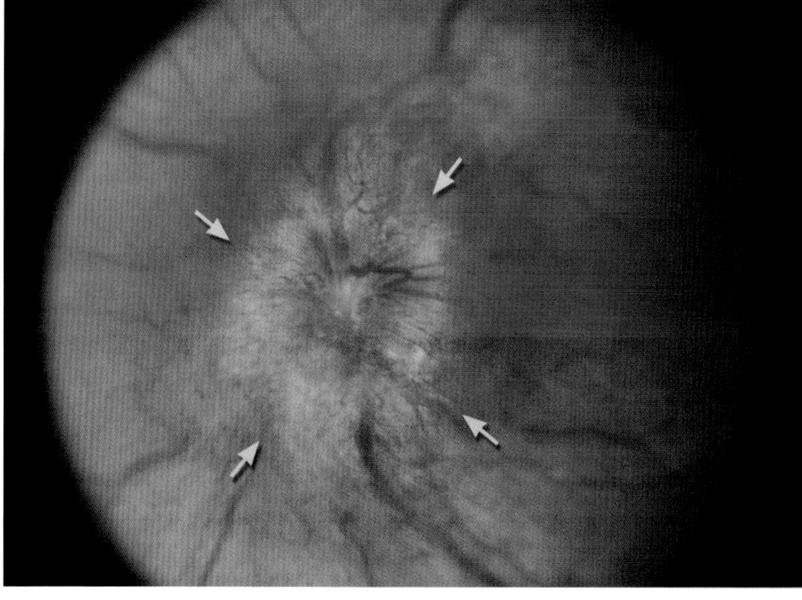

Color Plate 4. Papilledema (typical "champagne cork" configuration [*arrows*]) from increased intracranial pressure.

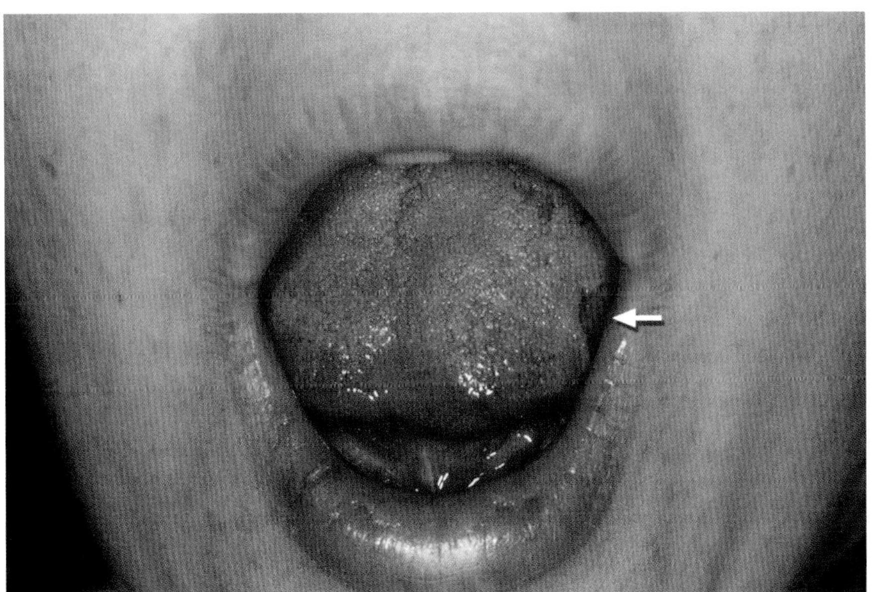

Color Plate 5. Tongue bite after seizures.

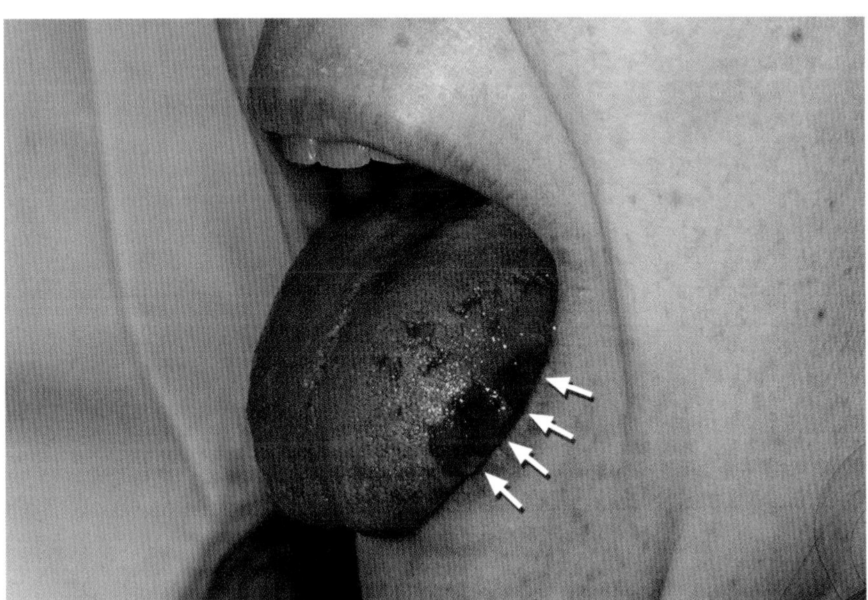

Color Plate 6. Tongue bite after seizures is much more evident when the tongue is pushed out.

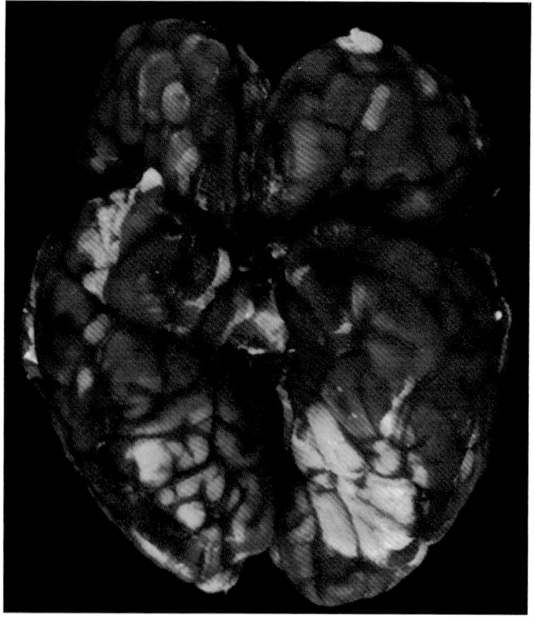

Color Plate 7. Pathologic specimen showing typical blood clots in basal cistern and subarachnoid space.

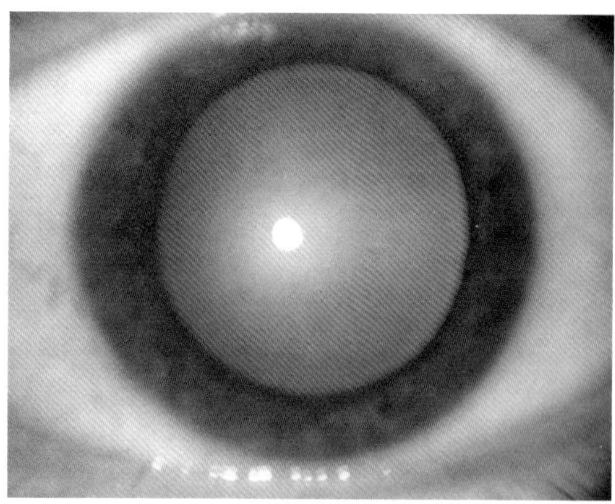

Color Plate 8. Normal red reflex, shown by retroillumination with fundus camera.

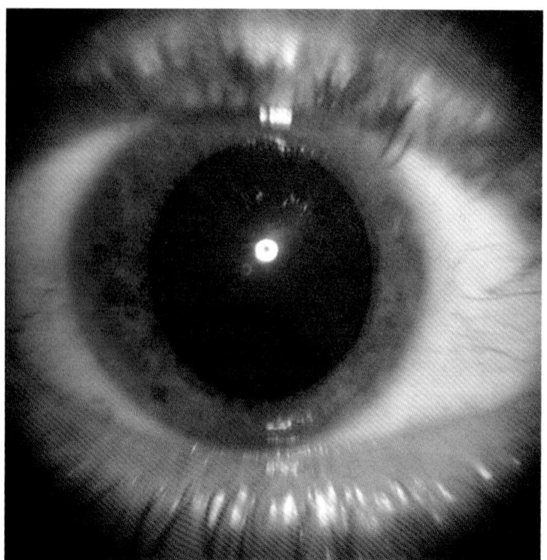

Color Plate 9. Absent red reflex due to vitreous hemorrhage ("black eye"). Same photographic technique as Color Plate 8.

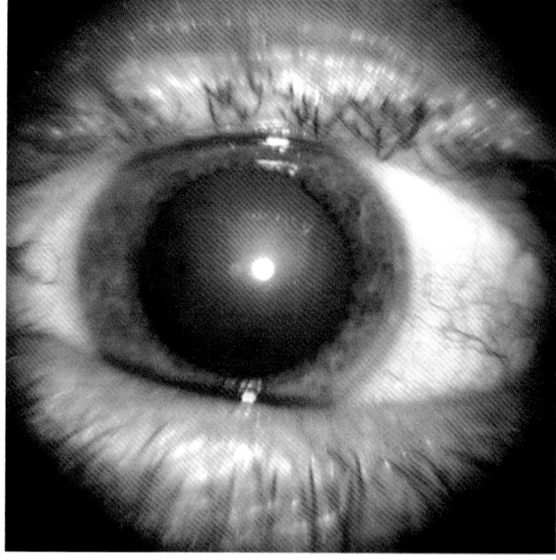

Color Plate 10. One year later, the patient in Color Plate 9 has marked impovement in vision, and red reflex is beginning to reappear. After vitrectomy, vision improved considerably.

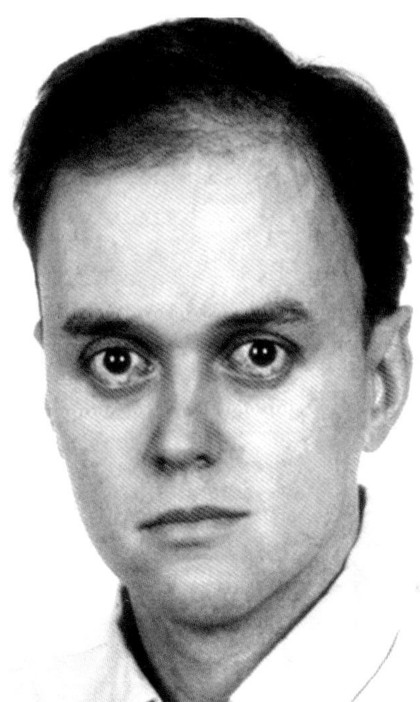

Color Plate 11. Ehlers-Danlos syndrome. The patient has characteristic expressive eyes, thin nasal bridge, thin lips, lobeless ears, and prematurely aged appearance (patient is 28 years old). (Courtesy of Dr. Schievink.)

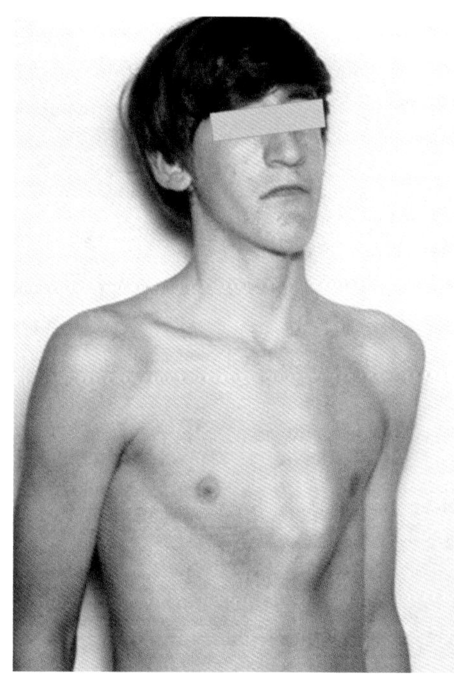

Color Plate 12. Marfan syndrome. The patient has tall stature, anterior chest deformity (pectus carinatum), and long head and face (dolichocephaly). (Courtesy of Dr. Schievink.)

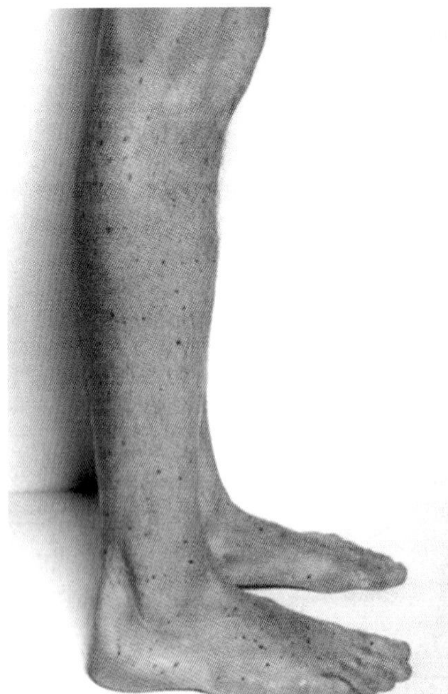

Color Plate 13. Melanotic spots (lentiginosis). A recently discovered familial syndrome with arterial dissections. (From Schievink et al.[47] By permission of the Massachusetts Medical Society.)

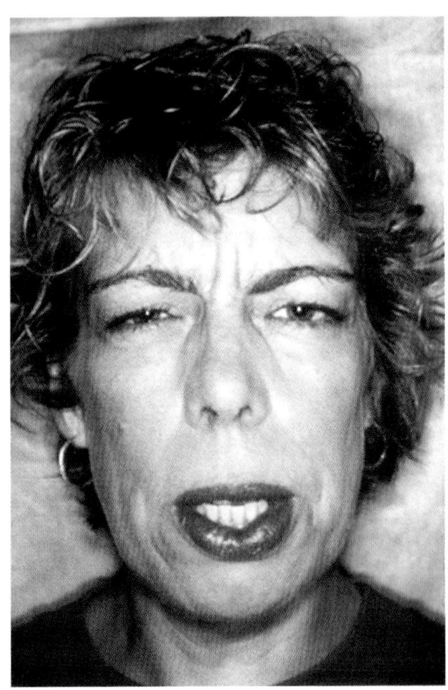

Color Plate 14. Phenotypes in patients with dissection. Loose skin (cutis laxa) in a patient with dissection. Ehlers-Danlos syndrome was suspected, but results of collagen analysis were normal. Many patients with dissection have a habitus suggesting a collagen disorder. (Courtesy of Dr. Schievink.)

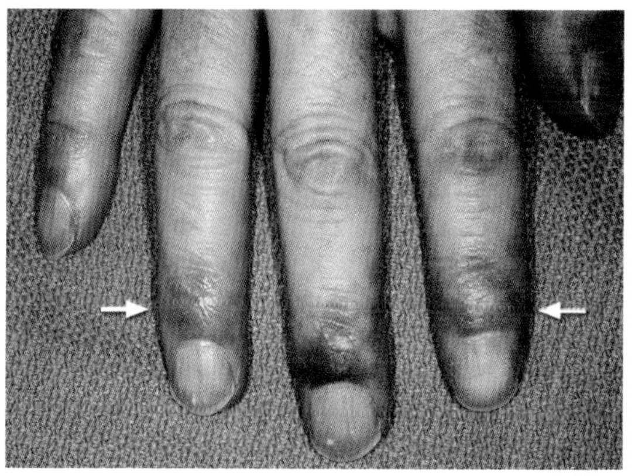

Color Plate 15. Extremities in a patient with antiphospholipid antibody syndrome.

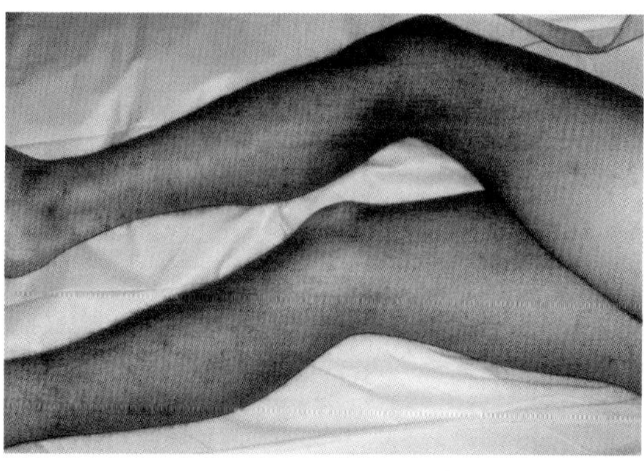

Color Plate 16. Example of skin lesions associated with meningococcemia. Pustulous vesicular rash.

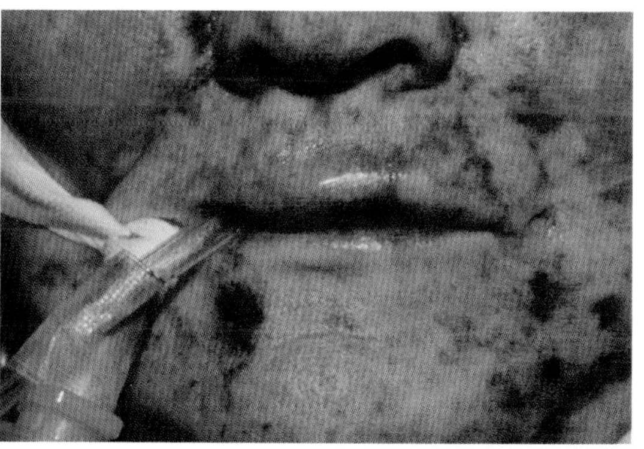

Color Plate 17. Typical patchy purple rash on face and lips in meningococcal meningitis.

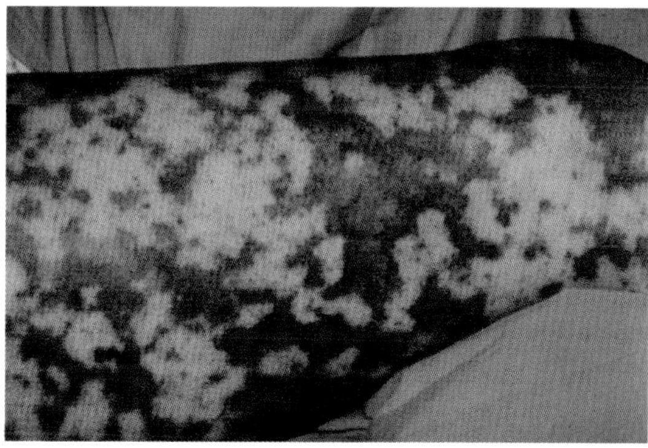

Color Plate 18. Typical patchy purple rash leg in meningococcal meningitis.

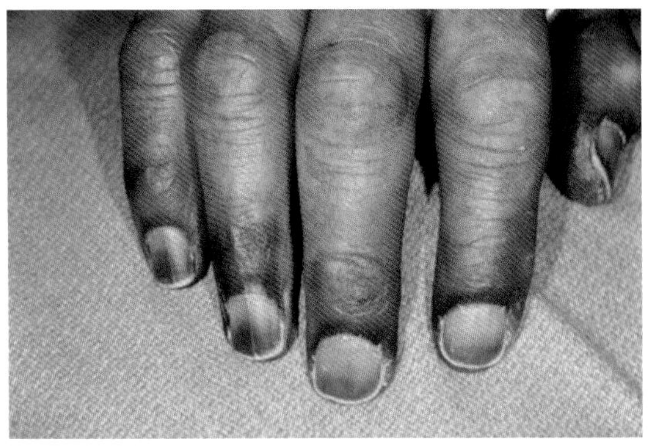

Color Plate 19. Typical patchy purple fingers in meningococcal meningitis.

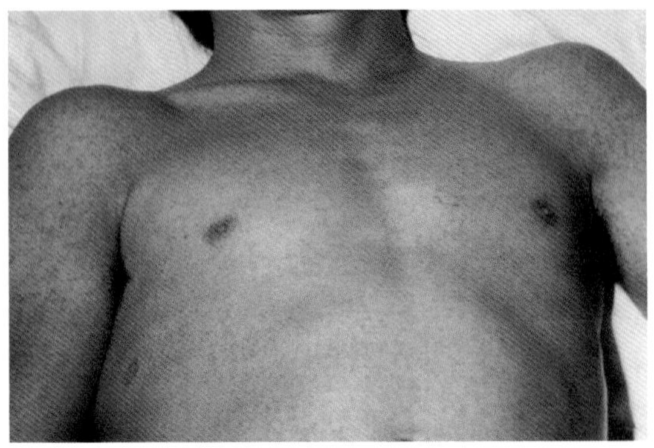

Color Plate 20. Generalized purpuric rash in patient with Rocky Mountain spotted fever.

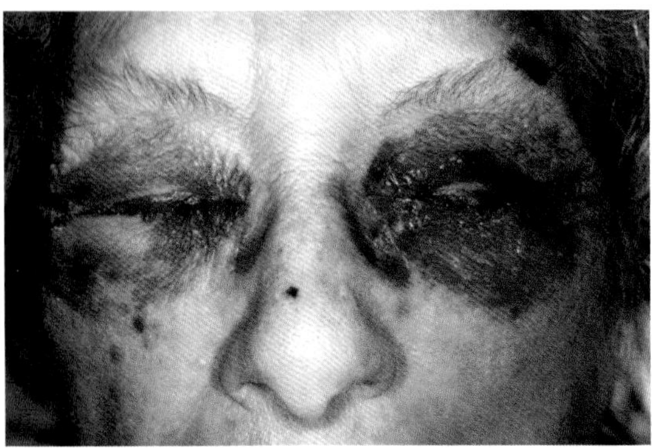

Color Plate 21. Ecchymosis of the eyelids indicative of orbital roof, midface, or zygomatic fracture.

Chapter 8
Major Ischemic Stroke Syndromes

Emergency treatment of acute ischemic stroke has gained the limelight with the first documented positive results of intravenous thrombolytic agents. Patients with an ischemic stroke and candidates for such aggressive management usually present with a major neurologic deficit, often involving the entire function of an arm and a leg, speech, perception of the left side of the body, and, if the lesion is localized in the brain stem or cerebellum, stance, swallowing, and vision. These deficits can be quantified by use of the National Institutes of Health stroke scale (Table 8.1), and grading is practical when interventional therapies are under consideration.

The causes of ischemic stroke are numerous, but only a few are common. Controversies and uncertainties remain about the use of thrombolytic agents, because many patients still do not qualify for intravenous or intra-arterial thrombolysis,[1] and the time window for intravenous administration of tissue-type plasminogen activator remains within 3 hours and cannot be extended to 6 hours.[2–4] This chapter discusses the most commonly encountered clinical presentations and the problems in management. Some of the less frequently encountered disorders are mentioned, particularly when different therapies are recommended. The approach to this vast diagnostic field is by the arterial system.

Large Vessel Occlusions

Ischemic stroke embodies a diverse group of patients with different modes of onset, progression, and outcome. More aggressive evaluation of ischemic stroke has resulted in a better definition of its mechanism.

Clinical Presentation

Characteristic clinical presentations should be familiar to any physician managing acute stroke, but the fine points can be addressed only by neurologists. The essence is combining the clinical features found through neurologic evaluation with findings of neuroimaging studies to allow quick triage.

Middle Cerebral Artery Occlusion

Catastrophic cerebral infarction often is caused by an occlusion of the middle cerebral artery (MCA). Its arterial system can be occluded at the M1 segment (proximal MCA), proximal to the lateral lenticulostriatal arteries, and at the M2 segment. The M2 segment is further divided by the superior and inferior trunks that supply the perisylvian area of the frontal and temporal lobes, respectively. The M2 MCA segment then is divided into the M3, or operculum, segment and the M4, or cortical, branches.

The most devastating MCA occlusion is at M1 or the stem, with a thrombus possibly extending into the carotid artery. Occlusion at the origin of the MCA may lead to gaze preference, hemianopsia, and flaccid hemiplegia of the arm, with some

Table 8.1. Stroke Scale of the National Institutes of Health and National Institute of Neurological Disorders and Stroke (the NIH Stroke Scale)*

Level of consciousness		Motor leg right	
Alert	0	No drift	0
Drowsy	1	Drift	1
Stuporous	2	Cannot resist gravity	2
Coma	3	No effort against gravity	3
Level of consciousness, questions		No movement	4
Answers both correctly	0	Motor leg left	
Answers one correctly	1	No drift	0
Incorrect	2	Drift	1
Level of consciousness, commands		Cannot resist gravity	2
Obeys both correctly	0	No effort against gravity	3
Obeys one correctly	1	No movement	4
Incorrect	2	Limb ataxia	
Gaze		Absent	0
Normal	0	Present in either upper or lower	1
Partial gaze palsy	1	Present in both upper and lower	2
Forced deviation	2	Sensory	
Visual		Normal	0
No visual loss	0	Partial loss	1
Partial hemianopsia	1	Dense loss	2
Complete hemianopsia	2	Neglect	
Bilateral hemianopsia	3	No neglect	0
Facial palsy		Partial neglect	1
Normal	0	Complete neglect	2
Minor	1	Dysarthria	
Partial	2	Normal articulation	0
Complete	3	Mild to moderate dysarthria	1
Motor arm right		Nearly unintelligible or worse	2
No drift	0	Language	
Drift	1	No aphasia	0
Cannot resist gravity	2	Mild to moderate aphasia	1
No effort against gravity	3	Severe aphasia	2
No movement	4	Mute	3
Motor arm left			
No drift	0		
Drift	1		
Cannot resist gravity	2		
No effort against gravity	3		
No movement	4		

*A sum score of 10 or greater is strongly indicative of a large vessel occlusion, predominantly in the middle cerebral artery. Examination may take only 5 minutes.

Modified from T Brott, HP Adams Jr, CP Olinger, et al. Measurements of acute cerebral infarction: a clinical examination scale. Stroke 1989;20:864. By permission of the American Heart Association.

sparing of movement in the leg. Global aphasia and speech apraxia occur if the left MCA is involved and left body neglect if the right MCA is involved. Hemisensory loss with no grimacing or withdrawal to pinprick is typical. A multimodulary speech deficit is common in left MCA occlusion: The patient has eyes open and may look about but is unable to follow any command or does so in an inappropriate manner. There is an inability to move the lips and tongue and to blow out the cheeks. Speech may be characterized by repetitive stopping and starting and fumbling words.[5] Other patients are mute. Occlusion of the superior trunk of the left MCA produces exactly the same characteristics and therefore cannot be differentiated clinically. However, occlusion of the inferior trunk of the left MCA produces a Wernicke-type aphasia and a superior homonymous quadrant anopsia ("pie in the sky").

An infarct may preferentially involve the perforating arteries of the MCA (lenticulostriate arteries) when the collateral supply from the anterior circulation and posterior cerebral artery is sufficient to protect the remainder of the hemisphere from infarction. A comma-shaped infarct, or so-called striatal capsular infarct, occurs with hemiplegia equally severe in the arm and leg and with fairly mild sensory symptoms.

In many patients, the defect may further evolve or fluctuate and in some may disappear dramatically. Decrease in deficit may occur in patients with large territorial MCA occlusions ("spectacular shrinking deficit").[6] It is explained by fragmentation of the obstructing clot.

Anterior Cerebral Artery Occlusion

Most anterior cerebral artery (ACA) distribution infarctions are caused by a cardioembolic source or by artery-to-artery embolization from internal carotid artery stenosis with a diameter reduction of more than 70%.[7] The clinical symptoms of acute ACA occlusion are complex and may not be obvious. Usually occlusion involves severe weakness of the leg in combination with other frontal lobe symptoms, such as abulia, loss of vitality, and incontinence. Transcortical motor and sensory aphasia, characterized by lack of spontaneous speech and comprehension but the ability to repeat phrases, has been reported in an infarction involving the ACA territory. Apraxia of the left arm with normal use of the right arm is typical, and this dissociation can be explained by corpus callosum infarction interrupting connecting fibers and can occur irrespective of occlusion of the right or left ACA. The disorder is revealed when patients can name objects placed in the right hand but are unable to recognize and name objects in the left hand.

An important artery that may become occluded is the recurrent artery of Heubner. Infarction of this territory produces weakness in the contralateral arm and side of the face, with dysarthria and hemichorea. If bilateral occlusions occur, a syndrome of akinetic mutism may evolve.

Basilar Artery Occlusion

The basilar artery gives off several paramedian vessels to the pons, as well as short circumference vessels, and two major cerebellar arteries, the proximal anterior inferior cerebellar artery (AICA) and, more distally, the superior cerebellar artery (SCA). The basilar artery divides into both posterior cerebellar arteries. Occlusions are possible at several levels, most often from artery-to-artery embolization. Occlusion of the basilar artery or its branches may produce several ischemic syndromes. Lodging of an embolus at the tip of the basilar artery results in infarction of the brain stem, thalamus, and occipital and medial temporal lobes. Cerebellar infarction may involve each or both of the feeding arteries to the cerebellum (posterior inferior cerebellar artery [PICA]-AICA and SCA). Less dramatic syndromes of brain stem infarction, many carrying French eponyms, are shown in Table 8.2 for easy reference, but they are rarely seen in its original presentation. (These syndromes remain interesting exercises in localization and are thus favorites of neurologists.)

Occlusion of the basilar artery results in a profound neurologic deficit but may start with any of these brain stem syndromes. However, a recent study of patients with basilar artery occlusion and thromboembolization found that sudden disturbance of consciousness was a predominant clinical symptom and was followed by brain stem signs without a clear unifying syndrome. In many patients, ophthalmoparesis and bulbar weakness develop early after onset.[8] Sudden vertigo, dysarthria, and quadriparesis are presenting features. Intranuclear ophthalmoplegia is common, explained by interruption of the intranuclear connections through the medial lemniscus fasciculus, and cold water irrigation may bring this on in a comatose patient (see Chapter 1). Patients may have hemiparesis mimicking a hemispheric lesion. Brief rhythmical shaking movements, most likely a forme fruste of extensor posturing, can be observed and are commonly misinterpreted as seizures, again leading to false localization in the hemisphere. An occluding embolus at the junction of the basilar artery and posterior cerebral artery may further interrupt the thalamic perforating artery and result in infarction of the thalamus bilaterally, midbrain, and occipital lobes. Vertical gaze palsy, abnormal convergence, skew deviation, behavioral disturbances, and visual hallucinations strongly suggest "top-of-the-basilar syn-

Table 8.2. Synopsis of Brain Stem Syndromes

Eponym	Lesion	Features
	Midbrain	
Weber	Cerebral peduncle	Ipsilateral III nerve palsy Contralateral hemiparesis
Benedict	Tegmentum red nucleus	Ipsilateral III nerve palsy Contralateral tremor, chorea
Parinaud	Quadrigeminal	Paralysis of upward gaze
Chiary-Foix-Nicolesco	Lateral	Hemiataxia Hemichorea Decreased vibration and proprioception Arm and leg weakness with or without facial weakness
	Pons	
Raymond	Paramedian area	Ipsilateral lateral rectus, muscle paresis, contralateral hemiplegia
Millard-Gubler	Medial lower	Ipsilateral facial palsy with contralateral hemiplegia (often also VI palsy)
Foville	Medial lower	Ipsilateral VII Ipsilateral paralysis of lateral gaze Contralateral hemiparesis
Raymond-Cestan	Medial	Quadriplegia Anesthesia Nystagmus
	Medulla oblongata	
Wallenberg	Lateral	Horner's ataxia (ipsilateral) IX, X Crossed hemianesthesia
Avellis	Nucleus ambiguus tractus solitarius Spinothalamic tract	X, XI bulbar palsy Contralateral dissociated hemianesthesia
Schmidt	Vagal nuclei Bulbar and spinal nuclei of accessory fibers	X, XI
Jackson	Nuclear vagus accessory; hypoglomus nerve	X, XI, XII
Tapia	Motor nuclei vagus and hypoglossus	X, XII

Roman numerals refer to the cranial nerves.

drome." Cortical blindness or polyopia (multiple images stacked up) due to bilateral occipital lobe ischemia may be a prominent presenting feature.

Many patients have progression to coma, with quadriplegia and pathologic withdrawal or extensor motor responses to pain. In our series of 25 patients with basilar artery occlusion who required mechanical ventilation, one-third lost all brain stem reflexes within the first 24 hours.[9] Failure to trigger the ventilator often occurs.

It is important to recognize "locked-in syndrome," which is the result of occlusion of the perforating arteries of the paramedian basilar artery, leading to dysfunction of the corticospinal tract, corticobulbar tract, and exiting sixth nerve fibers. The level of consciousness is normal, and the patient can communicate only with vertical eye movements and blinking (Chapter 1). Thalamic involvement or extension to the dorsal mesencephalon, thus affecting the reticular formation, may cause intermittent drowsiness and failure to consistently answer questions.

Cerebellar infarctions may involve the PICA, SCA, and, much less commonly, AICA. PICA occlusions may have different clinical presentations depending on the area of involvement, which may include the lateral medulla. Mainly, these occlusions are manifested by acute headache, vertigo, ataxia of gait, or limb ataxia, but isolated vertigo due to involvement of the vestibular portion of the vermis may be seen.

SCA occlusions may be the most frequent cerebellar infarcts, and acute dysarthria and ipsilateral dysmetria may be very prominent. This type of occlusion may closely mimic dysarthria clumsy hand lacunar syndrome. Vertigo is much less apparent.

AICA occlusions are manifested by characteristic acute deafness or profound unilateral hearing loss, but facial paralysis, Horner's syndrome, facial numbness, and loss of sensitivity to pain and temperature may occur as well.

Evolving cerebellar swelling may displace the pons or compress the medulla from tonsillar herniation (see Chapter 1). Impairment of consciousness occurs after a delay of 2 to 4 days, but patients may have cerebellar swelling at the time of admission to the emergency department.

Posterior Cerebral Artery

The posterior cerebral artery (PCA) produces characteristic neurobehavioral syndromes that can be easily recognized in the emergency department. A proximal PCA occlusion involving the dominant hemisphere (most often the left side) leads to alexia without agraphia. This dissociation syndrome is caused by an infarction of the splenium of the corpus callosum; patients are unable to read, but the ability to write is preserved because of intact language centers. Color agnosia may accompany a dominant hemispheric lesion. This color-naming disturbance should be tested in patients with right homonymous hemianopsia. Infarction of the dominant angular gyrus results in Gerstmann's syndrome, which involves finger agnosia (inability to name the fingers), inability to calculate, right-left disorientation, and agraphia. Right nondominant PCA occlusion may lead to prosopagnosia (inability to recognize familiar faces, such as those of family members or celebrities) in addition to a visual field defect.

Bilateral PCA occlusion can lead to two relatively rare syndromes, such as cortical blindness in which the patients may not recognize that they are blind and may relate vivid descriptions of the emergency room and persons surrounding them, all untrue. Another disorder is Balint's syndrome, with bilateral involvement in the border zone areas between ACA and PCA territories, thus often occurring after an episode of severe hypotension. Patients complain of "blindness," are unable to describe a full scene, and cannot describe more than two components of a visual field at the same time (simultanagnosia). In this syndrome, ocular apraxia may be observed, that is, lack of quick focusing on a new stimulus, previously called "spasm of fixation." When a stimulus is entering a visual field and even when told this is occurring, patients are not immediately alert to the stimulus. In addition, there is optic ataxia, referring to difficulty pointing accurately at a target under visual guidance. This can be brought about with the simple finger-pointing test. Distal occlusion of the PCA produces only a visual defect, usually with sparing of the macula due to collateral supply from the MCA.

Interpretation of Diagnostic Tests

Computed Tomography Scanning and Magnetic Resonance Imaging

Before third-generation computed tomography (CT) scanners, CT scanning in a patient with possible ischemic stroke was performed only to "exclude a hemorrhage." The definition of brain structures has improved with the newer generation of CT scanners, and early ischemia can be recognized. The vascular territories should be known when one views CT scans (Figure 8.1). If no obvious hypodensity is present, the CT scan should be carefully scrutinized for the early CT scan signs of cerebral infarction: an obscured outline of the lentiform nucleus or decrease in tissue attenuation, and sulci effacement (Figure 8.2). The subtle differences between gray and white matter are more easily detected when several CT window settings are used. Obscuration of the lentiform nucleus is the most frequent earliest sign[10] and may appear within the first hour of infarction. Early abnormalities on the CT scan also involve the parenchyma, with loss of the precise delineation between gray and white matter and, particularly, loss of the insular ribbon.[11] The insular segment of the MCA supplies the insular ribbon, and with complete occlusion of the MCA, the insular region becomes a watershed arterial zone.[12] In

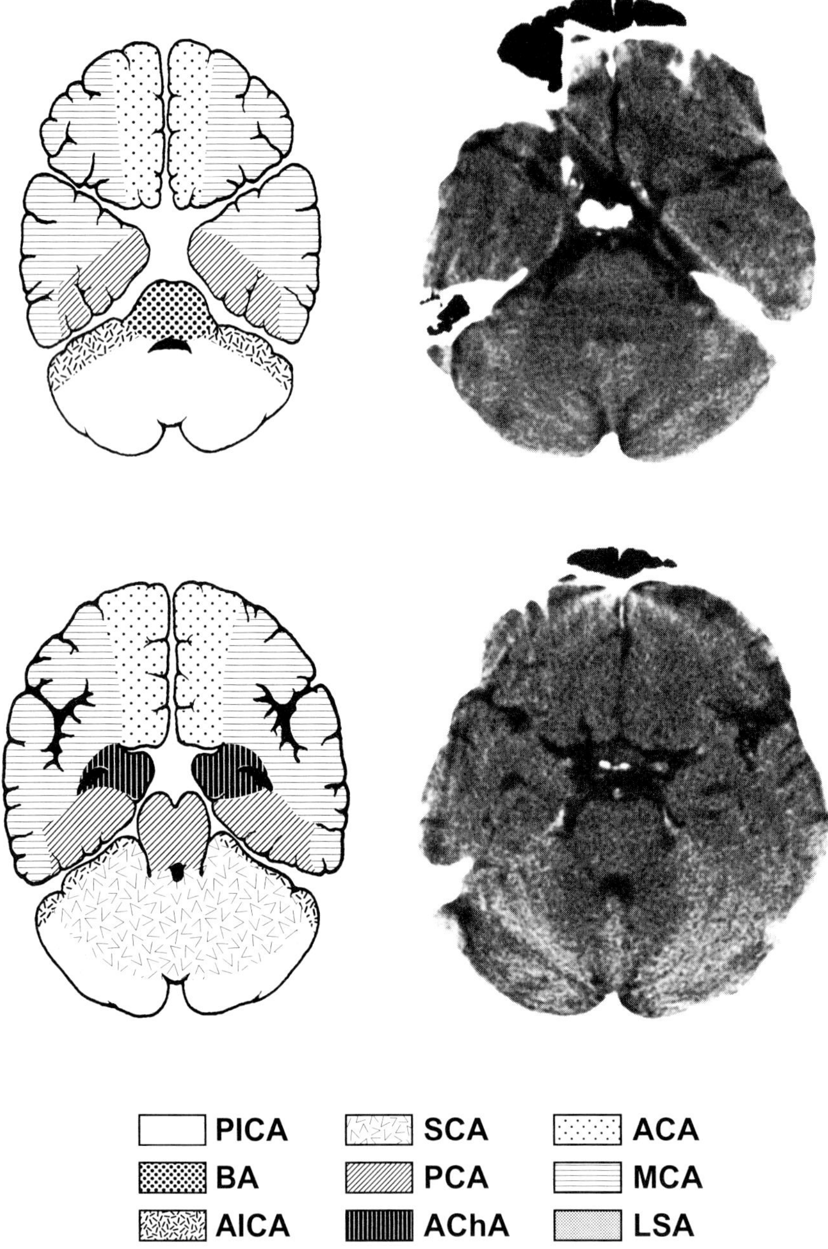

Figure 8.1. Vascular territories of the brain (computed tomography scans and corresponding arterial territories). (ACA = anterior cerebral artery; AChA = anterior choroidal artery; AICA = anterior inferior cerebellar artery; BA = basilar artery; LSA = left subclavian artery; MCA = middle cerebral artery; PCA = posterior cerebral artery; PICA = posterior inferior cerebellar artery; SCA = superior cerebellar artery.)

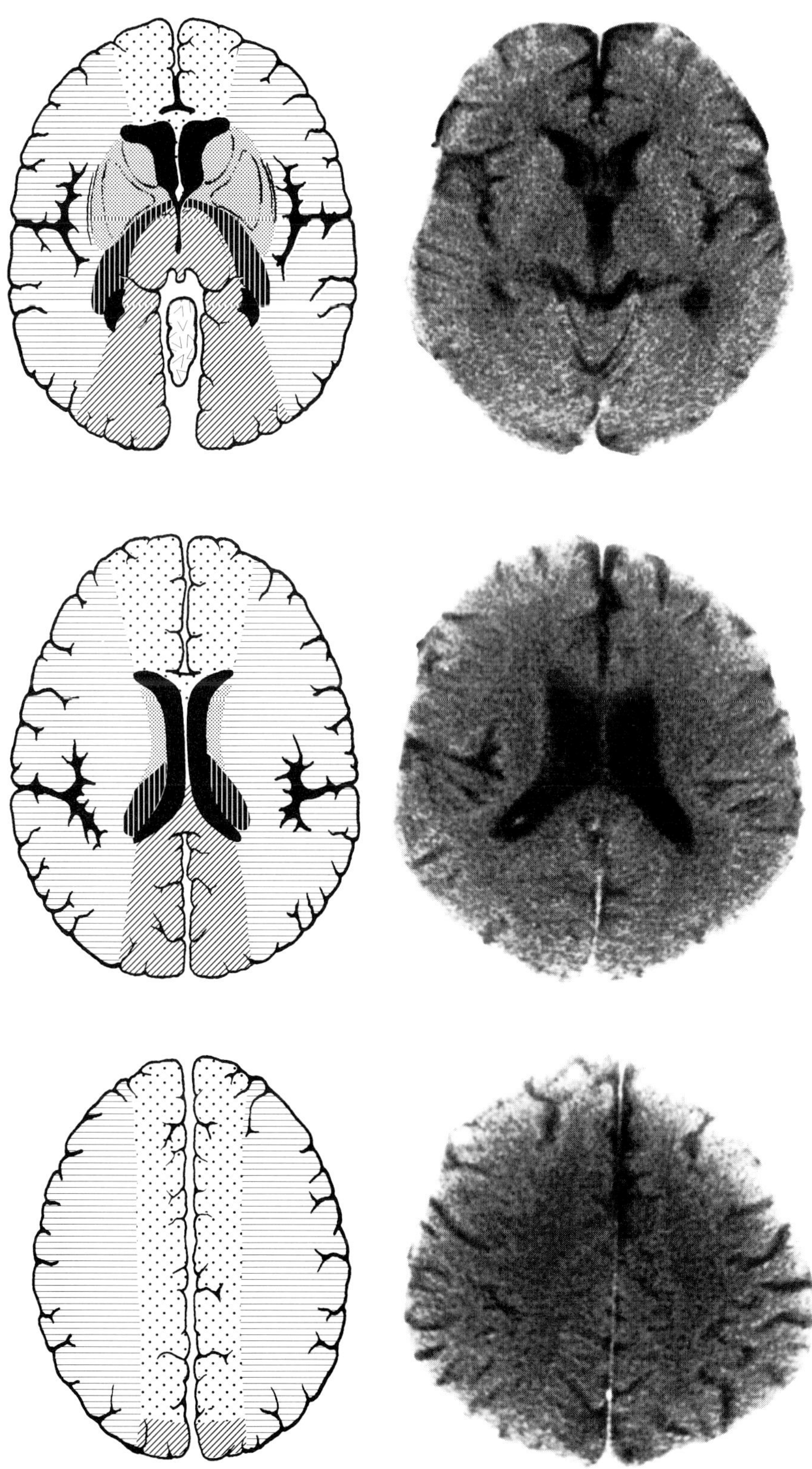

Figure 8.1. *Continued.*

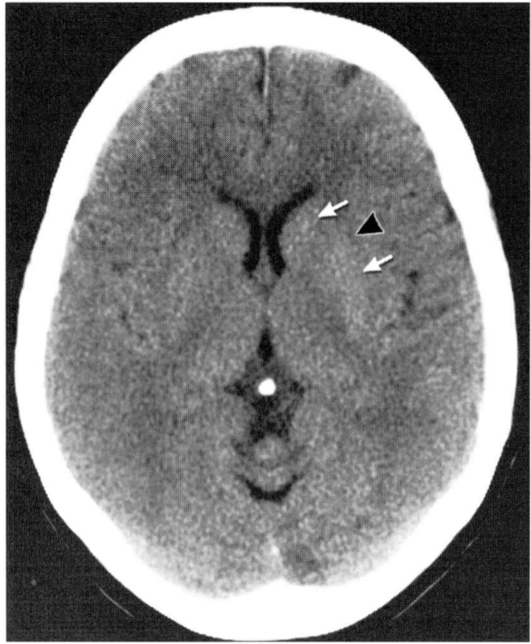

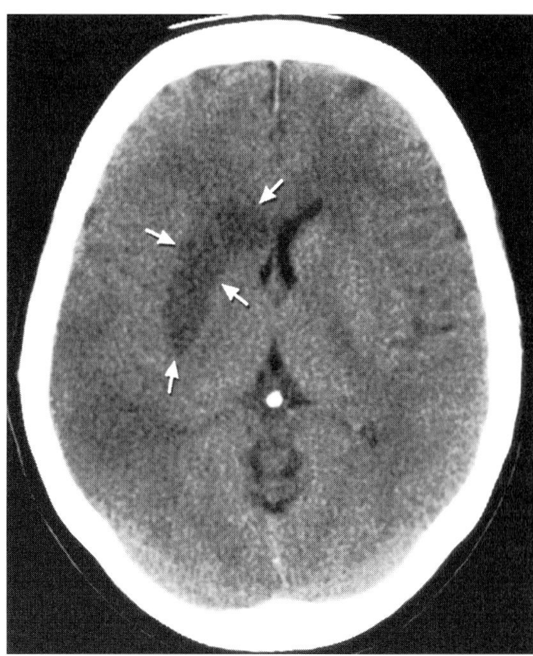

Figure 8.2. *Left*, Normal definition of the caudate nucleus, lentiform nucleus (*arrows*), and insular ribbon (*arrowhead*) in the left hemisphere has disappeared in the right hemisphere. *Right*, One day later, a computed tomography scan shows a hypodensity in that area (*arrows*).

addition, the insular cortex is the region most distant from the collateral flow from the ACA and PCA.

Hypodensity may involve the entire MCA territory (Figure 8.3A) but is usually evident days after onset. Hypodensity on CT scans may involve only the M2 territory (Figure 8.3B) or the lenticulostriate arteries (Figure 8.3C). A hypodensity can be seen within hours after MCA trunk occlusion.[13] In a small study of 25 patients, it appeared in 1 of 2 patients within an hour of the ictus, in 7 of 8 patients in the second hour, in all 3 patients in the third hour, in 7 of 8 patients in the fourth hour, and in all 4 patients scanned thereafter.[10] Transferred patients seen several hours after onset who had CT scanning during previous hospitalization at the time of the ictus should have a repeat CT scan, which may show a developing hypodensity.

A hyperdense MCA sign[14] actually indicates the clot in the MCA and has been recognized as a prognostic feature.[15] It may extend to the supraclinoid portion of the carotid artery, producing a T sign (Figure 8.4C). In our study, a hyperdense MCA together with early swelling (sulci effacement) predicted deterioration from further brain swelling.[16] In other studies, hemorrhagic transformation was deemed more likely in patients who had a hyperdense MCA sign.[14,17,18] When the clot fragments and breaks up, the hyperdense MCA sign disappears, often spontaneously or at times after intravenous administration of tissue-type plasminogen activator (tPA)[19] (Figures 8.4A and 8.4B). Swelling from MCA infarction often involves shift of the septum pellucidum followed by early trapping of the temporal horn. Involvement of the ACA circulation indicates a carotid occlusion, often from dissection (Figure 8.5).

Cerebral infarction is seen earlier on magnetic resonance imaging (MRI) than on CT scanning, but conventional CT scanning and T1- and T2-weighted MRI appear highly comparable in the detection of early signs of stroke.[20] Additional findings on MRI include lack of normal flow voids, which may represent direct visualization of the occluded vessel.[21] Arterial enhancement of the T1-weighted images in the ischemic zone after administration of gadolinium contrast material is caused by slow flow in an otherwise high-flow arterial system distal to the obstructing lesion.[22] This finding is seen in approximately 50% of patients with acute cortical infarcts.[21]

Newer MRI techniques using diffusion-weighted MRI or fluid-attenuated inversion recovery

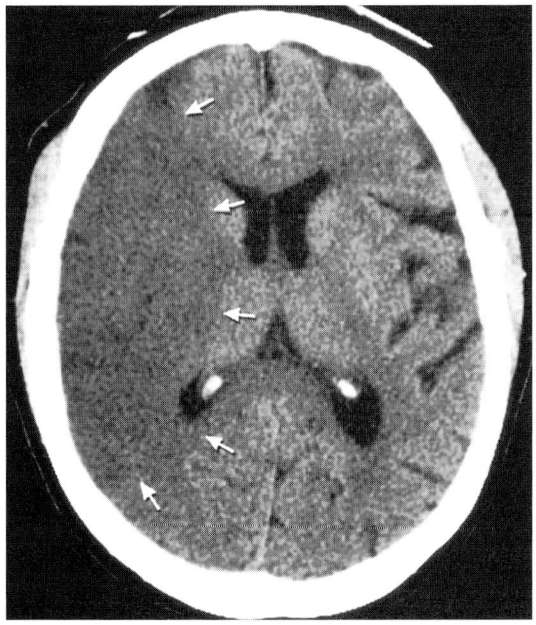

A

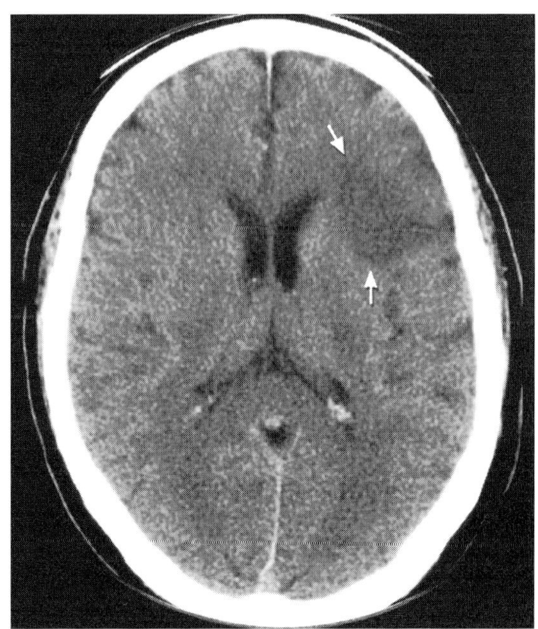

B

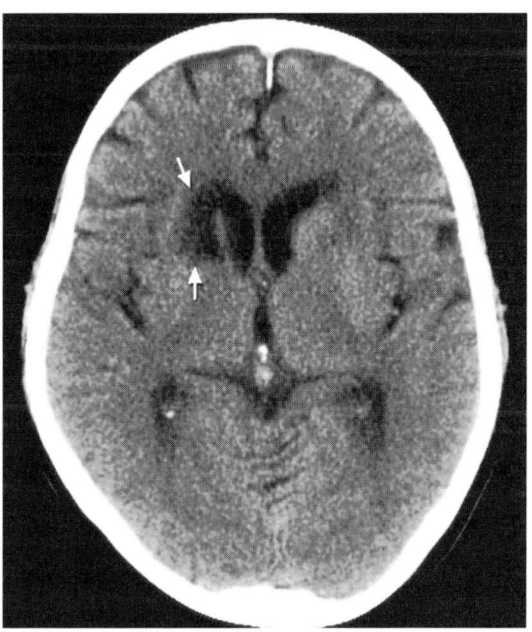

C

Figure 8.3. Computed tomography scans. **A.** Middle cerebral artery stem occlusion. **B.** Superior division occlusion. **C.** Capsulostriate infarct.

(FLAIR) are extremely sensitive for early infarction.[23] In diffusion-weighted imaging (DWI), areas of hyperintensity (bright areas) indicate decreased diffusion.[24,25] Several studies have shown that early infarction underlies the high signal intensity. It most likely reflects failure of water movement in tissue in this zone of infarction (Figure 8.6). The size of the lesion with this abnormality predicts future outcome, but the critical size for possible improvement is not known, and DWI cannot distinguish which lesions may be reversible after specific treatment (particularly thrombolytic therapy). Practical use of DWI in acute situations remains undefined, and most currently published studies on these magnetic

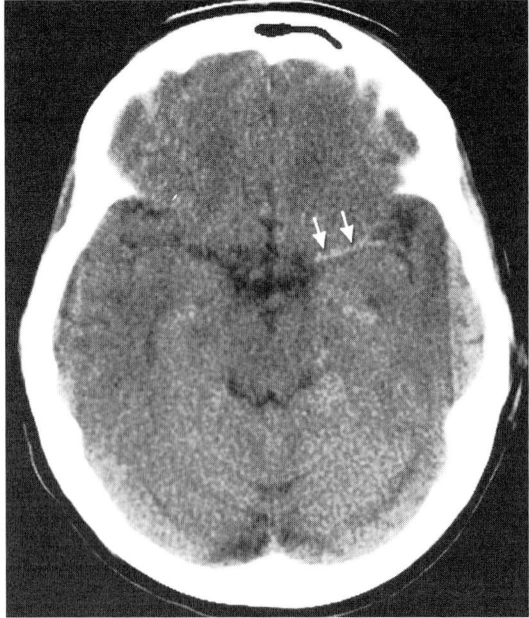
A

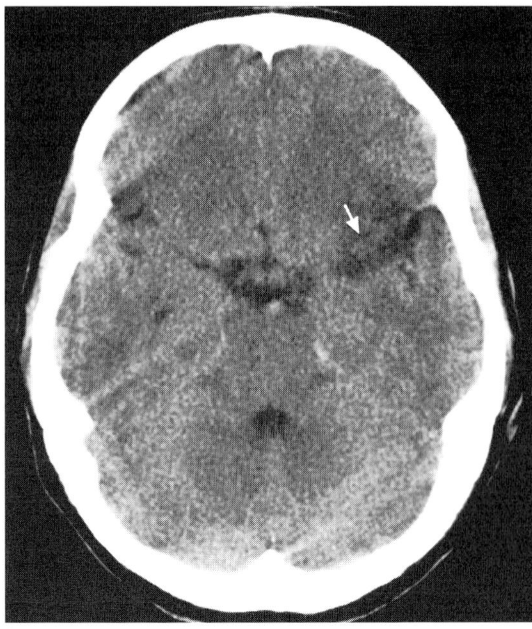
B

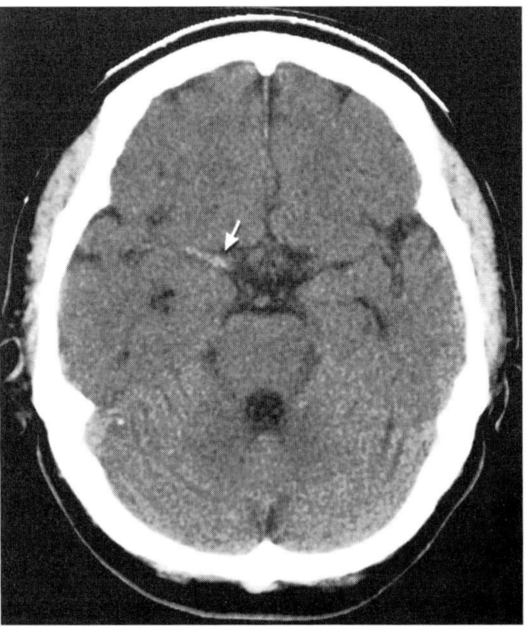
C

Figure 8.4. A–B. Hyperdense middle cerebral artery sign. The sign disappeared after administration of tissue-type plasminogen activator, but infarction developed. **C.** Hyperdense carotid sign ("T sign") involving the supraclinoid portion.

resonance sequences represent a fraction of the admitted patients with acute stroke. FLAIR sequences are also superior to routine magnetic resonance sequences, and a recent study comparing multimodulary magnetic resonance techniques found a sensitivity of 98% for DWI and 91% for FLAIR for detecting ischemic brain lesions within hours of the ictus.[26] The accuracy of DWI for subcortical infarcts is 95%.[27]

Currently, CT scanning remains the most important study and in most institutions without immediate 24-hour MRI services is not likely to be replaced soon

Figure 8.5. Signs of late swelling of middle cerebral artery infarct on computed tomography. Note sparing of the anterior cerebral artery and posterior cerebral artery territories (*black arrows*), shift, and contralateral hydrocephalus (*white arrows*).

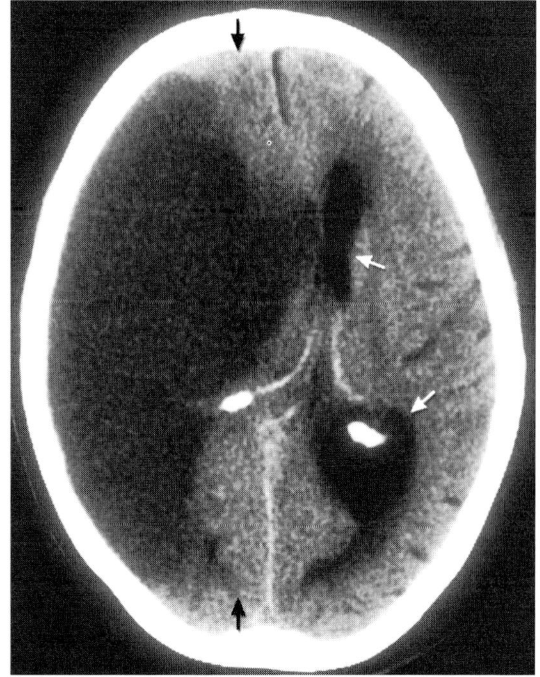

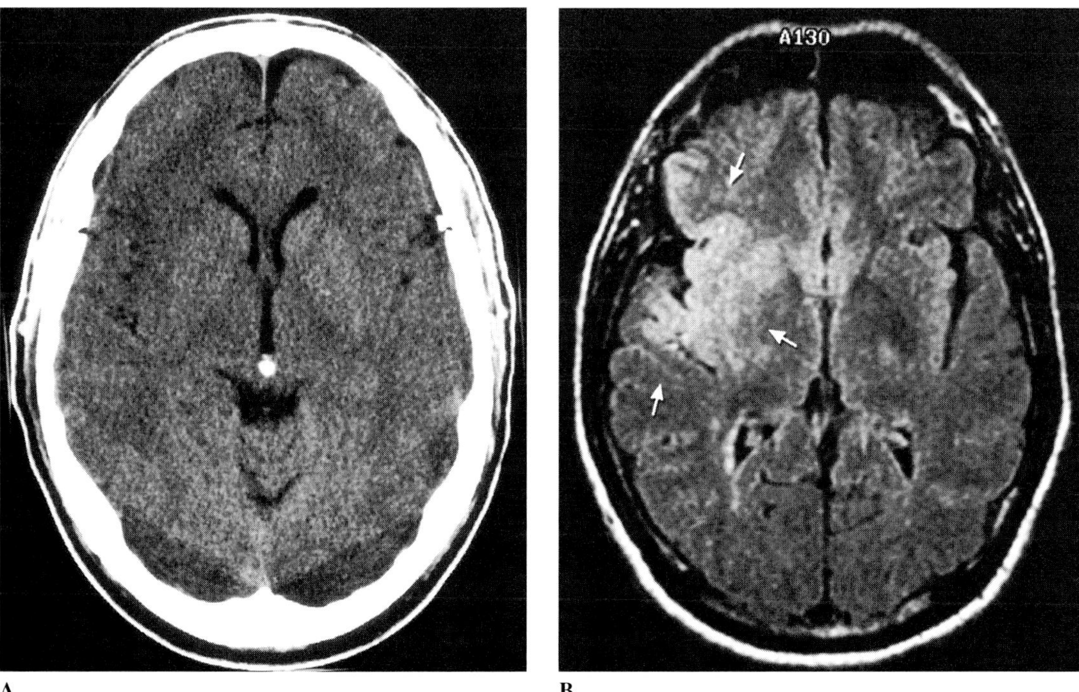

A B

Figure 8.6. A–B. Fluid-attenuated inversion recovery image of evolving right middle cerebral artery stroke compared with virtually normal computed tomography scan.

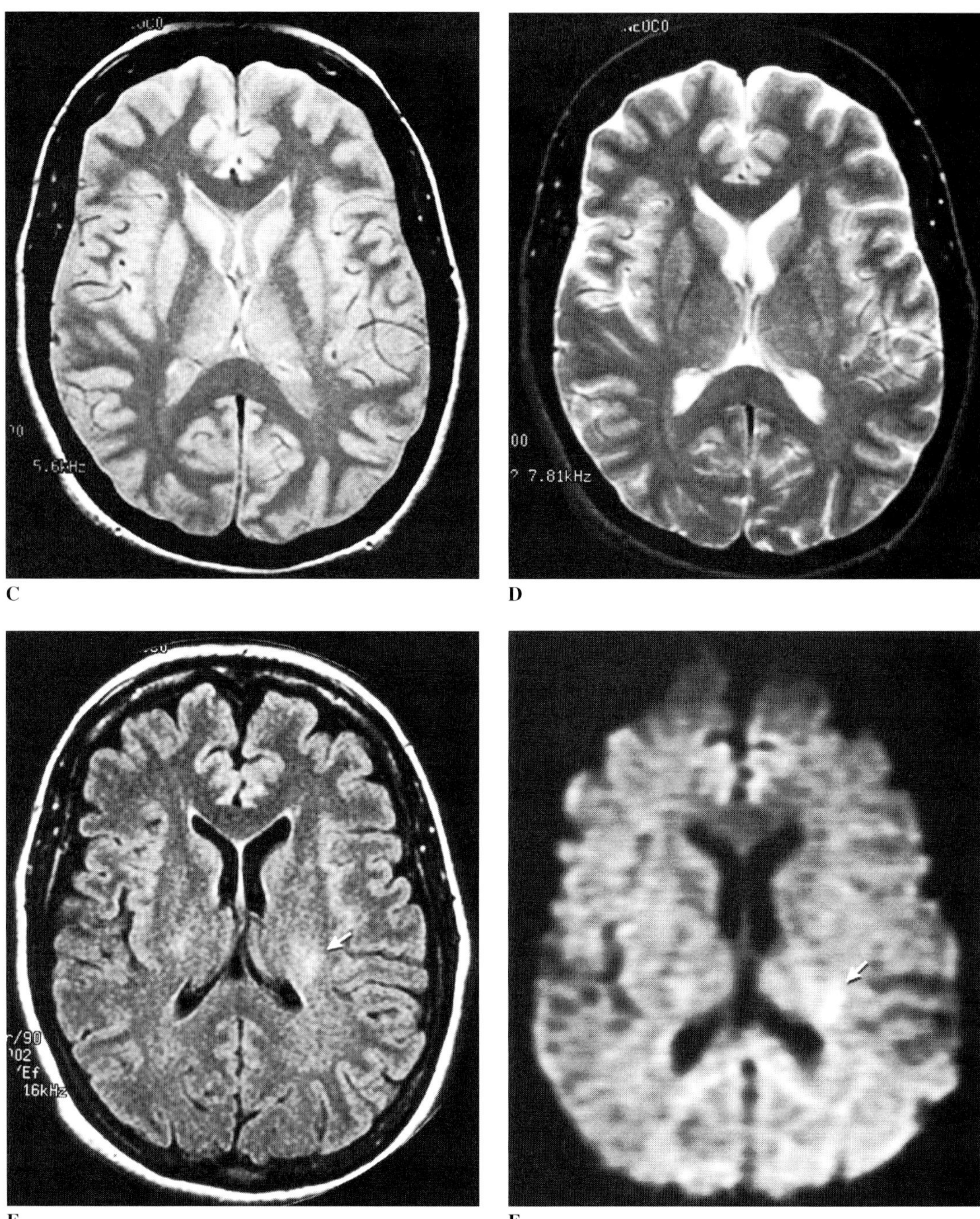

Figure 8.6. *Continued.* **C–F.** Recurrent hemiparesis and ischemic stroke with typical hyperintensity signal in capsule (all studies about 1 hour after onset). Intermediate and T2-weighted images are normal **(C, D)**, but fluid-attenuated inversion recovery **(E)** and diffusion-weighted imaging **(F)** document a new lesion in the posterior capsule (*arrow*).

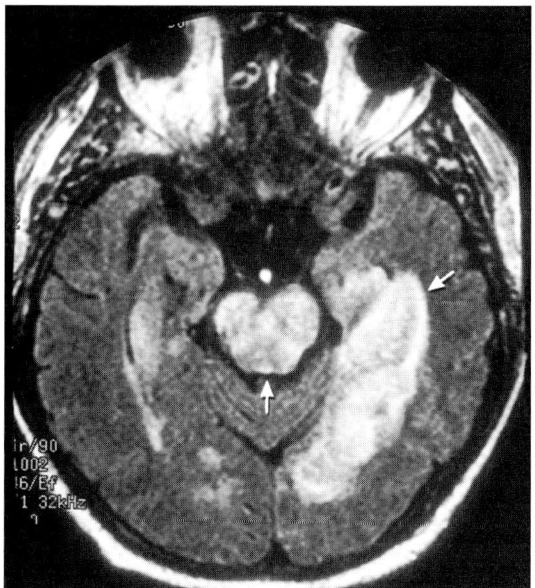

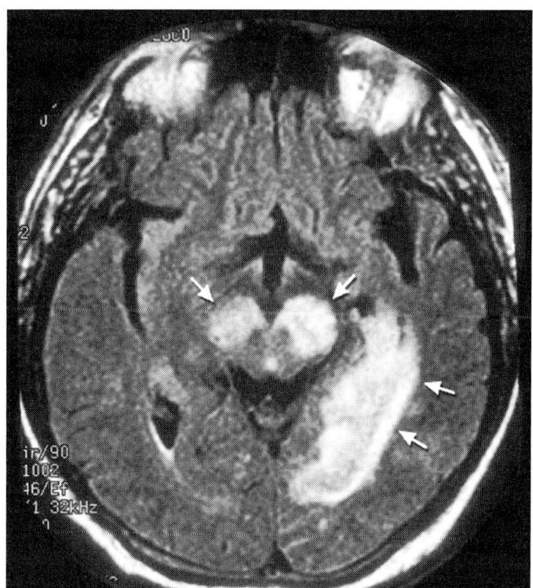

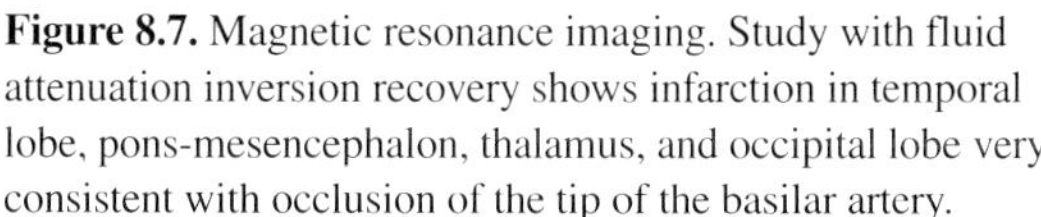

Figure 8.7. Magnetic resonance imaging. Study with fluid attenuation inversion recovery shows infarction in temporal lobe, pons-mesencephalon, thalamus, and occipital lobe very consistent with occlusion of the tip of the basilar artery.

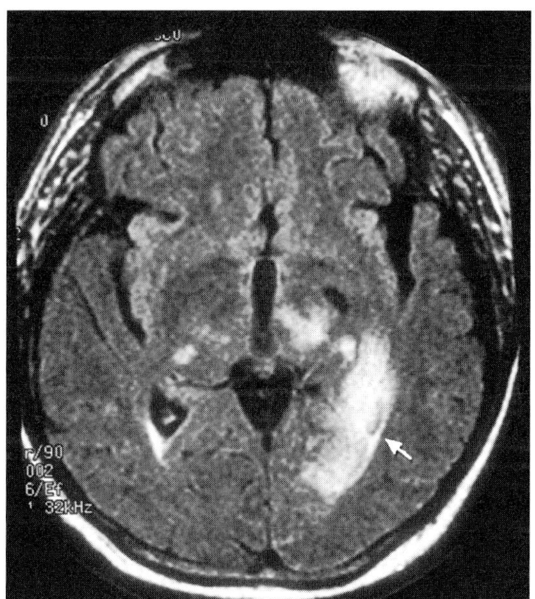

by these more sensitive, and undoubtedly superb, tests for the diagnosis of ischemic stroke. Until then, it is therefore of utmost importance that physicians treating ischemic stroke be familiar with the early signs of ischemic stroke on high-definition CT scans.[28]

Vertebrobasilar artery occlusion is diagnostic in virtually all cases, although the extent of the infarction may take some time to mature (Figure 8.7). A marked discrepancy between the initial CT scan (which may show only a hyperdense vascular artery sign) and the magnetic resonance images may be seen. CT scanning of cerebellar infarcts may be characterized by only a faintly developed hypodensity and distortion of the fourth ventricle. MRI is also the preferred test in cerebellar infarcts because it also defines the degree of compression and herniation (Figure 8.8). There is a marked discrepancy between CT and MRI findings in acute cerebellar infarcts.

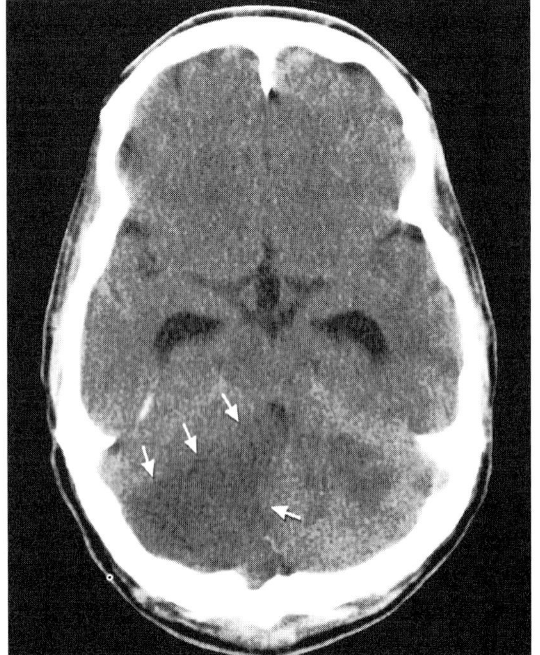

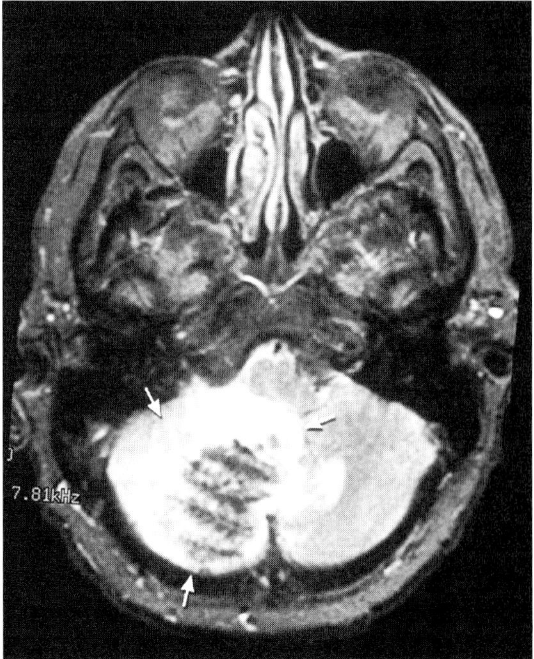

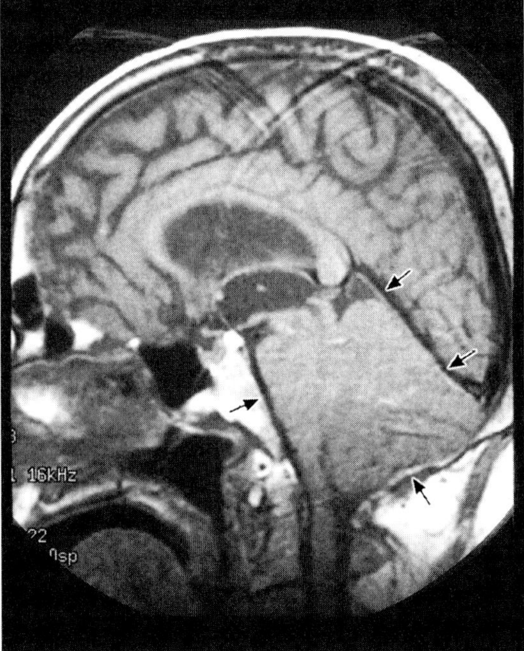

Figure 8.8. Cerebellar stroke with swelling and early hydrocephalus from fourth ventricle obstruction on computed tomography scan and magnetic resonance imaging.

Table 8.3. Absolute Exclusion Criteria for Intravenous or Intra-Arterial Thrombolysis

Computed tomography scan hypodensity ≥⅓ of volume of cerebral hemisphere
Rapidly resolving neurologic signs
Recent (within 30 days) surgery (including carotid endarterectomy); recent biopsy of a parenchymal organ or lumbar puncture
Recent hemorrhage or severe head injury
Advanced or terminal illness
Malignant hypertension (e.g., mean arterial pressure more than 140 mm Hg)
Stroke from infective endocarditis
Stroke from dissection of the ascending aorta
Stroke from carotid or vertebral dissection
Documented arteriovenous malformation
Pregnancy, lactation
Abnormal activated partial thromboplastin time or partial thromboplastin time
Abnormal platelet count

Computed Tomography Scan Angiography

CT scan angiography with a high dose of contrast medium is beginning to replace magnetic resonance angiographic studies.[29] It immediately provides the site of arterial occlusion and an estimate of the capacity of the collaterals. However, the introduction of a large amount of contrast material remains of concern in patients with increased serum creatinine levels, and the additional acquisition time may have an effect on the first 3-hour period in which intravenous tPA is used, particularly in institutions not yet equipped for the study.[30,31] In addition, observer agreement among neuroradiologists may be marginal in acute occlusion of the MCA, particularly in the assessment of symmetrical arterial enhancement.[32] Thus, the study may be less practical when used to assess vascular occlusion before the use of intravenous tPA.[30,31]

The role of CT scan angiography in basilar artery occlusion has not been determined, but the study may be useful in patients with fluctuating symptoms to assess whether occlusion is imminent, a finding that only then may lead to conventional cerebral angiography. It may also resolve problems with localization in patients with predominant hemiplegia.

Cerebral Angiography

Cerebral angiography remains the standard means of determining the extent of occlusion and collateral circulation. Its use in acute situations is defined by whether intra-arterial urokinase is considered and thus requires a certified interventional neuroradiologist to perform the procedure. In approximately one-third of patients, cerebral angiography done immediately after an ischemic stroke yields normal findings or shows a distal branch occlusion, a carotid occlusion, or a dissection unsuitable for thrombolysis.

First Priority in Management

Initial management should involve supportive stabilizing measures and consideration of thrombolysis. The contraindications for thrombolysis are shown in Table 8.3. Although CT scan findings should be normal, it is not known whether very early signs of infarction (effacement of the lentiform nucleus) preclude the use of tPA or urokinase. These signs may reduce the chance of recovery (indicators of permanent ischemia) or perhaps increase the risk of intracerebral hematoma. Obvious contraindications for thrombolysis are hypodensity (involving more than one-third of the MCA territory), sulci effacement, and other signs of brain swelling.

Intravenous thrombolysis with tPA can be started if symptoms have not abated within 3 hours after onset. Intravenous thrombolysis with tPA within 3 and 6 hours is not successful, and the risk of intracerebral hematoma increases. The ictus should be precisely known and not estimated. The administration of tPA is intravenous in a dose of 0.9 mg/kg (maximum, 90 mg), with 10% of the total dose given in a 1- to 2-minute bolus and 90% in a 1-hour infusion[33] (Capsule 8.1).

When patients are seen between 3 and 6 hours after onset, intra-arterial administration of urokinase should be considered.[34,35] A recent randomized study showed efficacy of clot lysis in patients eligible for this procedure.[36] Fluctuation often occurs in patients with an MCA (M1) occlusion, and some improvement may be related to improved collateral flow and partial dissolution of the thrombus. Cerebral angiography, however, should not be deferred for that reason, and in many patients an occluding thrombus is present that is suitable for thrombolysis. Combined therapy, that is, cerebral angiography after intravenous tPA and no improvement clinically

Capsule 8.1. Thrombolysis in Acute Stroke

Currently used fibrinolytic agents are plasminogen activators. Both tPA and urokinase catalyze plasmin formation from plasminogen. Plasmin degrades circulatory fibrinogen and the fibrin lattice of thrombi into soluble end products. Heparin enhances plasmin generation and thus enhances the tPA effect, which has a biologic half-life of 3 to 8 minutes. Urokinase has a plasma half-life of 9 to 12 minutes. In clinical use, these agents cause a marked decrease in or depletion of measurable circulating plasminogen and fibrinogen, resulting in prolongation of the partial thromboplastin time. The use of tPA for thrombolysis in acute stroke has been approved in the U.S., but major concerns remain. A recent review of 12 trials noted a substantial and significant excess of symptomatic and fatal hemorrhages (70 patients per 1,000 patients treated; 51 per 1,000 died).[3]

Table 8.4. Initial Management of Acute Ischemic Stroke in Anterior Circulation

Protect airway; endotracheal intubation if desaturation is noted on pulse oximeter
No antihypertensive medication; accept mean arterial pressure of ≤130 mm Hg; use 5 mg of labetalol intravenously if pressure is continuously elevated and no other cause is apparent
Rehydrate with 0.9% NaCl, 2 L/24 hours
Correct hyperglycemia (glucose >300 mg/dL) with insulin
Correct hyperthermia with cooling blanket
If computed tomography scans show swelling and coma is rapidly deepening, give mannitol 20–25%, 1 g/kg, and consider decompressive hemicraniectomy

followed by intra-arterial lysis of the clot if still present, is currently under investigation. Intravenous heparin is not used 24 hours after intravenous tPA but is recommended after intra-arterial urokinase.

Management of a massive ischemic stroke remains complex. Many therapeutic measures are unproven. The initial guidelines for stabilization are shown in Table 8.4. Options are intravenous heparin, blood pressure augmentation, and rehydration. It is important not to aggressively manage hypertension, because cerebral perfusion is marginal in the area of infarction. We discontinue any hypertensive agent and accept any mean arterial blood pressure less than 130 mm Hg in the first 24 hours. Patients should remain normovolemic, normoglycemic,[37] and normothermic. Mannitol can be considered when swelling leads to clinical deterioration, but decompressive hemicraniectomy to relieve intracranial pressure and reduce brain stem shift may be indicated for survival (Capsule 8.2).

The outcome of basilar artery occlusion is poor. Many series without the use of intra-arterial thrombolysis have reported 80% to 90% mortality or poor outcome. The management of basilar artery occlusion has been revolutionized by the use of intra-arterial thrombolysis within 12 hours of presentation.[35,39] MRI abnormalities showing early infarction in the cerebellum and pons probably should not preclude the use of intra-arterial thrombolysis, because they may indicate ischemia rather than permanent infarction.[35] Recanalization can be demonstrated in approximately 60% of patients, with clinical improvement in a similar proportion. However, the selection of patients potentially eligible for intra-arterial thrombolysis is not well defined. (Some centers have used thrombolysis in patients 14 to 79 hours after onset of symptoms, but most of these patients had fluctuating clinical courses interrupted by a sudden more severe deficit.[39]) The dose of urokinase varies. Usually, the urokinase solution prepared consists of 800,000 units mixed in physiologic saline for a total volume of 50 mL. At first, 250,000 units of urokinase is infused into the proximal aspect of the thrombus for 5 to 10 minutes. If no resolution of the thrombus occurs, an additional urokinase infusion of 320,000 units/hour is delivered into the proximal aspect of the thrombus. Up to 1,400,000 units of urokinase may be necessary to obtain full recanalization, at the risk, however, of systemic bleeding complications. Initial stabilization of vertebrobasilar artery occlusion is shown in Table 8.5.

Capsule 8.2. Decompressive Hemicraniectomy

Large hemispheric infarcts may be caused by carotid artery or middle cerebral artery occlusion. Swelling may occur after an interval of several days and cause a herniation syndrome.[38] Supportive therapies, such as hyperventilation and administration of mannitol, glycerol, barbiturates, and corticosteroids, have been unsuccessful. A large craniectomy with duraplasty to allow swelling outside the skull may be considered. This simple, but mutilating, procedure has significantly increased survival and has resulted in 30% to 50% functional outcome. The surgical procedure should be offered to patients irrespective of the involved hemisphere. Alternative therapies, such as moderate hypothermia (32°C or 33°C) or combined hypothermia and decompressive surgery, are currently being investigated. Randomized trials are needed to resolve many uncertainties about the outcome in patients with these interventions.

Predictors of Outcome

Large hemispheric infarcts have a poor prognosis when early swelling is evident on CT scans. Overall, mortality is 50%, but if signs of herniation occur, mortality approaches 80%. Indicators of poor prognosis are use of mechanical ventilation to protect the airway, gaze preference, and coma. Basilar artery occlusion is associated with major fluctuations in neurologic findings; thus, outcome remains difficult to predict early in the clinical course, certainly in the emergency department. The involvement of the thalamus in top-of-the-basilar artery occlusions can cause a devastating loss of memory despite frequent recovery from ataxia. Locked-in syndrome at presentation or coma virtually never is associated with functional outcome. The outcome in patients with acute basilar artery occlusion who have apnea is poor, and we and others have found no survivors.[9] However, dramatic reversals of coma and locked-in syndrome have been reported after urokinase injected intra-arterially but only within an ictus and treatment interval of 12 to 15 hours.[35] The cerebral angiogram has important prognostic features in basilar occlusion. Occlusion of the short restricted portion of the basilar artery has a higher probability of recanalization after intra-arterial thrombolysis than do longer occluded segments. In addition, collateral circulation predicted a good outcome after recanalization.[39]

Cerebellar infarcts may cause sudden deterioration from swelling and pontine compression. Outcome remains good, including in patients who have emergency surgical evacuation. Many patients of all ages may be able to ambulate with minimal assistance. Early withdrawal of care is not appropriate.

Table 8.5. Initial Management of Acute Ischemic Stroke in Posterior Circulation

Protect airway and intubate early if patient has marked bulbar symptoms
Maintain flat body position to optimize blood pressure
Perform immediate cerebral angiography of the posterior circulation if intra-arterial administration of urokinase is possible (<12 hours from onset)
Consider ventriculostomy or suboccipital craniectomy with cerebellar swelling from infarction

Triage

- ♦ If intra-arterial administration of urokinase is considered, cerebral angiography suite.
- ♦ Neurologic intensive care unit for monitoring brain swelling, hemorrhagic conversion, and, possibly, intracranial pressure.
- ♦ Patients with cerebellar infarcts who have normal Glasgow coma scores and early CT scan findings may go to the ward, but a repeat CT scan is needed within 12 hours to monitor early swelling.
- ♦ Operating room for suboccipital craniectomy or ventriculostomy, or both, in cerebellar infarcts when brain stem compression causes upward gaze palsy, deteriorating motor responses, and pupillary changes.

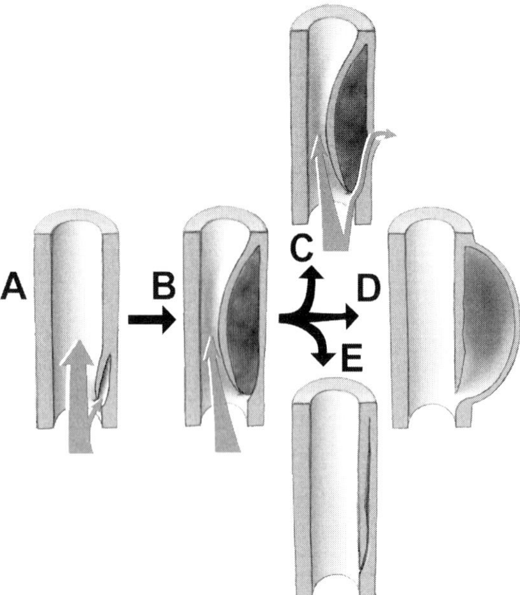

Figure 8.9. Process of arterial dissection (A) leading to occlusion (B), rupture (C), and pseudoaneurysm (D) or healing (E).

Arterial Dissection

A tear in the intima permits blood to dissect its way more distally into the muscular arterial wall and create a double lumen into the artery.[40,41] It occurs most commonly in the supraclinoid segment of the internal carotid artery.[42,43] The vast majority of vertebral artery dissections are at the level of the C1 and C2 vertebral bodies or at the intradural segment. The clot may dissect under the intima (subintimal) or throughout the media (subadventitial), causing distention of the vessel wall inward, producing occlusion, or outward, creating a pseudoaneurysm[41] (Figure 8.9). A false luminal channel can be created when intramural hemorrhage exits at a more distal site, but this is uncommon. Intracranial dissections may perforate the thin media and adventitia, causing subarachnoid hemorrhage with CT scan patterns similar to those of aneurysmal subarachnoid hemorrhage[44] (see Chapter 6 for management and illustrations). Pseudoaneurysms do not rupture but may become a nidus for emboli and thus may need surgical therapy if antiplatelet agents are ineffective.

Dissection of the internal carotid vertebral artery is mostly spontaneous and may represent 10% to 25% of ischemic strokes in adults aged 35 to 50.[42,43] Predisposing factors have been reported, and they may be more common in vertebral artery dissection than in carotid artery dissection. The dissection can be the result of a direct force to the artery, possibly triggered by strenuous activity, head turning, or chiropractic maneuvers but also by seemingly trivial insults, such as a brief Valsalva maneuver.[40] There is a seasonal predilection for autumn.[45] An increased incidence of upper respiratory infection during this period may suggest an inflammatory cause or insults from repeated flurries of cough. Dissections have been associated with congenital abnormalities of the wall of the artery, such as cystic medial necrosis, fibromuscular dysplasia,[46] Marfan's syndrome, Ehlers-Danlos syndrome type IV, alpha$_1$-antitrypsin deficiency, autosomal-dominant polycystic kidney disease, and familial lentiginosis[47] (Color Plates 11–14). In a recent prospective study of dissections at the Mayo Clinic, joint, skin laxity, and facial stigmata of an underlying vasculopathy were found but could not be characterized as typical arteriopathy.[48]

Dissection of the carotid or vertebral artery may be associated with head injury,[49] but in a recent report on five patients with traumatic dissections of the internal carotid arteries, cystic medial necrosis and marked lack of elastic fibers were found, suggesting a primary arteriopathy that increased the vulnerability of the arteries to trauma.[50]

Clinical Presentation

Headache or neck pain is present in approximately 60% of the patients. The headache can be sudden but infrequently is a typical "thunderclap headache" (see Chapter 6). Thunderclap headache should suggest subarachnoid hemorrhage from dissection through the entire wall in the intracranial portion. Headache may precede an ischemic stroke by several days and may not be clearly remembered or vocalized by the patient. The character of the headache is dull and seldom throbbing. Retro-orbital headache of sudden onset should point to carotid artery dissection. Carotid artery dissection might be associated with a new presentation of Horner's syndrome, pulsatile tinnitus, and lower cranial nerve involvement, particularly the twelfth cranial nerve, causing weakness of the tongue. Other lower cranial nerves can become compressed in the cervical parapharyngeal space.[42] The ninth to twelfth cranial nerves are in close proximity to the internal carotid artery and alone or in combination can become involved, producing dysarthria, dysphasia, dysphonia, and dysgeusia (metallic or nasty taste). Less common are a decreased sensation of the frontal division of the trigeminal nerve, oculomotor palsy, and abducens palsy.[51] Carotid dissection may be almost completely without any clinical neurologic deficits except for a new carotid bruit. This finding in a young patient with sudden facial or occipital headache should point to a dissection and prompt immediate neuroimaging studies.

Cerebral infarction involves MCA branch occlusions from propagated emboli. The interval between dissection and cerebral infarction varies widely, from minutes to 1 month, but is less than a week in most patients.[52] Low ("misery") flow infarction involving watershed areas is an uncommon mechanism[53,54] despite trickle flow with poor collateral compensation in some patients. Carotid occlusion may result in a malignant infarct with massive swelling involving the ACA and MCA territory.

A dissection of the extracranial vertebral artery is manifested almost immediately by signs of an ischemic stroke in the cerebellum involving, as expected, the territory of the PICA. Severe vertigo, vomiting, and appendicular ataxia might be presenting symptoms. In patients with vertebral artery dissection, the lateral medulla may become involved, causing typical Wallenberg's syndrome[55] (see Table 8.2). Swelling of the infarcted cerebellar tissue might cause considerable mass effect, displacement of the pons, and obstructive hydrocephalus.

Interpretation of Diagnostic Tests

Magnetic Resonance Imaging and Magnetic Resonance Angiography

MRI may replace conventional cerebral angiography as the first diagnostic test because it provides a definitive diagnosis in a large proportion of cases. Magnetic resonance angiography (MRA) is highly sensitive and specific in the diagnosis of internal carotid artery dissection but much less sensitive for a diagnosis of vertebral artery dissection.[56,57] Combined MRI and MRA compared with conventional arteriography has a sensitivity of 84% and specificity of 99% for the diagnosis of carotid dissection.[58] MRI also may show the typical dense crescent or double-lumen sign, which reflects an intramural thrombus, often at lower slices. Recanalization occurs within 3 to 6 months (Figures 8.10 and 8.11).

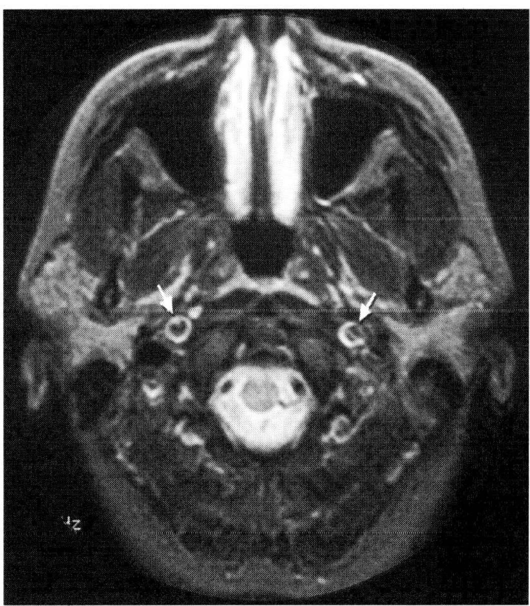

Figure 8.10. Magnetic resonance image showing double lumen phenomenon in bilateral carotid dissections.

Cerebral Angiography

Cerebral angiography remains the standard procedure. The most typical angiographic finding is relatively smooth, irregularly tapered luminal narrowing, often producing a very high stenosis (string sign)[57] (Figure 8.12). Dissections may occur in both vertebral arteries, in the carotid and vertebral arteries, or in all four arteries at the same time. A pseudoaneurysm might be found later, with typical fusiform appearance.

First Priority in Management

Carotid dissections might resolve within 6 weeks up to 3 months. Reconstitution to a normal lumen after 6 months is uncommon. Many physicians favor anticoagulation with intravenous heparin fol-

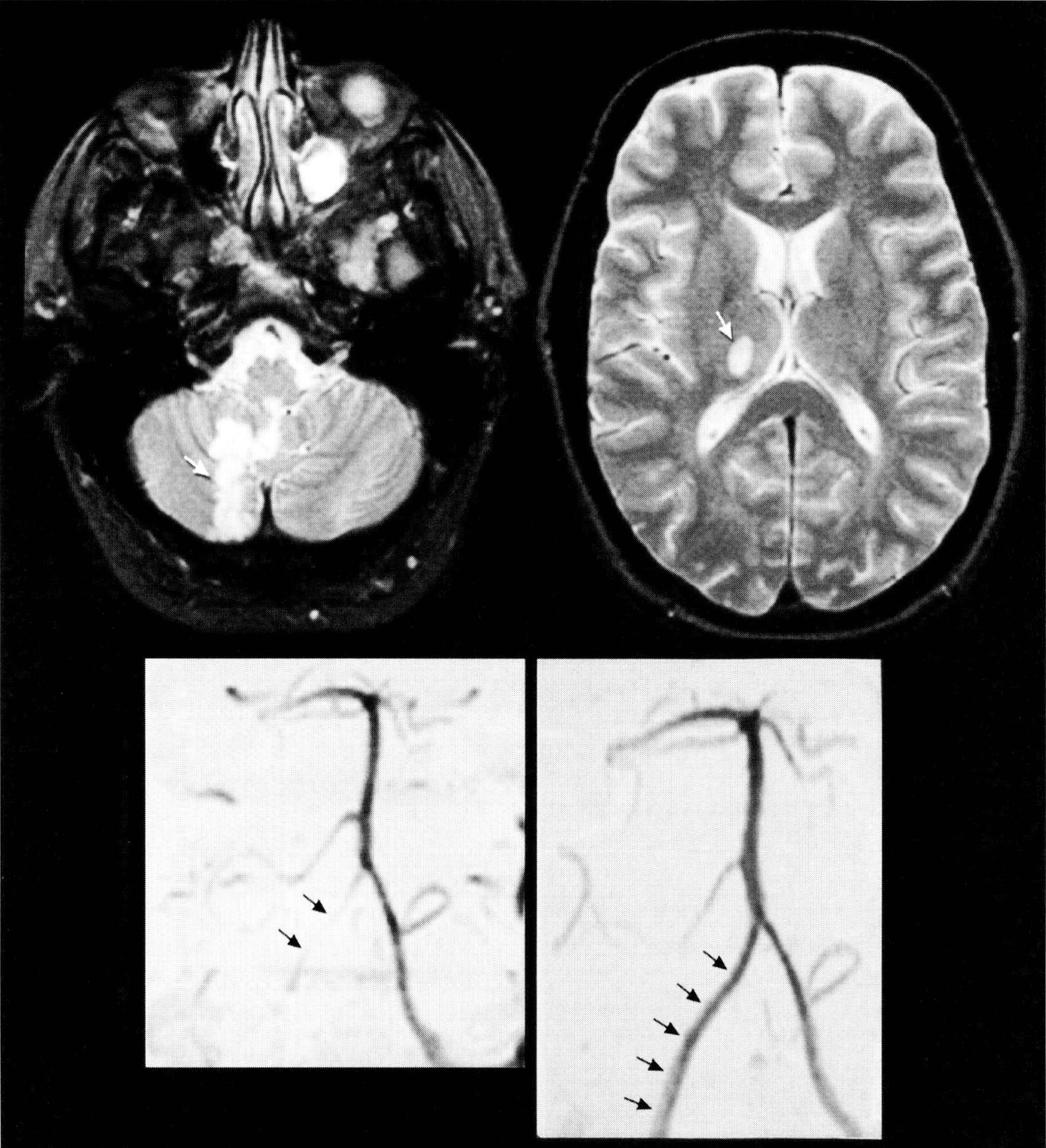

Figure 8.11. Magnetic resonance angiography shows a right vertebral artery dissection and cerebellar and thalamic infarcts (*arrows*). Recanalization of the right vertebral artery occurred in 3 months.

lowed by warfarin (aiming at an international normalized ratio between 2 and 3) until MRI and MRA show recanalization, but this is not done if the dissection involves the intracranial portion, because of the risk of causing subarachnoid hemorrhage (which in fact is very low [10%] in patients with intracranial dissection).[59] Antithrombotic therapy with aspirin, 325 mg daily, or clopidogrel, 75 mg daily, can be continued for another 3 months, but this period is arbitrary. Aneurysmal dilatation also may disappear spontaneously. However, it might become a source of recurrent transient ischemic attacks. If embolization occurs despite antiplatelet therapy, aneurysmal dilatation warrants surgical therapy or coil embolization of the artery with stenting of the occluded artery.[60]

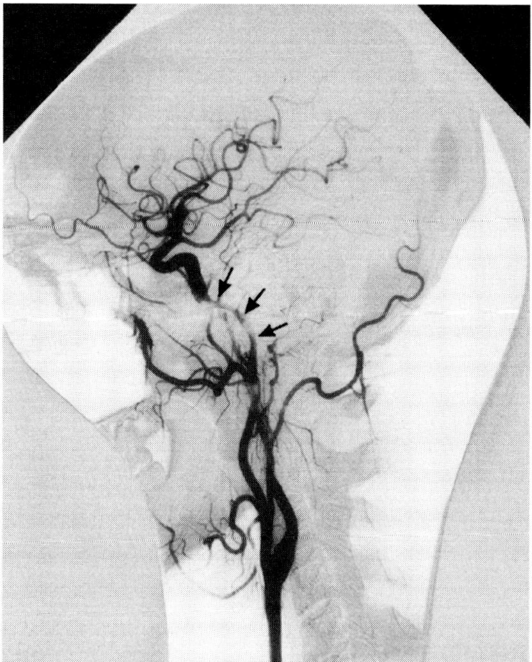

Figure 8.12. Cerebral angiogram of distal carotid artery dissection (*arrows*).

Predictors of Outcome

Dissection may recur in 1% per year (2% in the first month).[61] Patients with associated hereditary disorders do not have a higher incidence of recurrence of dissection. However, a history of dissection in a family member does increase the incidence of recurrence. Outcome from infarction due to dissection appears more favorable (approximately three-fourths of the patients) in younger patients than in elderly patients with similar infarcts; the explanation is not known. Massive swelling may occur because of involvement of the anterior circulation; mortality is high without treatment by decompressive craniectomy. Half our patients survived brain swelling with medical management alone.

Triage

- ♦ Admission to the ward for intravenous administration of heparin in patients with extracranial dissections.
- ♦ Admission to the neurologic-neurosurgical intensive care unit when early hemispheric brain swelling is evident on CT scans.

Table 8.6. Further Diagnostic Considerations in Patients with Multiple Cerebral Infarctions

Cerebral angiitis	Primary isolated angiitis (granulomatous) of the central nervous system
	Giant cell arteritis
	Associated systemic or collagen vascular disease (sarcoidosis, Behçet's disease, polyarteritis nodosa, Wegener's disease, systemic lupus erythematosus, Sneddon's syndrome)
	Associated infection (herpes zoster, cytomegalovirus, neurosyphilis)
	Drug-induced (amphetamines, heroin)
Endocarditis	Subacute bacterial infections
	Nonbacterial inflammation in advanced cancer
Coagulopathies	Protein C deficiency
	Antiphospholipid antibody syndrome
	Protein S deficiencies
	Antithrombin III deficiencies
Hemoglobin disorders	Sickle-cell syndromes
Platelet disorders	Thrombotic thrombocytopenic purpura
	Antiphospholipid antibody syndrome
	Hemolytic-uremic syndrome
	Diffuse intravascular coagulation
	Malignant angioendotheliomatosis (intravascular lymphomatosis)

- ♦ Admission to the neurologic-neurosurgical intensive care unit for patients who have vertebral dissections with cerebellar infarct.

Multiple Small Vessel Occlusions

Multiple cerebral infarctions represent a separate entity but with multiple different causes. The differential diagnosis is particularly complex in younger persons, and extensive evaluation of underlying coagulopathies or intrinsic vasculopathies is needed. The diagnostic considerations in patients with multiple infarctions who are examined in the emergency room are shown in Table 8.6. Only the disorders that are clinically the most relevant because of early specific features are discussed here.

Vasculitis of the Central Nervous System

Granulomatous vasculitis or isolated angiitis of the central nervous system (CNS) is an emergency and may rapidly lead to permanent devastating ischemic strokes or, less commonly, to intracranial hematomas or subarachnoid hemorrhage.[62,63] Progressive or recurrent neurologic symptoms are common, but because of the infrequent occurrence of this disorder, they may not be recognized as typical features of CNS vasculitis until the destruction is permanent. Delay in diagnosis has been established as an unfortunate fact.[64]

The presentation of CNS vasculitis as subarachnoid hemorrhage is discussed in Chapter 6 and as a consequence of herpes zoster encephalitis in Chapter 10.

Clinical Presentation

Two-thirds of the patients present with severe, persistent headache overriding any other symptom. Profound aphasia, apraxia, or hemiparesis may occur, but acute confusion and, most typically, emotional lability with crying or bizarre hysterical or childish behavior are more common. Some patients become dull and abulic, particularly with preferential involvement of the anterior cerebral circulation. Multifocal neurologic findings can be expected, because the pattern involves scattered inflammation of the medium- and small-sized arteries.[64]

CNS vasculitis may be secondary to a systemic illness or drug abuse. Skin lesions, joint swelling, or additional evidence of a mononeuritis multiplex or progressive polyneuropathy may point to a connective tissue disorder or systemic vasculitis. The use of amphetamine often can be inferred only from a careful history of drug use, which is not volunteered by most patients with strokes.[65–67]

Infectious causes can produce CNS vasculitis, but other localizations should be evident (e.g., retina for cytomegalovirus, painful crusty skin lesions for herpes zoster, pulmonary manifestations associated with *Histoplasma* or *Coccidioides immitis*, or systemic manifestations of human immunodeficiency virus infection). Finally, lymphoproliferative disorders (Hodgkin's lymphoma) may be associated with vasculitis.[68]

Moore's criteria for the diagnosis of isolated angiitis of the CNS are (1) recent severe onset of headaches, confusion, or multifocal neurologic deficits that are recurrent or progressive; (2) typical angiographic findings; (3) exclusion of systemic disease or infection; and (4) leptomeningeal and parenchymal biopsy findings that confirm vascular inflammation and exclude infection, neoplasia, and noninflammatory vascular disease.[63,69,70]

Interpretation of Diagnostic Tests

Computed Tomography Scanning and Magnetic Resonance Imaging. The sensitivity of CT scanning in isolated angiitis is low, but occasionally subarachnoid hemorrhage can be found[71] (see Chapter 6). CT scanning may help diagnose Wegener's granulomatosis, characterized by bone thickening and focal erosive changes of the nasal septum and soft tissue masses in the sinuses. MRI abnormalities should reveal infarction involving several vascular territories, producing effacement of sulci and hyperintense signals following the gyri (Figure 8.13). Lesions deep in the white matter that spare the overlying cortex are less common.[72] Meningeal enhancement alone has been reported.[14] Conversely, it can be generally stated that normal MRI findings, certainly with FLAIR sequences, virtually exclude widespread CNS vasculitis.[73] MRA may be useful as an initial screening test, but it overestimates narrowing, may not visualize abnormalities in medium-sized or smaller arteries due to current poor resolution, and, therefore, does not match conventional cerebral angiography.

Cerebral Angiography. The sensitivity of cerebral angiography in CNS vasculitis is high, approximately 95% to 99%, but specificity is low. A cerebral angiogram with negative findings has been described in biopsy-proven CNS vasculitis. Suggestive findings are changed vessel caliber, with constriction, occlusion ("cutoffs"), irregularities, and dilatation showing a characteristic beading pattern (see Figure 8.13). Alternative explanations for the angiographic findings include cerebral vasospasm (very unusual on the day of onset of hemorrhage), advanced atherosclerosis (proximal carotid artery abnormalities or irregularities in the proximal verte-

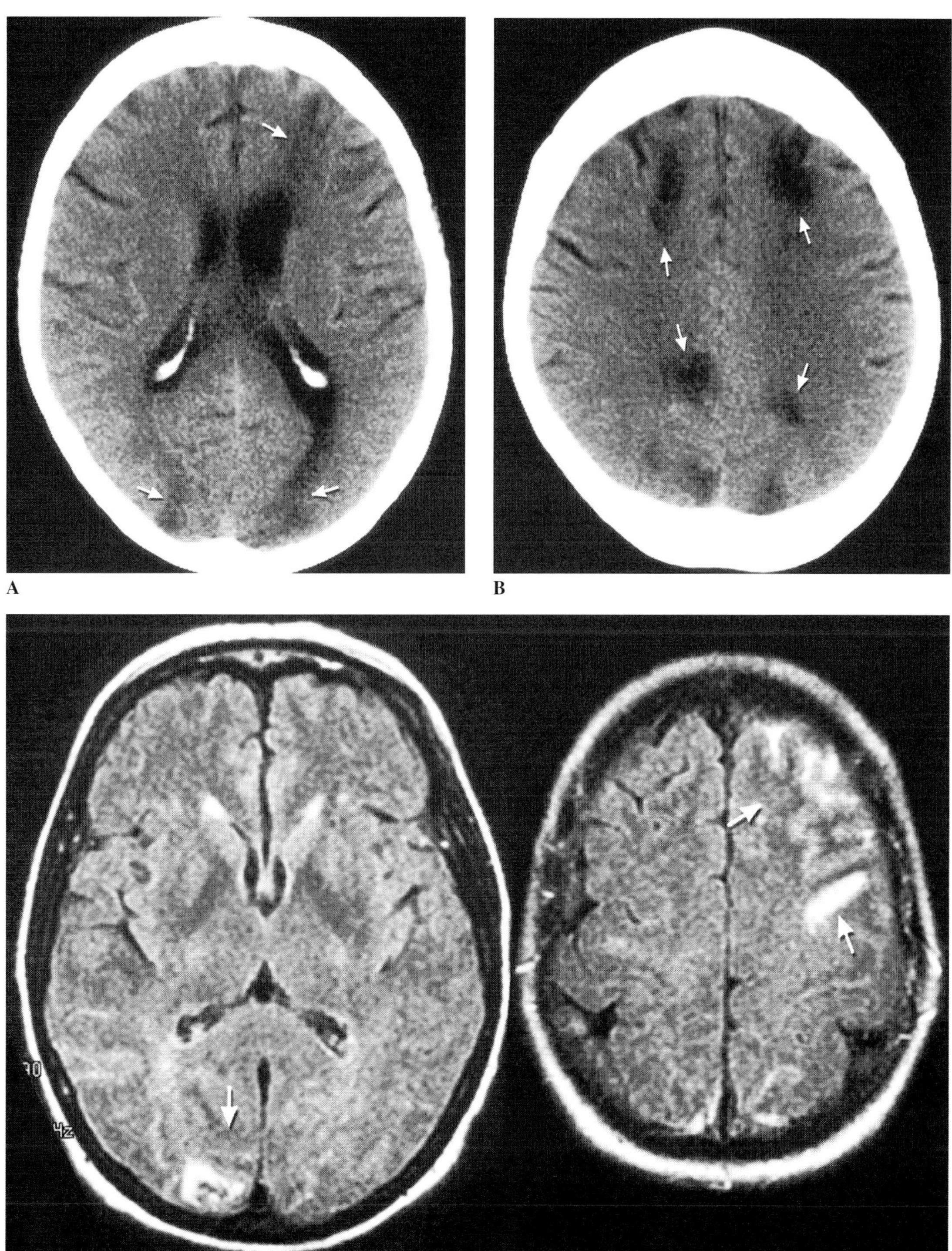

C

Figure 8.13. Computed tomography **(A–B)** and magnetic resonance imaging **(C)** show multiple infarcts associated with central nervous system vasculitis.

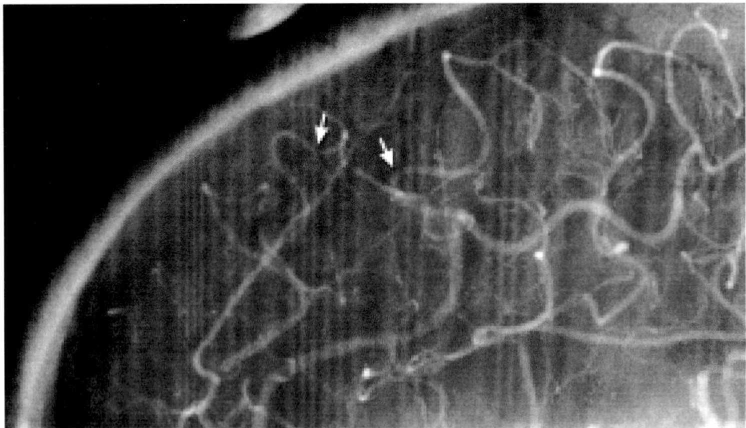

Figure 8.13. *Continued.* **D.** Cerebral angiographic findings of segmental stenosis and beading are typical.

brobasilar system may be suggestive of atheromatous disease), and radiation-induced occlusive vasculopathy (abnormalities inside the radiation field).[74,75] The inflammatory changes in the wall eventually lead to fibrosis and may lead to fixed angiographic narrowing.[76]

Blood and Serology. It is important to exclude a connective tissue disorder by measurement of antinuclear antibody, rheumatoid factor, antineutrophil cytoplasmic antibodies, sedimentation rate, and serology against human immunodeficiency virus, herpes zoster virus, cytomegalovirus, syphilis, and *Toxoplasma*. It is also important to obtain a urinary sample for amphetamines.

Cerebrospinal Fluid. A profound inflammatory response is usually absent, including in patients with progressive disease. Mildly increased protein may be the only sign. Mild pleocytosis ($\leq$20 lymphocytes/mm^3) has been found in fewer than 50% of cases.[77]

Brain Biopsy. Biopsy should involve the area that is abnormal on MRI, and available series claim 70% sensitivity. Random brain biopsy has a very low yield and probably should be deferred if angiographic findings are diagnostic and the cerebrospinal fluid is normal. The biopsy specimen, which should include the dura, leptomeninges, cortex, and white matter, is fixed in 10% buffered formalin for light microscopy.[78] Tissue samples should be frozen or stored with dry ice for later interpretation by electron microscopy. The pathologic hallmark is an infiltrate consisting of lymphocytes, histiocytes, and plasma cells involving the intima or media, with occasional necrosis of both leptomeningeal and intracerebral vessels.[79] Giant cells may be seen in areas of fragmented internal elastic lamina. Prominent necrosis should suggest polyarteritis nodosa. (Unfortunately, less characteristic or ambiguous pathologic findings may be the only result after a brain biopsy.)

First Priority in Management

Only aggressive treatment with corticosteroids, 1.5 mg/kg per day, and cyclophosphamide, 2 mg/kg per day orally, can reverse CNS vasculitis, and it should be started early. Corticosteroid administration can be tapered after 4 weeks, but cyclophosphamide, which has very low side effects with this dose, should be given for 1 year. The patient should be familiar with a 20% risk of infertility from cyclophosphamide, and egg or sperm harvesting should be offered. Famotidine should be added for stomach ulcer protection, and liberal hydration and frequent monitoring of the white blood cell count are respectively needed to reduce the risk of hemorrhagic cystitis and change the dose in case of neutropenia.

Predictors of Outcome

Recurrence is common when patients are treated with corticosteroids only. Outcome can be very good after aggressive combination therapy with administration of cyclophosphamide for at least 1 year (the estimated relapse rate then is <10%). Corticosteroid doses can be tapered after 6 months. Mortality is uncommon, and functional outcome is good.

Triage

- Urgent cerebral angiography and neurosurgical consultation for possible cerebral biopsy.
- Neurology ward.

Hematologic Disorders

Albeit unusual, disorders of coagulation, disorders of the structure of red blood cells, and platelet dysfunction may cause multiple cerebral infarcts in rapid succession.[80,81] These disorders may not be apparent with routine automated laboratory evaluation in the emergency department, which measures only white blood cell count, platelet count, and sedimentation rate. Both small and large arteries may become occluded, and neurologic deficits may vary. Noteworthy clinical features of these hematologic disorders are discussed in this section.

Clinical Presentation

Red Blood Cell Disorder. Sickle cell syndromes are rather prevalent, in most instances caused by a single amino acid substitution in the globin beta chains (valine instead of glutamic acid). Sickle cell disease or sickle cell tract (heterozygotic state) is more prevalent in African-American patients, often manifested after a hypoxemic trigger, cold, or excessive alcohol consumption. Sickled masses of red blood cells occlude arterial and venous systems, but other mechanisms, such as vasculopathy or fat embolization from infarcted bone marrow, may be operative. Stroke as a first presentation of sickle cell disease has rarely been documented, but earlier ischemic strokes, predominantly those localized in the subcortical white matter, may be silent. One should inquire about previous episodes of *Streptococcus pneumoniae* infections, osteomyelitis by *Salmonella* species, painless hematuria, painful priapism, retinal-vitreous hemorrhage, or crises resulting in chest and abdominal pain.

Polycythemia vera, a more complex disorder of increased erythrocytes and platelets, causes increased viscosity. It should be considered in patients with plethora, generalized pruritus, splenomegaly, headaches, and paresthesias. With a prevalence of 5 cases per 1 million persons, it is very uncommon.

Polycythemia may occur as a consequence of hypoxemia with cyanotic heart disease or obstructive pulmonary disease, but its association with ischemic stroke is less evident, also because precise understanding of the mechanism is lacking.

Platelet Disorders. Thrombotic thrombocytopenic purpura should be considered in multiple strokes of undetermined cause when patients present with a documented gradual decrease in platelet count. Middle-aged women are predominantly affected. Characteristic additional clinical signs are hematuria, myalgia, bloody diarrhea, fever, and, in some patients, rapidly developing renal failure. These symptoms, caused by systemic platelet microthrombi, may not appear in 25% of cases, and ischemic stroke may be the defining illness. Seizures are comparatively frequent, and nonconvulsive status epilepticus may be a presenting feature. Headache, acute confusional episodes, and hemiparesis may progress to coma if not aggressively treated with plasma exchange.

Thrombocytosis may occur in many underlying disorders, often chronic myeloid leukemia and myelofibrosis, or as a myeloproliferative disorder itself. Cerebrovascular manifestations, although recognized as a complication of myeloproliferative disorders, are not well studied.

Antiphospholipid Antibody Syndrome. This increasingly recognized syndrome associated with antiphospholipid antibodies is a common manifestation in younger patients.[82,83] Both anticardiolipin antibodies and lupus anticoagulants can be demonstrated, but they may not be linked to each other. Evidence of arterial occlusions (ocular, peripheral artery, pulmonary, or mesenteric artery) or venous occlusions (deep venous thrombosis), miscarriages, and prior unexplained pulmonary hypertension are clues to the diagnosis. In 20% of patients, ischemic stroke is part of this syndrome. Inappropriate treatment results in a high rate of recurrence of cerebral infarction.[82–84] Clinical features may include cardiac bruit (from associated mitral valve lesions or, possibly, Libman-Sacks endocarditis) and livedo reticularis.[84] Blotchy hands and feet should point to the diagnosis (Color Plate 15).

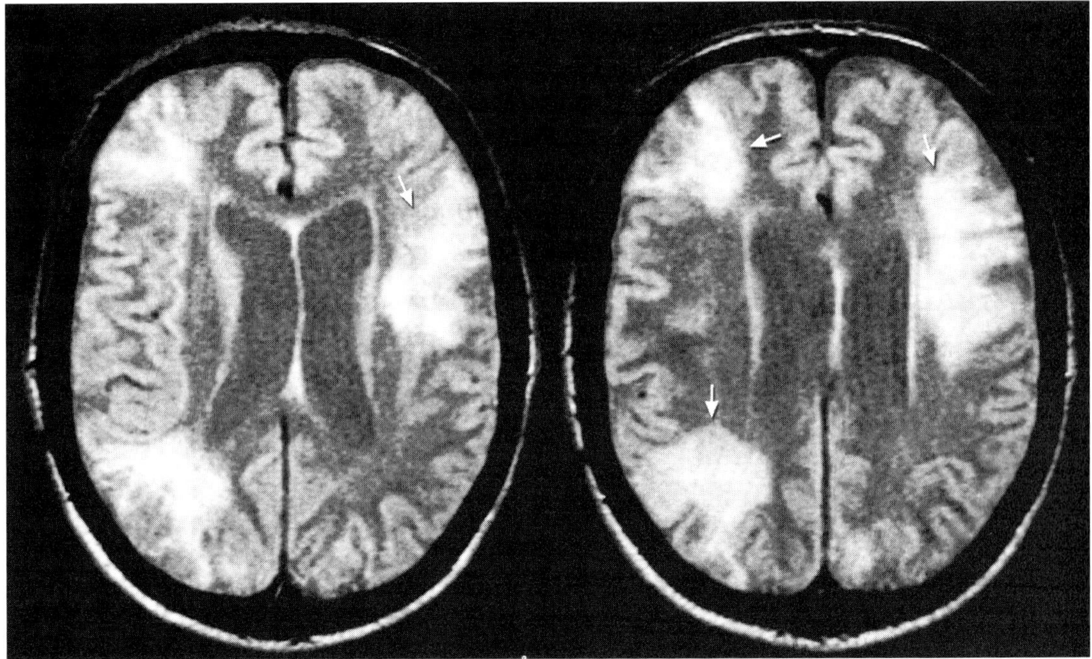

Figure 8.14. Magnetic resonance images showing multiple ischemic infarcts (*arrows*) in antiphospholipid antibody syndrome.

Interpretations of Laboratory Tests

Blood and Serum. Hemoglobin electrophoresis yields the diagnosis in sickle cell disease. Associated findings are increased leukocyte count, recent decrease in hemoglobin concentration (hemolytic anemia), and hyperbilirubinemia.

Polycythemia vera is diagnosed by increases in hematocrit and white cell count and, at later stages, bone marrow metaplasia. Laboratory criteria (minor criteria) are platelets >400,000/μL, leukocytes >12,000/μL, leukocyte alkaline phosphatase score >100, and vitamin B_{12} >900 pg/mL.

Thrombotic thrombocytopenic purpura is considered when the following laboratory findings are present: fragmented red blood cells (schistocytes, or helmet cells), increased reticulocytes, unconjugated bilirubinemia with normal prothrombin time and partial thromboplastin time, and normal fibrin degradation products differentiating it from disseminated intravascular coagulation and antiphospholipid antibody syndrome. Lactate dehydrogenase is greatly increased. Haptoglobin should be low or even unmeasurable.

Anticardiolipid antibodies can be determined, but only a high titer of IgG is diagnostic[85] (many laboratories define high titer as 20 to 100 IgG phospholipid units or more). IgM titers may vary significantly and can be increased by nonspecific stimuli, such as fever, infection, and pharmaceutical agents. Activated partial thromboplastin time is a good screening test. Prolonged thrombocytopenia may occur in one-third of the patients with antiphospholipid antibody syndrome.

Magnetic Resonance Imaging. Multiple cerebral infarcts, often involving branches of the ACA and MCA territory, are nonspecific but can be visualized on MRI with much higher sensitivity. The study is particularly diagnostic in thrombotic thrombocytopenic purpura and antiphospholipid antibody syndrome (Figure 8.14).

First Priority in Management

The recommended management options for specific hematologic disorders are summarized in Table 8.7. Specific treatment in these disorders is seldom started

Table 8.7. Management of Stroke in Unusual Hematologic Disorders

Disorder	Management
Sickle-cell disease	Exchange transfusion Oral folate
Polycythemia vera	Phlebotomy, 500 mL (aim at hematocrit ≤42%) Hydroxyurea, 500 mg twice daily
Thrombotic thrombocytopenic purpura	Plasma exchange (up to three exchanges) Prednisone, 60 mg Alternatively, intravenous immunoglobulin, 1–2 g/kg
Thrombocytosis (any cause)	Plateletpheresis Avoid anticoagulation
Antiphospholipid antibody syndrome	Heparin and long-term warfarin (international normalized ratio, 3 or 4) Cyclophosphamide (when associated with systemic lupus erythematosus)

immediately in the emergency room because of the necessary delay for diagnostic tests. Administration of corticosteroids in patients with presumed clinical CNS vasculitis is advised, and it should begin if no other causes are evident and if the patient is known to have collagen vascular disease. Brain biopsy within days in corticosteroid-treated patients should not mask inflammation and certainly not necrosis.

Predictors of Outcome

Outcome is difficult to predict because of the rarity of the disorders; thus, general rules apply. Multiple small vessel occlusions may result in full recovery. Untreated, the disorders may lead to multi-infarct dementia, disabling hemiplegia, and speech and language disorders.

Triage

- Neurologic ward.
- Intensive care unit in life-threatening thrombotic thrombocytopenic purpura, sickle cell crises, and evidence of other sites of vascular occlusion.
- Concomitant medical illnesses may warrant admission to a medical or surgical intensive care unit.
- Hematology consultation and consideration of bone marrow biopsy.

Cerebral Venous Thrombosis

Cerebral venous sinus thrombosis is rare, equally distributed in males and females; however, the incidence rises steeply in the second and third decades in women, because of its association with the use of oral contraceptives. The clinical spectrum of cerebral venous sinus thrombosis varies from a mild headache to progressive papilledema with rapidly deteriorating multiple hemorrhagic infarcts. The disorder is an acute neurologic emergency that may have a catastrophic outcome if not timely treated with intravenous heparin and, if available, endovascular lysis of the propagating thrombus within the cerebral venous system. Many conditions can be associated with cerebral venous thrombosis; however, despite extensive laboratory tests and increasingly sophisticated evaluation of coagulopathies, up to one-third of the cases remain entirely unexplained. Causes associated with cerebral venous thrombosis are oral contraceptive use, pregnancy, the puerperium, antiphospholipid antibody syndrome and lupus anticoagulant, congenital coagulopathies, and damage to the jugular vein associated with surgical trauma, sacrifice, or direct cannulation. Infectious causes, such as acute sinusitis, mastoiditis, infections involving the facial skin, and dental abscesses, need immediate recognition and treatment.

Clinical Presentation

The common early feature is headache refractory to commonly prescribed pain medication. The headache is related to increased intracranial pressure, which in turn is associated with venous hypertension. Venous hypertension reduces the reabsorption of cerebrospinal fluid and results in papilledema. The progression of headache, seizures, and focal neurologic deficits is rapid, in days, but in approximately one-third of the patients, the course may be protracted.[86] Cerebral infarction is typically hemorrhagic and may involve multiple territories. When multiple cerebral infarcts cause substantial swelling, herniation can occur.[87] A large intracranial temporal hematoma may progress to uncal herniation syndrome. Involvement of a cortical vein alone is rare. Commonly, the vein of Labbé is involved in these types of cortical infarcts, which are located in the parietal temporal region. (This vein is the largest superficial vein and mostly drains the posterior temporal region.) Cortical vein thrombosis may be manifested by focal or generalized seizures evolving into focal neurologic findings such as aphasia and hemiparesis.[88]

Interpretation of Diagnostic Tests

Neuroimaging

A typical CT scan feature is the cord sign, representing clot in the transverse sinus (Figures 8.15 and 8.16). CT scanning may show multiple hemorrhagic infarcts with early swelling. MRI and MRA usually are diagnostic and reveal the extent of venous thrombosis. Flow void is absent, and thrombus appears hyperintense on T1-weighted and hypointense on T2-weighted images[89,90] (Figure 8.17). In a recent study of transcranial Doppler ultrasonography, increased flow velocities or asymmetries in venous flow velocities were noted,[91] but the practical value of the technique in the emergency department is not known, and extent can be better defined by MRI and magnetic resonance venography.

Serum

A propensity toward thrombosis should be examined by measuring antithrombin III, protein C and protein S deficiencies,[92] lupus anticoagulant, and antiphospholipid antibodies. Factor V Leiden and the recently discovered 20210A allele mutation of the prothrombin gene may increase the risk of cerebral venous thrombosis.[86,93,94]

First Priority in Management

There is a current shift in the management of cerebral venous thrombosis. Intravenous heparin has substantially reduced morbidity and mortality, even in patients with already developed hemorrhagic infarcts.[95] Low-molecular-weight heparin was not more effective in a small randomized trial.[96] Nonetheless, thrombosis may progress despite adequate anticoagulation. Recanalization with thrombolytic agents through a catheter in the thrombosed vein has been successful in some case series.[86,97]

Predictors of Outcome

In a large group of patients, 86% had good recovery, and patients with involvement of only a portion of the venous system had even better recovery.[86] Coma at presentation, seizures, and intracerebral hematomas do not predict poor outcome. A major discrepancy exists between the devastation seen on MRI and the outcome, and neuroimaging should not be a major factor in deciding on future care. Blindness from papilledema or seizures may become persistent sequelae.

Triage

- ♦ Patients receiving intravenous heparin who have progression: to the radiology suite for endovascular lysis of the clot (if expertise is available).
- ♦ Neurologic intensive care unit to consider evacuation of hemorrhagic mass.
- ♦ Treatment of increased intracranial pressure if multiple hemorrhagic infarcts and edema occur.

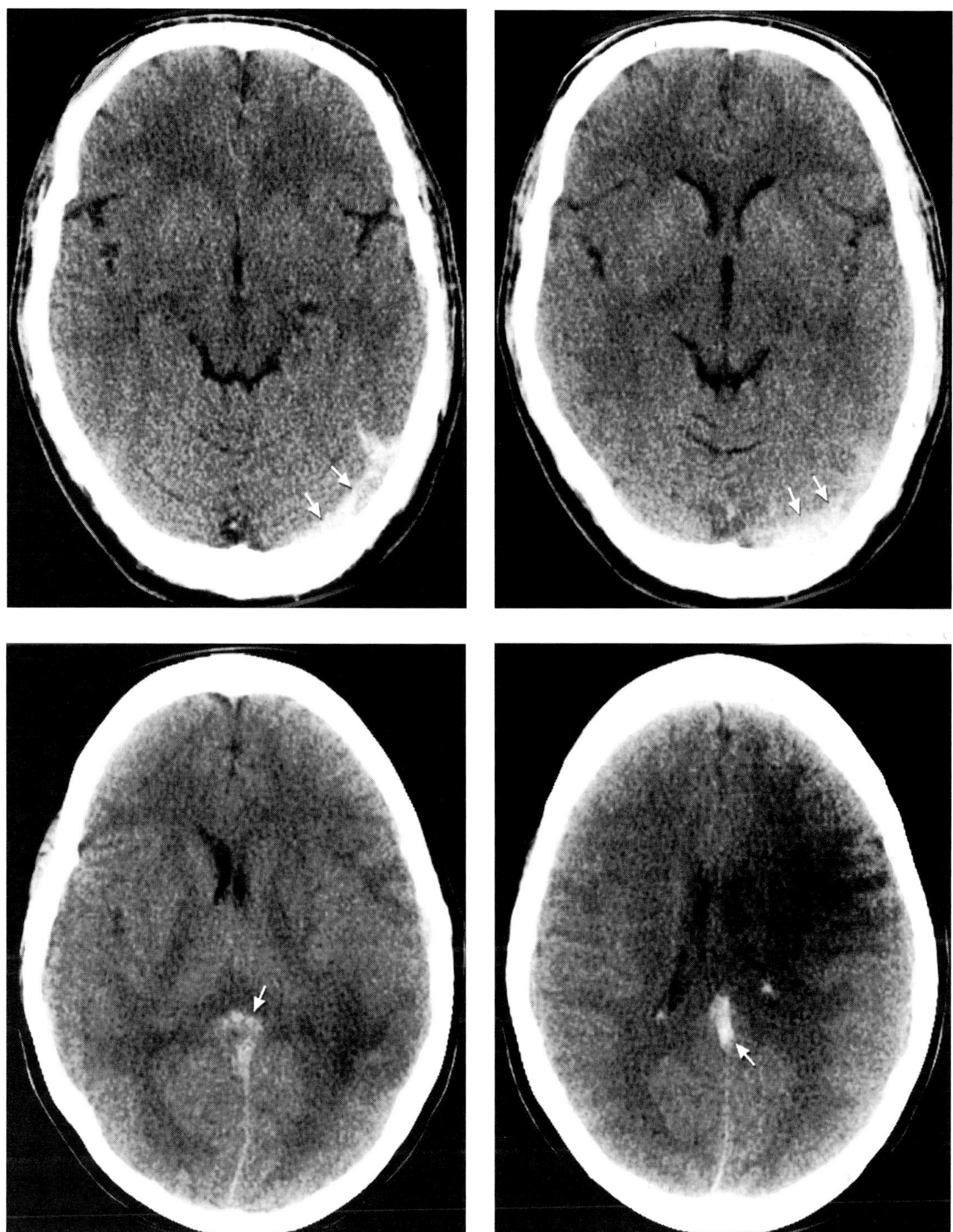

Figure 8.15. Computed tomography scan with "string sign" (transverse sinus). Note hyperdensity in sigmoid sinus, transverse sinus, and vein of Galen and straight sinus (*arrows*).

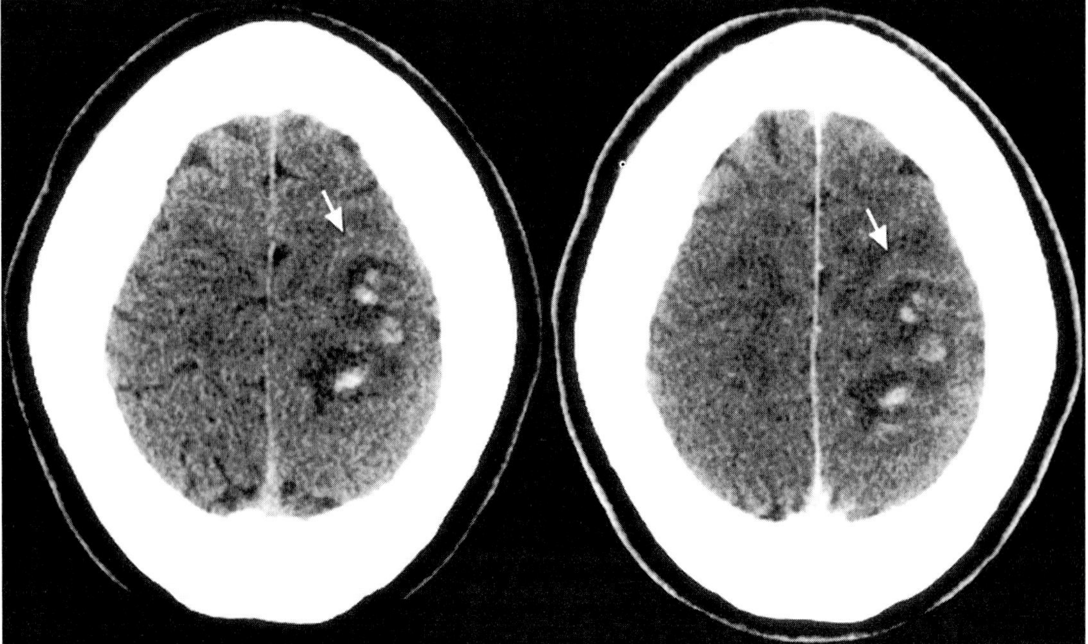

A

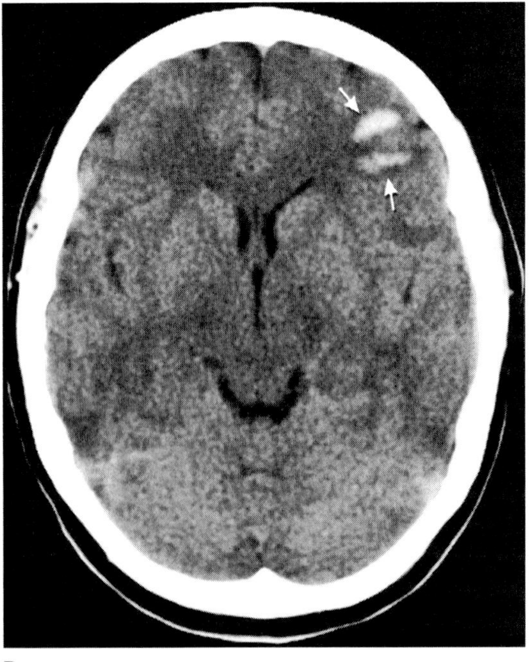

B

Figure 8.16. Hemorrhagic infarct from sagittal sinus thrombosis **(A)** and cortical venous thrombosis **(B).**

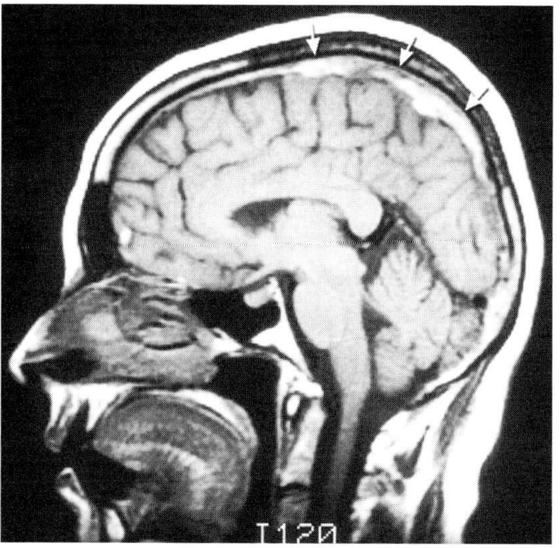

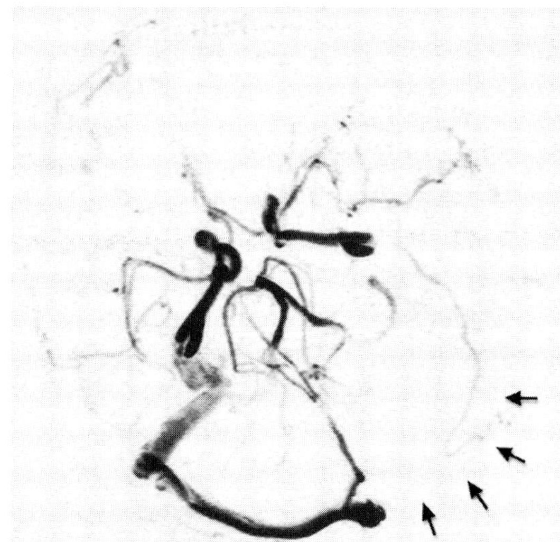

Figure 8.17. Magnetic resonance imaging and magnetic resonance angiography diagnosis of sagittal sinus and left transverse sinus thrombosis.

References

1. Caplan LR, Mohr JP, Kistler JP, Koroshetz W. Should thrombolytic therapy be the first-line treatment for acute ischemic stroke? Thrombolysis—not a panacea for ischemic stroke. N Engl J Med 1997;337:1309.
2. Hacke W, Kaste M, Fieschi C, et al. Randomised double-blind placebo-controlled trial of thrombolytic therapy with intravenous alteplase in acute ischaemic stroke (ECASS II). Lancet 1998;352:1245.
3. Wardlaw JM, Warlow CP, Counsell C. Systematic review of evidence on thrombolytic therapy for acute ischaemic stroke. Lancet 1997;350:607.
4. Hankey GJ. Thrombolytic therapy in acute ischaemic stroke: the jury needs more evidence. Med J Aust 1997;166:419.
5. Saito I, Segawa H, Shiokawa Y, et al. Middle cerebral artery occlusion: correlation of computed tomography and angiography with clinical outcome. Stroke 1987; 18:863.
6. Minematsu K, Yamaguchi T, Omae T. 'Spectacular shrinking deficit': rapid recovery from a major hemispheric syndrome by migration of an embolus. Neurology 1992;42:157.
7. Bogousslavsky J, Regli F. Anterior cerebral artery territory infarction in the Lausanne Stroke Registry. Clinical and etiologic patterns. Arch Neurol 1990;47:144.
8. Schwarz S, Egelhof T, Schwab S, Hacke W. Basilar artery embolism. Clinical syndrome and neuroradiologic patterns in patients without permanent occlusion of the basilar artery. Neurology 1997;49:1346.
9. Wijdicks EFM, Scott JP. Outcome in patients with acute basilar artery occlusion requiring mechanical ventilation. Stroke 1996;27:1301.
10. Tomura N, Uemura K, Inugami A, et al. Early CT finding in cerebral infarction: obscuration of the lentiform nucleus. Radiology 1988;168:463.
11. Russell EJ. Diagnosis of hyperacute ischemic infarct with CT: key to improved clinical outcome after intravenous thrombolysis? (Editorial.) Radiology 1997; 205:315.
12. Truwit CL, Barkovich AJ, Gean-Marton A, et al. Loss of the insular ribbon: another early CT sign of acute middle cerebral artery infarction. Radiology 1990; 176:801.
13. von Kummer R, Nolte PN, Schnittger H, et al. Detectability of cerebral hemisphere ischaemic infarcts by CT within 6 h of stroke. Neuroradiology 1996; 38:31.
14. Negishi C, Sze G. Vasculitis presenting as primary leptomeningeal enhancement with minimal parenchymal findings. AJNR Am J Neuroradiol 1993;14:26.
15. von Kummer R, Allen KL, Holle R, et al. Acute stroke: usefulness of early CT findings before thrombolytic therapy. Radiology 1997;205:327.
16. Wijdicks EFM, Diringer MN. Middle cerebral artery territory infarction and early brain swelling: progression and effect of age on outcome. Mayo Clin Proc 1998;73:829.
17. Motto C, Aritzu E, Boccardi E, et al. Reliability of hemorrhagic transformation diagnosis in acute ischemic stroke. Stroke 1997;28:302.
18. Tomsick T, Brott T, Barsan W, et al. Prognostic value of the hyperdense middle cerebral artery sign and stroke scale score before ultraearly thrombolytic therapy. AJNR Am J Neuroradiol 1996;17:79.
19. Wildenhain SL, Jungreis CA, Barr J, et al. CT after intracranial intraarterial thrombolysis for acute stroke. AJNR Am J Neuroradiol 1994;15:487.

20. Kertesz A, Black SE, Nicholson L, Carr T. The sensitivity and specificity of MRI in stroke. Neurology 1987;37:1580.
21. Bryan RN, Levy LM, Whitlow WD, et al. Diagnosis of acute cerebral infarction: comparison of CT and MR imaging. AJNR Am J Neuroradiol 1991;12:611.
22. Katz BH, Quencer RM, Kaplan JO, et al. MR imaging of intracranial carotid occlusion. AJR Am J Roentgenol 1989;152:1271.
23. Fisher M, Prichard JW, Warach S. New magnetic resonance techniques for acute ischemic stroke. JAMA 1995;274:908.
24. Lutsep HL, Albers GW, DeCrespigny A, et al. Clinical utility of diffusion-weighted magnetic resonance imaging in the assessment of ischemic stroke. Ann Neurol 1997;41:574.
25. Zivin JA. Diffusion-weighted MRI for diagnosis and treatment of ischemic stroke (editorial). Ann Neurol 1997;41:567.
26. van Everdingen KJ, van der Grond J, Kappelle LJ, et al. Diffusion-weighted magnetic resonance imaging in acute stroke. Stroke 1998;29:1783.
27. Singer MB, Chong J, Lu D, et al. Diffusion-weighted MRI in acute subcortical infarction. Stroke 1998;29:133.
28. Bahn MM, Oser AB, Cross DT III. CT and MRI of stroke. J Magn Reson Imaging 1996;6:833.
29. Shrier DA, Tanaka H, Numaguchi Y, et al. CT angiography in the evaluation of acute stroke. AJNR Am J Neuroradiol 1997;18:1011.
30. Brant-Zawadzki M. CT angiography in acute ischemic stroke: the right tool for the job? AJNR Am J Neuroradiol 1997;18:1021.
31. Knauth M, von Kummer R, Jansen O, et al. Potential of CT angiography in acute ischemic stroke. AJNR Am J Neuroradiol 1997;18:1001.
32. Na DG, Byun HS, Lee KH, et al. Acute occlusion of the middle cerebral artery: early evaluation with triphasic helical CT—preliminary results. Radiology 1998;207:113.
33. The National Institute of Neurological Disorders and Stroke rt-PA Stroke Study Group. Tissue plasminogen activator for acute ischemic stroke. N Engl J Med 1995;333:1581.
34. Gönner F, Remonda L, Mattle H, et al. Local intra-arterial thrombolysis in acute ischemic stroke. Stroke 1998;29:1894.
35. Wijdicks EFM, Nichols DA, Thielen KR, et al. Intra-arterial thrombolysis in acute basilar artery thromboembolism: the initial Mayo Clinic experience. Mayo Clin Proc 1997;72:1005.
36. del Zoppo GJ, Higashida RT, Furlan AJ, et al. PROACT: a phase II randomized trial of recombinant pro-urokinase by direct arterial delivery in acute middle cerebral artery stroke. Stroke 1998;29:4.
37. Scott JF, Robinson GM, French JM, et al. Prevalence of admission hyperglycaemia across clinical subtypes of acute stroke (letter to the editor). Lancet 1999;353:376.
38. Hacke W, Schwab S, Horn M, et al. 'Malignant' middle cerebral artery territory infarction: clinical course and prognostic signs. Arch Neurol 1996;53:309.
39. Cross DT III, Moran CJ, Akins PT, et al. Relationship between clot location and outcome after basilar artery thrombolysis. AJNR Am J Neuroradiol 1997;18:1221.
40. Caplan LR, Baquis GD, Pessin MS, et al. Dissection of the intracranial vertebral artery. Neurology 1988;38:868.
41. Fisher CM, Ojemann RG, Roberson GH. Spontaneous dissection of cervico-cerebral arteries. Can J Neurol Sci 1978;5:9.
42. Mokri B, Houser OW, Sandok BA, Piepgras DG. Spontaneous dissections of the vertebral arteries. Neurology 1988;38:880.
43. Mokri B, Sundt TM Jr, Houser OW, Piepgras DG. Spontaneous dissection of the cervical internal carotid artery. Ann Neurol 1986;19:126.
44. Mizutani T, Aruga T, Kirino T, et al. Recurrent subarachnoid hemorrhage from untreated ruptured vertebrobasilar dissecting aneurysms. Neurosurgery 1995;36:905.
45. Schievink WI, Wijdicks EFM, Kuiper JD. Seasonal pattern of spontaneous cervical artery dissection. J Neurosurg 1998;89:101.
46. Houser OW, Baker HL Jr. Fibromuscular dysplasia and other uncommon diseases of the cervical carotid artery: angiographic aspects. Am J Roentgenol Radium Ther Nucl Med 1968;104:201.
47. Schievink WI, Michels VV, Mokri B, et al. Brief report: a familial syndrome of arterial dissections with lentiginosis. N Engl J Med 1995;332:576.
48. Schievink WI, Wijdicks EFM, Michels VV, et al. Heritable connective tissue disorders in cervical artery dissections: a prospective study. Neurology 1998;50:1166.
49. Mokri B, Piepgras DG, Houser OW. Traumatic dissections of the extracranial internal carotid artery. J Neurosurg 1988;68:189.
50. Mokri B, Meyer FB, Piepgras DG. Primary arteriopathy in traumatic cervicocephalic arterial dissections (abstract). Ann Neurol 1997;42:433.
51. Schievink WI, Mokri B, Garrity JA, et al. Ocular motor nerve palsies in spontaneous dissections of the cervical internal carotid artery. Neurology 1993;43:1938.
52. Biousse V, D'Anglejan-Chatillon J, Touboul PJ, et al. Time course of symptoms in extracranial carotid artery dissections. A series of 80 patients. Stroke 1995;26:235.
53. Steinke W, Schwartz A, Hennerici M. Topography of cerebral infarction associated with carotid artery dissection. J Neurol 1996;243:323.
54. Lucas C, Moulin T, Deplanque D, et al. Stroke patterns of internal carotid artery dissection in 40 patients. Stroke 1998;29:2646.
55. Yamaura A, Watanabe Y, Saeki N. Dissecting aneurysms of the intracranial vertebral artery. J Neurosurg 1990;72:183.
56. Kitanaka C, Tanaka J, Kuwahara M, Teraoka A. Magnetic resonance imaging study of intracranial vertebrobasilar artery dissections. Stroke 1994;25:571.
57. Provenzale JM. Dissection of the internal carotid and vertebral arteries: imaging features. AJR Am J Roentgenol

1995;165;1099.

58. Levy C, Laissy JP, Raveau V, et al. Carotid and vertebral artery dissections: three-dimensional time-of-flight MR angiography and MR imaging versus conventional angiography. Radiology 1994;190:97.
59. Hosoya T, Adachi M, Yamaguchi K, et al. Clinical and neuroradiological features of intracranial vertebrobasilar artery dissection. Stroke 1999;30:1083.
60. Schievink WI, Piepgras DG, McCaffrey TV, Mokri B. Surgical treatment of extracranial internal carotid artery dissecting aneurysms. Neurosurgery 1994;35:809.
61. Schievink WI, Mokri B, O'Fallon WM. Recurrent spontaneous cervical-artery dissection. N Engl J Med 1994;330:393.
62. Biller J, Loftus CM, Moore SA, et al. Isolated central nervous system angiitis first presenting as spontaneous intracranial hemorrhage. Neurosurgery 1987; 20:310.
63. Calabrese LH, Duna GF. Evaluation and treatment of central nervous system vasculitis. Curr Opin Rheumatol 1995;7:37.
64. Hankey GJ. Isolated angiitis/angiopathy of the central nervous system. Cerebrovasc Dis 1991;1:2.
65. Citron BP, Halpern M, McCarron M, et al. Necrotizing angiitis associated with drug abuse. N Engl J Med 1970;283:1003.
66. Martin K, Rogers T, Kavanaugh A. Central nervous system angiopathy associated with cocaine abuse. J Rheumatol 1995;22:780.
67. Matick H, Anderson D, Brumlik J. Cerebral vasculitis associated with oral amphetamine overdose. Arch Neurol 1983;40:253.
68. Giang DW. Central nervous system vasculitis secondary to infections, toxins, and neoplasms. Semin Neurol 1994;14:313.
69. Moore PM. Diagnosis and management of isolated angiitis of the central nervous system. Neurology 1989;39:167.
70. Moore PM, Cupps TR. Neurological complications of vasculitis. Ann Neurol 1983;14:155.
71. Kumar R, Wijdicks EFM, Brown RD Jr, et al. Isolated angiitis of the CNS presenting as subarachnoid haemorrhage. J Neurol Neurosurg Psychiatry 1997;62:649.
72. Greenan TJ, Grossman RI, Goldberg HI. Cerebral vasculitis: MR imaging and angiographic correlation. Radiology 1992;182:65.
73. Harris KG, Tran DD, Sickels WJ, et al. Diagnosing intracranial vasculitis: the roles of MR and angiography. AJNR Am J Neuroradiol 1994;15:317.
74. Brant-Zawadzki M, Anderson M, DeArmond SJ, et al. Radiation-induced large intracranial vessel occlusive vasculopathy. AJR Am J Roentgenol 1980;134:51.
75. Devinsky O. Radiation-induced cerebral vasculitis revisited (letter to the editor). Stroke 1988;19:784.
76. Alhalabi M, Moore PM. Serial angiography in isolated angiitis of the central nervous system. Neurology 1994;44:1221.
77. Stone JH, Pomper MG, Roubenoff R, et al. Sensitivities of noninvasive tests for central nervous system vasculitis: a comparison of lumbar puncture, computed tomography, and magnetic resonance imaging. J Rheumatol 1994;21:1277.
78. Parisi JE, Moore PM. The role of biopsy in vasculitis of the central nervous system. Semin Neurol 1994; 14:341.
79. Vollmer TL, Guarnaccia J, Harrington W, et al. Idiopathic granulomatous angiitis of the central nervous system. Diagnostic challenges. Arch Neurol 1993; 50:925.
80. Greaves M. Coagulation abnormalities and cerebral infarction (editorial). J Neurol Neurosurg Psychiatry 1993;56:433.
81. Hart RG, Kanter MC. Hematologic disorders and ischemic stroke. A selective review. Stroke 1990; 21:1111.
82. Levine SR, Brey RL, Sawaya KL, et al. Recurrent stroke and thrombo-occlusive events in the antiphospholipid syndrome. Ann Neurol 1995;38:119.
83. Levine SR, Deegan MJ, Futrell N, Welch KM. Cerebrovascular and neurologic disease associated with antiphospholipid antibodies: 48 cases. Neurology 1990;40:1181.
84. Lockshin MD. Antiphospholipid antibody syndrome. JAMA 1992;268:1451.
85. Tanne D, Triplett DA, Levine SR. Antiphospholipid-protein antibodies and ischemic stroke: not just cardiolipin any more. Stroke 1998;29:1755.
86. Bousser M-G, Russell RR. Cerebral venous thrombosis. Major Probl Neurol 1997;33:1.
87. Villringer A, Einhaupl KM. Dural sinus and cerebral venous thrombosis. New Horiz 1997;5:332.
88. Jacobs K, Moulin T, Bogousslavsky J, et al. The stroke syndrome of cortical vein thrombosis. Neurology 1996;47:376.
89. Corvol JC, Oppenheim C, Manai R, et al. Diffusion-weighted magnetic resonance imaging in a case of cerebral venous thrombosis. Stroke 1998;29:2649.
90. Perkin GD. Cerebral venous thrombosis: developments in imaging and treatment. J Neurol Neurosurg Psychiatry 1995;59:1.
91. Stolz E, Kaps M, Dorndorf W. Assessment of intracranial venous hemodynamics in normal individuals and patients with cerebral venous thrombosis. Stroke 1999;30:70.
92. Lefebvre P, Lierneux B, Lenaerts L, et al. Cerebral venous thrombosis and procoagulant factors—a case study. Angiology 1998;49:563.
93. Ludemann P, Nabavi DG, Junker R, et al. Factor V Leiden mutation is a risk factor for cerebral venous thrombosis: a case-control study of 55 patients. Stroke 1998; 29:2507.
94. Biousse V, Conard J, Brouzes C, et al. Frequency of the 20210 G—>A mutation in the 3'-untranslated region of the prothrombin gene in 35 cases of cerebral venous thrombosis. Stroke 1998;29:1398.

95. Wingerchuk DM, Wijdicks EFM, Fulgham JR. Cerebral venous thrombosis complicated by hemorrhagic infarction: factors affecting the initiation and safety of anticoagulation. Cerebrovasc Dis 1998;8:25.
96. de Bruijn SFTM, Stam J, for the Cerebral Venous Sinus Thrombosis Study Group. Randomized, placebo-controlled trial of anticoagulant treatment with low-molecular-weight heparin for cerebral sinus thrombosis. Stroke 1999;30:484.
97. Frey JL, Muro GJ, McDougall CG, et al. Cerebral venous thrombosis: combined intrathrombus rtPA and intravenous heparin. Stroke 1999;30:489.

Chapter 9

Acute Bacterial Infections of the Central Nervous System

Bacterial seeding of the brain may exert its destructive effect at an early stage in the clinical course. Delay in diagnosis due to difficulty to appreciate nonspecific symptoms or, equally common, failure to act timely when signs become apparent contributes to later morbidity.[1] Indeed, the vexing concern for any physician is to recognize a bacterial infection when obvious signs, such as fever, confusion, skin rash, and recent sinusitis or otitis, are absent. Intracranial abscesses may be first unmasked only after a single seizure without fever. In adults, the most common causative organisms in community-acquired meningitis are *Streptococcus pneumoniae*, *Neisseria meningitidis*, *Listeria monocytogenes*, and *Haemophilus influenzae*.[2,3] From the onset, it is clear that the priorities in evaluation (computed tomography [CT] or cerebrospinal fluid [CSF]) of a presumed bacterial meningitis are complicated.[4] Also, management in bacterial meningitis caused by *S. pneumoniae* or *N. meningitidis* has become problematic with the emergence of organisms resistant to penicillin and cephalosporin. Without question, a medical debacle may evolve rapidly in the first hour after entry to the emergency department. This chapter focuses on early aggressive management of common bacterial infections of the central nervous system. It emphasizes avoidance of pitfalls and provides guidelines to make clinical decisions simple and straightforward.

Acute Bacterial Meningitis

The pathophysiology of bacterial meningitis involves many pathways that may, at least in the most severe cases, lead to cerebral edema, brain tissue displacement, and, probably most important, cerebral infarction. The consequences of meningeal inflammation are discussed in Capsule 9.1.

Clinical Presentation

In most adults, a healthy state is first interrupted by an upper respiratory tract infection or ear infection, and antibiotic therapy does not make any major progress. Thus, potential sources for acute bacterial meningitis, such as pneumonia, paranasal sinusitis, and middle ear infection, should be sought. These sources are more prevalent in patients with profound comorbidity, such as diabetes mellitus, prior transplantation, long-term dialysis, splenectomy, or alcoholism.

Characteristic symptoms and signs of acute bacterial meningitis are fever, headache, and reduced alertness. The degree of fever in bacterial meningitis may vary. Most patients have so-called hectic temperature, with an increase to 39°C or 40°C, but low-grade fever may be present in the elderly, immunosuppressed patients, or patients who have been taking oral antibi-

Capsule 9.1. Pathogenesis of Bacterial Meningitis and Its Consequences

A common sequence in the development of bacterial meningitis is as follows: Nasopharyngeal colonization occurs and is dependent on fimbriae and specific surface cell receptors. Attachment may be facilitated by previous viral infection. It is followed by development of bacteremia. The polysaccharide capsule should counter the classic complement pathway or alternative complement pathway (common in patients with underlying sickle cell disease and splenectomy) and defy phagocytosis. Next is meningeal invasion and entrance into the cerebrospinal fluid through the choroid plexus, again facilitated by receptors. The bactericidal activity in the subarachnoid space is poor because the complement activity needed to initiate phagocytosis is low. Then an inflammatory response is mounted by components of the lysed bacterial cell mass (teichoic acid endotoxin), which induce production of inflammatory cytokines (tumor necrosis factor, interleukin-1, and macrophage inhibitory protein). Neutrophils invade, and blood-brain barrier permeability increases, finally causing vasogenic brain edema. The toxic oxygen metabolites cause cytotoxic edema, and cerebrospinal fluid outflow resistance from protein-rich exudate in the subarachnoid space produces interstitial edema and hydrocephalus.

Cerebral infarcts from vasculitis, vasospasm of basal arteries, or thrombosis of the major venous sinuses may occur, possibly only in the most fulminant cases with virulent pathogens.[5–8]

otics or antipyretic drugs, all of whom may have greatly reduced mechanisms to mount this febrile response.[2] Temperature is usually constantly elevated, and marked temperature oscillations may therefore suggest a localized collection of pus (e.g., tonsillar, mastoid, or middle ear abscess).

More than 75% of patients with bacterial meningitis are confused, irritable, or stuporous. Most patients can be roused with a forcible command or painful stimulus. Elderly patients may simply have a blank expression and be motionless and withdrawn.[9,10]

Nuchal rigidity is common in bacterial meningitis. Flexion of the neck causes flexion in the hips and knees (Brudzinski's sign of meningismus). Cranial nerve involvement may include abducens nerve palsy as a false localizing sign of increased intracranial pressure, facial nerve palsy associated with mastoiditis, and, most worrisome, inflammation of the cochlear nerve leading to permanent hearing loss.

Seizures are more prevalent in children and young adults but may approach 10% in adults or the elderly. Seizures, particularly focal, can be attributed to focal edema, early cortical venous thrombosis, and cerebral infarction from occlusion of penetrating branches encased by the basal purulent exudate.

Generalized myoclonus may occur and should immediately prompt measurement of the level of penicillin or cephalosporin. It is common in patients with coexistent renal disease, which reduces excretion and allows penicillin or cephalosporins to accumulate to toxic levels.[11]

Rapidly developing coma with pathologic motor responses is uncommon in adults, but when present, it signals a fulminant variant with diffuse cerebral edema or multiple cerebral infarcts from secondary inflammatory vasculitis.[12] Increased intracranial pressure leading to cerebral herniation syndromes occurs in approximately 10% of patients. Rarely, meningeal veins become necrotic or thrombosed, a condition leading to extensive hemorrhagic cortical infarction and bihemispheric swelling.

Meningococcal meningitis may progress to shock from adrenal hemorrhages. Petechiae, widespread purpuric rash with patches of necrotic skin (Color Plates 16 through 19), conjunctival hemorrhage, and punctate lesions inside the mouth and on the lips are seen in conjunction with shock, profound hyponatremia, hyperkalemia (Addison's disease), and laboratory evidence of intravascular coagulation.

Tuberculous meningitis should be suspected in patients with human immunodeficiency virus (HIV) infection, malnutrition, drug abuse, homelessness, or any immunosuppressed state. Prodromal symptoms of coughing, weight loss, and night sweats followed by confusion and rapidly developing coma with cranial nerve deficits are frequent but nonspecific. Tubercles in the choroidea at ophthalmoscopy, hilar adenopathy on chest radiographs, and hydrocephalus on CT scans are additional indicators for tuberculous meningitis. In a recent series, 32 of 48 patients with adult tuberculous meningitis had an extrameningeal tuberculous location.[13]

Interpretation of Diagnostic Tests

Computed Tomography and Magnetic Resonance Imaging

CT scanning should precede CSF examination, because images can be acquired very quickly with modern CT scanners. The nonspecific presentation of fever, seizures, and neck stiffness may indicate a subdural empyema or an intracranial abscess with ventricular rupture rather than bacterial meningitis. When CT scanning is deferred, either of these conditions may theoretically worsen with lumbar puncture.

If diffuse cerebral edema is present, herniation may occur with lumbar puncture despite removal of a small amount of CSF (e.g., 5 mL) or the use of a smaller needle (e.g., 22 gauge), but herniation from fulminant meningitis may occur irrespective of lumbar puncture. CT scan images are typically normal in bacterial meningitis. Mild obstructive hydrocephalus (see Chapter 3), cerebral edema, and hypodensities from ischemic strokes have been reported in a small proportion of patients.[3,14] However, CT scan findings are abnormal in 51% of patients with tuberculous meningitis. Ventricular dilatation, superficial meningeal enhancement, and hypodensity representing cerebral infarcts are common in tuberculous meningitis.

Magnetic resonance imaging (MRI), particularly fluid-attenuated inversion recovery sequences, may reveal important findings in any type of bacterial meningitis because of its superb sensitivity; cerebral infarcts (Figure 9.1) or the inflammatory exudate[15] (Figure 9.2) may be detected. MRI may also document involvement of vestibular and cochlear structures in patients with hearing loss.[16]

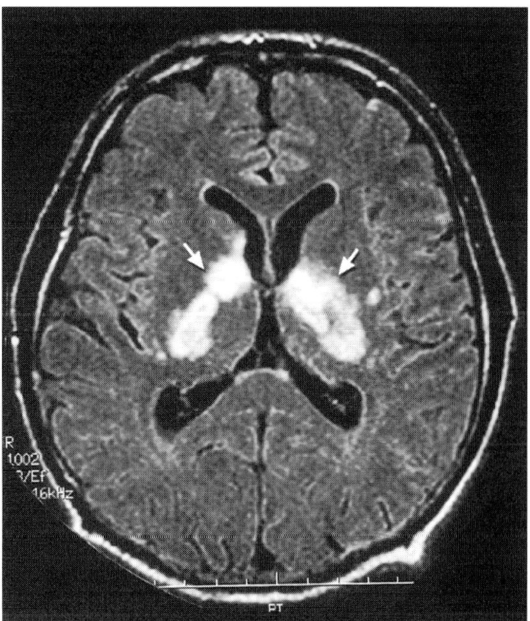

Figure 9.1. Magnetic resonance image with fluid-attenuated inversion recovery (FLAIR) sequences in patient with fulminant pneumococcal meningitis. Bilateral thalamic infarcts from penetrating branch occlusions are producing coma. (From Vernino et al.[15] By permission of the American Academy of Neurology.)

Cerebrospinal Fluid

The CSF in acute bacterial meningitis is typically turbid or xanthochromic, with increased opening pressure (>200 cm H_2O) and polymorphonuclear pleocytosis (cell count >1,000 cells/mm^3). Higher CSF leukocyte counts are less common in *S. pneumoniae* than in *N. meningitidis*, possibly a reflection of a poor immunocompetent state.[17] In addition, increased protein (often >100 mg/dL) and decreased glucose concentration (<40 mg/dL) are typical findings. CSF glucose should be compared with serum glucose, which may be increased as a stress response to the acute neurologic illness (normal ratio of CSF glucose to serum glucose is 0.6). Decreased CSF glucose concentration is typical of bacterial meningitis but may occur in fungal, tuberculous, or carcinomatous meningitis, in neurosarcoidosis, or, rarely, as a reflection of marked hypoglycemia. When CSF is bloody, the total white blood cell count is falsely increased, complicating interpretation. Red blood cells from a traumatic puncture increase the total cell count of 1 white blood cell per 700 red blood cells.

CSF lymphocytosis is most compatible with viral, fungal, and tuberculous meningitis. However, initial CSF lymphocytosis in bacterial meningitis was found in 6% of 428 patients and in 24% of patients with CSF leukocyte counts of fewer than 1,000 cells/mm^3, irrespective of previous antibiotic use.[17] A predomi-

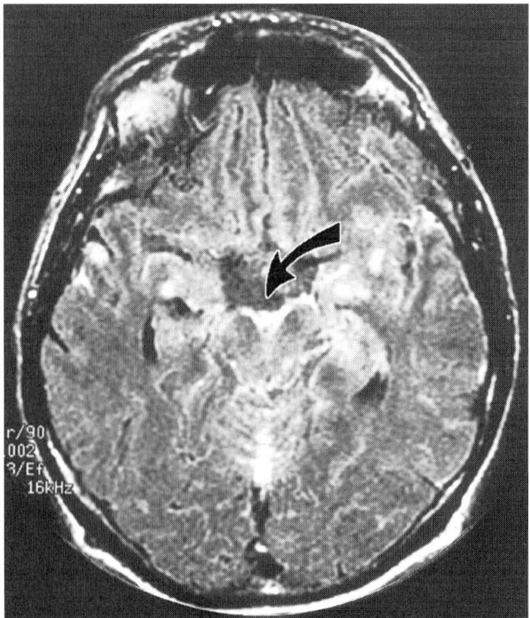

Figure 9.2. Magnetic resonance image with fluid-attenuated inversion recovery (FLAIR) sequences demonstrates purulent exudate (*arrow*) not visible on routine sequences or after gadolinium T1 enhancement. (From Vernino et al.[15] By permission of the American Academy of Neurology.)

nant CSF lymphocytosis may occur early in the ictus, most often associated with *L. monocytogenes* meningitis in immunosuppressed patients. If glucose concentration is decreased, predominant lymphocytes in the CSF formula should strongly point to the possibility of tuberculous or fungal meningitis.[18] At least three CSF samples are needed to obtain material for a smear; an enzyme-linked immunosorbent assay may visualize the tuberculous bacilli in 40% of smears. CSF cultures require up to 6 weeks for growth. On the other hand, fungal meningitis may not be detected with any of these tests, and meningeal biopsy may be needed. Other diagnostic tests are available to complement CSF cultures (Capsule 9.2).

First Priority in Management

Cephalosporins and vancomycin should be given intravenously at once, before any further diagnostic tests are ordered and, in fact, when the first purulent spinal fluid drops appear in the test tube. Recommended empirical therapy is shown in Figure 9.3. The addition of vancomycin is important to intermediately preempt cephalosporin-resistant *Streptococcus pneumoniae*, which has become increasingly frequent. Vancomycin administration should be closely monitored (aiming at a trough of 10 mg/mL and a peak serum level of 50 mg/mL) and continued for 14 days, if indicated. (Vestibular damage is uncommon from vancomycin and is much more likely from direct inflammation of the vestibular nerve due to meningitis.) Antibiotic therapy for specific organisms is summarized in Table 9.1. A combination of three antituberculous drugs is additionally needed if tuberculous meningitis is likely on the basis of the initial CSF formula and clinical presentation.[21] Dexamethasone is reserved for fulminant variants (e.g., brain edema, impending brain herniation), including tuberculous meningitis,[22] but its use is unproven in adult-onset bacterial meningitis.[23] Dexamethasone may seriously reduce penetration of cephalosporins and, particularly, vancomycin (Capsule 9.3).

Chemoprophylaxis is indicated in meningococcal meningitis and is administered to any person who had close contact with the patient. Recommendations

Capsule 9.2. Rapid Diagnostic Tests

Latex particle agglutination tests can rapidly detect bacterial antigens in purulent cerebrospinal fluid. The specificity is close to 100%; the sensitivity depends on the organism (*Haemophilus influenzae*, 78% to 86%; *Streptococcus pneumoniae*, 69% to 100%; *Neisseria meningitidis*, 33% to 70%). Experience with polymerase chain reaction in acute bacterial infection is limited. The technique is useful in certain unusual causes of bacterial infections, but processing takes from 12 hours to 3 days. It has a sensitivity of 70% to 80% in Lyme disease.

Gram's stain has a positive yield in 60% to 80% of patients, but the yield is much lower (40% to 50%) with previous antibiotic use. Acid-fast stain may diagnose tuberculosis in 35% to 80% of cases.[19,20]

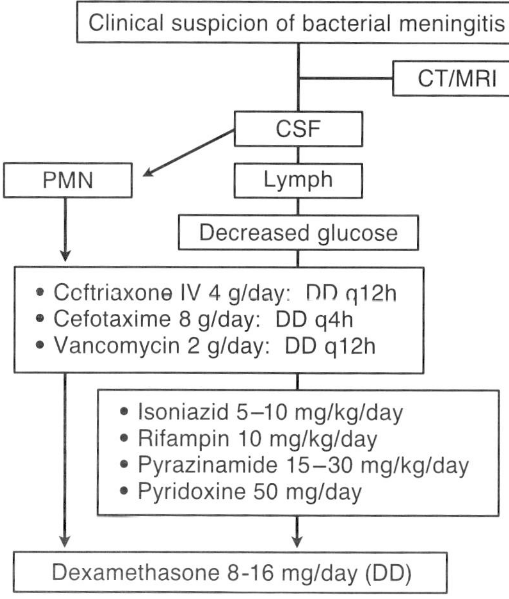

Figure 9.3. Empirical therapy for acute bacterial meningitis. (CSF = cerebrospinal fluid; CT = computed tomography; DD = divided dose; IV = intravenously; MRI = magnetic resonance imaging; PMN = polymorphonuclear cells.)

for chemoprophylaxis, which should be discussed in the emergency department, are shown in Table 9.2.

Predictors of Outcome

S. pneumoniae meningitis continues to cause sequelae such as hearing loss, seizures, personality change, and cognitive deficits.[26] Drug-resistant strains of pneumococci cause significantly higher mortality than other pneumococcal bacteria. Coma at onset or focal seizures increase the risk of death. Acute complications, such as brain edema and cerebral infarcts, significantly increase the chance of a persistent vegetative state. Many predictors of poor outcome have been identified in tuberculous meningitis, including extremes of age, malnutrition, miliary disease, hydrocephalus, documented ischemic stroke, and low total CD4 cell count in a subset with HIV infection.[18]

Triage

- Consider otolaryngologic evaluation before transport.

Table 9.1. Recommended Antimicrobial Therapy for Bacterial Meningitis

Organism	Antibiotic, total daily dose (dosing interval)
Neisseria meningitidis	Penicillin G, 20–24 million U/day IV (divided doses q4h) *or* Ampicillin, 12 g/day IV (q4h)
Streptococcus pneumoniae	Ceftriaxone *or* cefotaxime *plus* vancomycin
Gram-negative bacilli (except *Pseudomonas aeruginosa*)	Ceftriaxone, 2–4 g/day IV (q12h) *or* Cefotaxime, 8 g/day IV (q4h)
Pseudomonas aeruginosa	Ceftazidime, 6–12 g/day IV (q8h), and gentamicin, 5 mg/kg IV (divided doses q8h)
Haemophilus influenzae type b	Ceftriaxone *or* cefotaxime
Staphylococcus aureus (methicillin-sensitive)	Oxacillin, 9–12 g/day IV (q4h)
Staphylococcus aureus (methicillin-resistant)	Vancomycin, 2 g/day IV (q12h)
Listeria monocytogenes	Ampicillin, 12 g/day IV (q4h)
Enterobacteriaceae	Cefotaxime, 12 g/day (q4h), or ceftriaxone, 4–6 g/day (q12h)

Modified from Roos KL, Tunkel AR, Scheld WM. Acute bacterial meningitis in children and adults. In WM Scheld, RJ Whitley, DT Durack (eds). Infections of the Central Nervous System, 2nd ed. Philadelphia: Lippincott–Raven Publishers, 1997;335. By permission of the publisher.

- Admission to a neurologic intensive care unit is indicated to monitor the development of cerebral edema or, more commonly, hydrocephalus.
- If seizures have occurred, loading with fosphenytoin or phenytoin, 20 mg/kg intravenously, is advised before transport.

Subdural Empyema and Epidural Abscess

Sinusitis, recent sinus surgery, and, less commonly, otitis or traumatic brain injury are sources that may cause infection of the subdural space. Infection may spread directly, through erosion of the posterior

Capsule 9.3. Dexamethasone in Bacterial Meningitis

Dexamethasone reduces the production of cytokines and thus reduces the inflammatory response. Dexamethasone may reduce permeability of the blood-brain barrier and thus reduce cerebral edema. However, reduction of meningeal inflammation may reduce the penetration of antibiotics that require an impaired blood-brain barrier.

Dexamethasone reduces mortality, deafness, and neurologic deficits in children with bacterial meningitis caused by *Haemophilus influenzae*. Dexamethasone also reduces morbidity in tuberculous meningitis, but only in the most severe cases. In fulminant bacterial meningitis, dexamethasone is arbitrarily recommended for 4 days. Preferably, dexamethasone should be administered 30 minutes or less prior to the first antibiotic dose. Antibiotic therapy causes bacteriolysis and release of endotoxin. Dexamethasone may preempt production of tumor necrosis factor initiated after release of endotoxin.[22–25]

Table 9.2. Chemoprophylaxis for Meningococcal Meningitis

Antibiotic	Dose
Rifampin (oral agent)	Adults: 600 mg q12h for 2 days Children >1 year: 10 mg/kg q12h for 2 days Children <1 year: 5 mg/kg q12h for 2 days
Ceftriaxone (intramuscular injection)	Adults: 250 mg Children: 125 mg
Ciprofloxacin (oral agent)	Single dose of 750 mg
Sulfisoxazole (oral agent)	Adults: 1 g q12h for 2 days Children 1–12 years: 500 mg q12h for 2 days Children <1 year: 500 mg daily for 2 days

Data from Cuevas LE, Hart CA. Chemoprophylaxis of bacterial meningitis. J Antimicrob Chemother 1993;31(Suppl B):79; Feigin RD, McCracken GH Jr, Klein JO. Diagnosis and management of meningitis. Pediatr Infect Dis J 1992;11:785; Gaunt PN, Lambert BE. Single dose ciprofloxacin for the eradication of pharyngeal carriage of *Neisseria meningitidis*. J Antimicrob Chemother 1988;21:489; Schwartz B, Al-Tobaiqi A, Al-Ruwais A, et al. Comparative efficacy of ceftriaxone and rifampicin in eradicating pharyngeal carriage of group A *Neisseria meningitidis*. Lancet 1988;1:1239.

wall of the frontal sinus or tegmen tympani of the middle ear, or indirectly, through retrograde extension of thrombophlebitis.[27] This complication of meningitis is very rare in adults and is often mistakenly diagnosed at first as bacterial meningitis.[28]

Epidural abscess is produced by sources similar to those in subdural empyema, but in this condition, the suppurative infection is localized between the dura and bone. Continuous infection is most common, and the abscess creates a mass effect, gradually lifting the dura from the overlying skull.

Clinical Presentation

Patients (often males in the second or third decade) with subdural empyema are very ill with fever, vomiting, excruciating headache, and, most commonly, localizing neurologic deficits, such as aphasia, apraxia, or visuospatial neglect, hemiparesis, and focal seizures.[29] Most of these seizures arise in the premotor area of the frontal lobe (adversive seizures), with turning of the head and eyes, abduction of the contralateral arm, and flexion in the elbow with raised arm similar to the posture of a fencer. Other patients have speech arrest without impairment of consciousness or jacksonian seizures (the spread of the seizure reflects the cortical topography, beginning in the hand and moving to the face, the leg, and the foot).[30]

Clinical presentation is insidious and directly related to the mass effect, which may take weeks to become prominent and critical. Papilledema may be observed in patients with a comparatively slow-growing abscess. This allows time for increased intracranial pressure to be transmitted to the optic nerve sheaths, with subsequent venous stasis and resultant disk swelling. Nuchal rigidity is present, and if localizing neurologic signs are absent and the

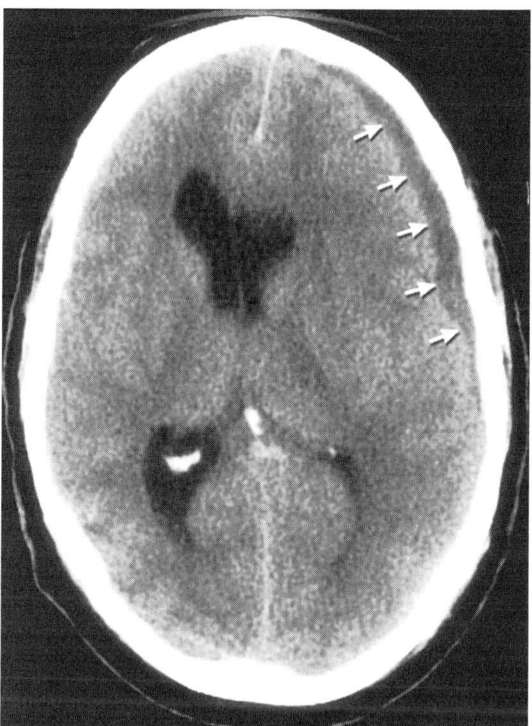

Figure 9.4. Computed tomography scan showing subdural empyema with mass effect.

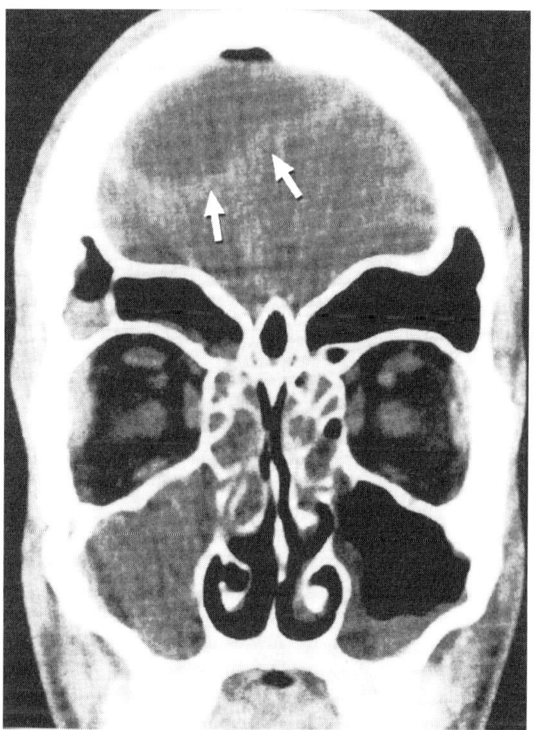

Figure 9.5. Coronal postcontrast computed tomography image depicting bilateral sinusitis and a low-density epidural collection (*arrows*) with a small amount of air. (From Gallagher RM, Gross CW, Phillips CD. Suppurative intracranial complications of sinusitis. Laryngoscope 1998;108:1635. By permission of the American Laryngological, Rhinological and Otological Society.)

classic association with recent pyogenic sinusitis or surgery is not appreciated, bacterial meningitis is often incorrectly diagnosed. Misdiagnosis may also be more prevalent when the epidural empyema overlies or collects between the hemispheres. Headache and fever may be the only symptoms in these patients. An uncommon but localizing symptom complex of facial pain (trigeminal nerve involvement), facial palsy, and abducens paresis can be observed if the petrous bone is involved in the process (Gradenigo's syndrome).

Interpretation of Diagnostic Tests

Computed Tomography and Magnetic Resonance Imaging

CT scans or MRI demonstrates a fairly characteristic lesion (Figure 9.4), usually supratentorially. Small collections may also be seen in the posterior fossa.[31] Noncontrast CT scanning shows a hypodensity over or between the hemispheres along the falx, but enhancement of the pus collection after contrast administration reveals the characteristic crescent shape of the mass. Imaging of the mastoid and paranasal sinuses to seek a potential source is imperative.[32,33]

MRI with gadolinium is superior to contrast CT because bone artifacts that may limit detection are absent.[34] MRI also clearly distinguishes between hydroma (similar T1- and T2-weighted signals to CSF) and pus (hyperintensive to CSF on T2-weighted image and hypointense to CSF on T1).[35] MRI may also detect parenchymal involvement and development of cerebral venous thrombosis, but a separate magnetic resonance venogram may be needed.

In a patient with an epidural abscess, a lentiform mass overlying the cerebral convexity without hemispheric involvement is clearly evident on CT scans with contrast (Figure 9.5), but MRI may further localize small locations and their extent.[36] Lack of gadolinium enhancement of the dura below the mass strongly favors epidural localization.[37]

Cerebrospinal Fluid

Lumbar puncture is relatively contraindicated, but when available (as mentioned earlier, often when bacterial meningitis was suspected), the findings include variable total cell counts (10 to 500/mm^3), increase in polymorphonucleated cells (<10 white blood cells may occur in 10% of patients), increased protein (60% to 80% of patients), normal glucose in CSF (at least 50% of cases), but often negative Gram's stain and sterile culture (>90% of patients).[27,30] The CSF isolates are often *Streptococcus milleri* (otorhinogenic source), *Staphylococcus aureus*, or coagulase-negative staphylococcus (sinus, trauma, or surgery). When pneumonia is concomitantly present, *S. pneumoniae*, *Escherichia coli*, and *H. influenzae* are common infectious agents. Blood cultures are seldom diagnostic.

First Priority in Management

Surgical evacuation and immediate antibiotic coverage are therapeutic interventions in the first hours of presentation. Antibiotic therapy in the emergency department should start with a combination of a third-generation cephalosporin and metronidazole. However, anaerobic isolates are uncommon. Alternatively, a combination of piperacillin sodium and tazobactam sodium (Zosyn) can be considered (Table 9.3). Craniotomy rather than aspiration over multiple bur holes is preferred.[38–40] In a patient with an epidural abscess, grafting may be needed if the dura is destroyed or penetrated by the inflammation. Parenteral antibiotic therapy should continue for 2 to 6 weeks. Conservative management is seldom considered and perhaps an option only in the remote clinical situation of full alertness, tiny fluid collections (<1 cm in diameter), and rapid clinical improvement after intravenous antibiotics.[40] However, clinical deterioration may occur suddenly.

Predictors of Outcome

Subdural empyema is a potential calamity if not quickly acted on.[41] Complacency leads to death in a matter of days, often from cerebral venous thrombosis as a result of cortical thrombophlebitis. Surgical drainage and intravenous antibiotics are mandatory, resulting in the greatest chance of recovery with a minimal neurologic deficit. In a review of 102 patients with subdural empyema, treatment before the patients lapsed into stupor increased the chance of survival, reducing mortality to 10%.[42]

Triage

- ♦ Otolaryngologic evaluation before transport.
- ♦ Direct transport to the operating room.
- ♦ Consider mannitol, 1 g/kg, if CT scan shows a significant mass effect before transport.
- ♦ Intravenous loading with phosphenytoin or phenytoin, 20 mg/kg, if seizures have occurred.

Brain Abscess

In referral hospital emergency departments, the incidence of brain abscess may approximate 1 in 10,000 hospital admissions.[43] The causes are listed in Table 9.4. The paranasal sinuses, middle ear, and teeth remain the most common sources of entry. One should expect the cause in 30% of patients with a bacterial brain abscess to remain unresolved.

Clinical Presentation

Brain abscess most often is manifested by dull headache and rarely by fever or papilledema.[44]

Neurologic signs depend on localization of the abscess and, as expected because of a lack of symptoms, on localization in the frontal or occipital lobe. Clinical findings may become more evident if edema surrounds the mass and certainly if rupture into the ventricular system occurs. Sudden worsening of headache and stupor may then be common clinical features. Level of consciousness depends on the timing of referral, and now significantly more patients seen in the emergency department are fully alert, with headache alone.[45] Seizures due to cerebral abscess are often generalized tonic-clonic seizures and have an estimated incidence of 40%.

Localization of an abscess in the cerebellum and brain stem is rare. The signs are ataxia, vomiting, appendicular dysmetria, and nystagmus.

Table 9.3. Initial Empirical Antibiotic Therapy in Subdural Empyema and Epidural Abscess

Likely source	Covers	Antimicrobial therapy
Otitis media or mastoiditis	Streptococci	Cefotaxime, 8–12 g/day IV q4h, divided doses
	Anaerobes	Metronidazole, 15 mg/kg loading, 7.5 mg/kg q4h
	Enterobacteria	
Sinusitis	Streptococci	*or*
	Anaerobes	
	Enterobacteria	Piperacillin sodium and tazobactam sodium, 3.375 g q6h
	Staphylococcus aureus	
	Haemophilus species	

Table 9.4. Brain Abscess: Predisposing Conditions, Site of Abscess, Microbiology, and Antibiotics

Predisposing condition	Site of abscess	Usual microbial isolates
Contiguous focus or primary infection		
Otitis media or mastoiditis	Temporal lobe or cerebellum	Streptococci (anaerobic or aerobic), *Bacteroides fragilis*, Enterobacteriaceae
Frontoethmoidal sinusitis	Frontal lobe	Predominantly streptococci (anaerobic or aerobic), *Bacteroides* spp, Enterobacteriaceae, *Staphylococcus aureus*, *Haemophilus* spp
Sphenoidal sinusitis	Frontal or temporal lobe	Same as frontoethmoidal sinusitis
Dental sepsis	Frontal lobe	Mixed *Fusobacterium*, *Bacteroides*, and *Streptococcus* spp
Penetrating head injury or postsurgical infection	Near the laceration	*S. aureus*, streptococci, Enterobacteriaceae, *Clostridium* spp
Hematogenous spread or distant site of infection		
Congenital heart disease	Multiple sites	Streptococci (aerobic, anaerobic, or microaerophilic), *Haemophilus* spp
Lung abscess, empyema, bronchiectasis	Multiple sites	*Fusobacterium* spp, *Actinomyces* spp, *Bacteroides* spp, *Streptococcus* spp, *Nocardia asteroides*
Bacterial endocarditis	Multiple sites	*S. aureus*, *Streptococcus* spp

Modified from Wispelwey B, Scheld WM. Brain abscess. In GL Mandell, RG Douglas Jr, JE Bennett (eds), Principles and Practice of Infectious Diseases, 3rd ed. New York: Churchill Livingstone, 1990;778. By permission of the publisher.

Interpretation of Diagnostic Tests

CT scanning is diagnostic[46] (Figure 9.6). A common misinterpretation of the abnormality in a noncontrast CT scan image is a cerebral infarct. MRI may further define mass effect and demonstrate additional lesions. In T1-weighted sequences, a hypodense center consisting of pus with a ring at the periphery is characteristic and may become evident only after contrast enhancement. T2-weighted images show a hyperintense signal with edema, which should be separated from the actual lesion in assessment of its size.[47] MRI is also more sensitive in detecting newly developing lesions, particularly cerebritis, and it may demonstrate the proximity of the abscess to the ventricular system. Differentiation of brain abscess from cystic brain tumor remains difficult. In two preliminary studies, results from magnetic resonance spectroscopy suggested that brain abscess could be distinguished on the basis of amino acids and other components, including acetate, in spectra absent in the neoplasm.[48,49]

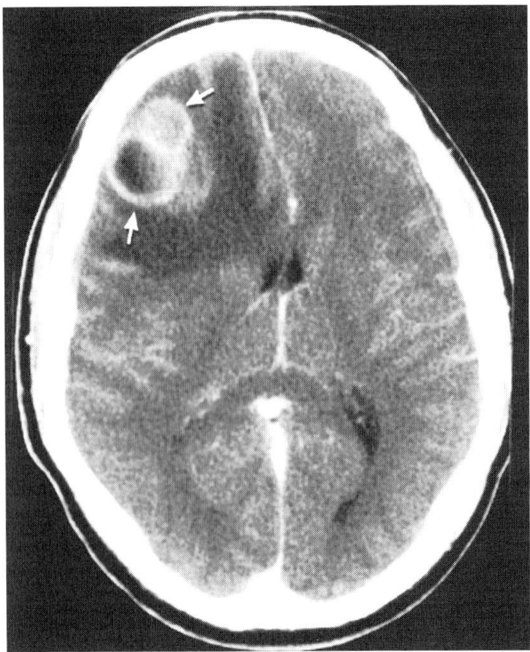

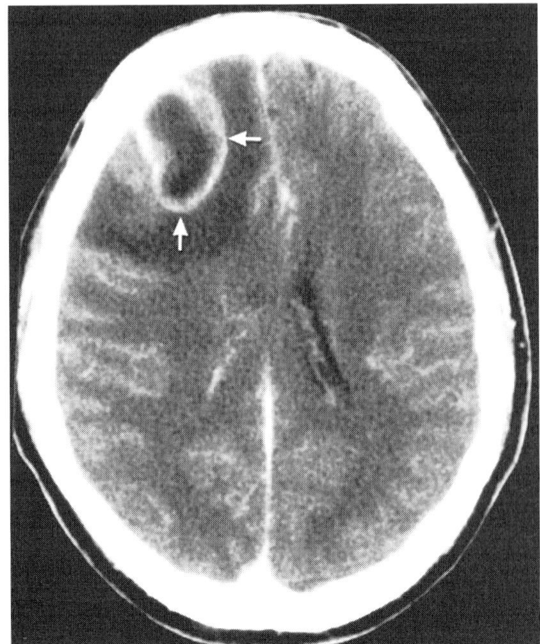

Figure 9.6. Computed tomography scans showing abscess in the frontal lobe with perilesional edema.

First Priority in Management

Antibiotic therapy aimed at a polymicrobial flora should be started immediately (Table 9.5). The decision to operate depends on several factors. Open craniotomy with debridement or stereotactic CT-guided aspiration is the first procedure in most cases. Early excision of an abscess should be considered if a thick, fibrotic capsule reduces the success of catheter drainage alone, predominantly in abscesses due to *Mycobacterium tuberculosis* and *Nocardia*. Impending rupture to the ventricular system is a reason for early surgical intervention.[50] However, surgery can be deferred if multiple abscesses are present, if the diameter of the abscess is less than 3 cm on CT scan images, or if *Toxoplasma* is considered. Corticosteroids (dexamethasone, 10 mg intravenously every 6 hours) with aggressive antibiotic coverage should be considered if edema is profound and signs of early herniation are developing. The dose should be tapered in 3 to 7 days. Aggressive ventricular drainage with intraventricular administration of antibiotics is needed in patients with ventricular pus from rupture into the ventricular system. If the abscess is localized in the brain stem, stereotactic drainage is more cumbersome. Empirical therapy with antibiotics lasting up to 3 months may be preferred to surgical drainage with identification of the organism, but both approaches are successful.

Predictors of Outcome

Important factors predicting poor outcome in cerebral abscess are symptoms of short duration, decreased consciousness, rapidly progressive neurologic deficit, number and size of abscesses, and ventricular rupture.[51] Mortality is closely linked to initial presentation in coma, which increases the frequency to 50% to 80% as opposed to a minimal risk of death in patients who are alert.

Triage

- To the operating room: patients with abscess and mass effect, close proximity to the ventricular system, or hydrocephalus.
- To the ward: patients with multiple small cerebral abscesses. Management is by intravenous administration of antibiotics with central venous catheter access.

Table 9.5. Suggested Empirical Therapy for Brain Abscess by Presumed Source

Putative source	Antibiotic therapy
Paranasal sinus	Cefotaxime, 1–2 g IV q4–8h (maximum dose, 12 g/day)
	Metronidazole, 500 mg IV q6h
Otogenic	Ceftazidime, 1–2 g IV q4–8h (maximum dose, 12 g/day)
	Metronidazole, 500 mg IV q6h
Spread from other sites	Nafcillin, 2 g IV q4h
	Cefotaxime, 1–2 g IV q4–8h (maximum dose, 12 g/day)
	Metronidazole, 500 mg IV q6h
Penetrating trauma	Nafcillin, 2 g IV q4h
	Cefotaxime, 1–2 g IV q4–8h
Surgical procedure	Vancomycin, 1 g IV q12h
	Ceftazidime, 1–2 g IV q4–8h

References

1. Aronin SI, Peduzzi P, Quagliarello VJ. Community-acquired bacterial meningitis: risk stratification for adverse clinical outcome and effect of antibiotic timing. Ann Intern Med 1998;129:862.
2. Sigurdardottir B, Bjornsson OM, Jonsdottir KE, et al. Acute bacterial meningitis in adults. A 20-year overview. Arch Intern Med 1997;157:425.
3. Durand ML, Calderwood SB, Weber DJ, et al. Acute bacterial meningitis in adults. A review of 493 episodes. N Engl J Med 1993;328:21.
4. Saha S, Saint S, Tierney LM Jr. Clinical problem-solving. A balancing act. N Engl J Med 1999;340:374.
5. Glimåker M, Kragsbjerg P, Forsgren M, Olcén P. Tumor necrosis factor-α (TNFα) in cerebrospinal fluid from patients with meningitis of different etiologies: high levels of TNFα indicate bacterial meningitis. J Infect Dis 1993;167:882.
6. Pfister HW, Borasio GD, Dirnagl U, et al. Cerebrovascular complications of bacterial meningitis in adults. Neurology 1992;42:1497.
7. Quagliarello V, Scheld WM. Bacterial meningitis: pathogenesis, pathophysiology, and progress. N Engl J Med 1992;327:864.
8. Saez-Llorens X, Ramilo O, Mustafa MM, et al. Molecular pathophysiology of bacterial meningitis: current concepts and therapeutic implications. J Pediatr 1990;116:671.
9. Behrman RE, Meyers BR, Mendelson MH, et al. Central nervous system infections in the elderly. Arch Intern Med 1989;149:1596.
10. Rasmussen HH, Sorensen HT, Moller-Petersen J, et al. Bacterial meningitis in elderly patients: clinical picture and course. Age Ageing 1992;21:216.
11. Herishanu YO, Zlotnik M, Mostoslavsky M, et al. Cefuroxime-induced encephalopathy. Neurology 1998; 50:1873.
12. Igarashi M, Gilmartin RC, Gerald B, et al. Cerebral arteritis and bacterial meningitis. Arch Neurol 1984;41:531.
13. Verdon R, Chevret S, Laissy JP, Wolff M. Tuberculous meningitis in adults: review of 48 cases. Clin Infect Dis 1996;22:982.
14. Cabral DA, Flodmark O, Farrell K, Speert DP. Prospective study of computed tomography in acute bacterial meningitis. J Pediatr 1987;111:201.
15. Vernino S, Wijdicks EFM, McGough PF. Coma in fulminant pneumococcal meningitis: new MRI observations. Neurology 1998;51:1200.
16. Dichgans M, Jager L, Mayer T, et al. Bacterial meningitis in adults: demonstration of inner ear involvement using high-resolution MRI. Neurology 1999;52:1003.
17. Arevalo CE, Barnes PF, Duda M, Leedom JM. Cerebrospinal fluid cell counts and chemistries in bacterial meningitis. South Med J 1989;82:1122.
18. Berenguer J, Moreno S, Laguna F, et al. Tuberculous meningitis in patients infected with the human immunodeficiency virus. N Engl J Med 1992;326:668.
19. Maxson S, Lewno MJ, Schutze GE. Clinical usefulness of cerebrospinal fluid bacterial antigen studies. J Pediatr 1994;125:235.
20. Jacobs MR. Drug-resistant *Streptococcus pneumoniae*: rational antibiotic choices. Am J Med 1999;106:48S.
21. Gropper MR, Schulder M, Sharan AD, Cho ES. Central nervous system tuberculosis: medical management and surgical indications. Surg Neurol 1995;44:378.
22. Girgis NI, Farid Z, Kilpatrick ME, et al. Dexamethasone adjunctive treatment for tuberculous meningitis. Pediatr Infect Dis J 1991;10:179.
23. Lebel MH, Freij BJ, Syrogiannopoulos GA, et al. Dexamethasone therapy for bacterial meningitis. Results of two double-blind, placebo-controlled trials. N Engl J Med 1988;319:964.
24. Mustafa MM, Lebel MH, Ramilo O, et al. Correlation of interleukin-1 beta and cachectin concentrations in cerebrospinal fluid and outcome from bacterial meningitis. J Pediatr 1989;115:208.
25. Mustafa MM, Ramilo O, Olsen KD, et al. Tumor necrosis factor in mediating experimental *Haemophilus influenzae* type B meningitis. J Clin Invest 1989;84:1253.
26. Wenger JD, Hightower AW, Facklam RR, et al. Bacterial meningitis in the United States, 1986: report of a multistate surveillance study. J Infect Dis 1990; 162:1316.
27. Dill SR, Cobbs CG, McDonald CK. Subdural empyema: analysis of 32 cases and review. Clin Infect Dis 1995;20:372.
28. Farkas AG, Marks JC. Subdural empyema: an important diagnosis not to miss. BMJ 1986;293:118.
29. Bhandari YS, Sarkari NB. Subdural empyema. A review of 37 cases. J Neurosurg 1970;32:35.

30. Brock DG, Bleck TP. Extra-axial suppurations of the central nervous system. Semin Neurol 1992;12:263.
31. Morgan DW, Williams B. Posterior fossa subdural empyema. Brain 1985;108:983.
32. Hoyt DJ, Fisher SR. Otolaryngologic management of patients with subdural empyema. Laryngoscope 1991;101:20.
33. Kaufman DM, Litman N, Miller MH. Sinusitis: induced subdural empyema. Neurology 1983;33:123.
34. Hodges J, Anslow P, Gillett G. Subdural empyema: continuing diagnostic problems in the CT scan era. Q J Med 1986;59:387.
35. Sadhu VK, Handel SF, Pinto RS, Glass TF. Neuroradiologic diagnosis of subdural empyema and CT limitations. AJNR Am J Neuroradiol 1980;1:39.
36. Weingarten K, Zimmerman RD, Becker RD, et al. Subdural and epidural empyemas: MR imaging. AJR Am J Roentgenol 1989;152:615.
37. Tsuchiya K, Makita K, Furui S, et al. Contrast-enhanced magnetic resonance imaging of sub- and epidural empyemas. Neuroradiology 1992;34:494.
38. Bok AP, Peter JC. Subdural empyema: burr holes or craniotomy? A retrospective computerized tomography-era analysis of treatment in 90 cases. J Neurosurg 1993;78:574.
39. Luken MG III, Whelan MA. Recent diagnostic experience with subdural empyema. J Neurosurg 1980;52:764.
40. Mauser HW, Ravijst RA, Elderson A, et al. Nonsurgical treatment of subdural empyema. Case report. J Neurosurg 1985;63:128.
41. Nathoo N, Nadvi SS, Van Dellan JR, Gouws E. Intracranial subdural empyemas in the era of computed tomography: a review of 699 cases. Neurosurgery 1999;44:529.
42. Mauser HW, Van Houwelingen HC, Tulleken CA. Factors affecting the outcome in subdural empyema. J Neurol Neurosurg Psychiatry 1987;50:1136.
43. Yen PT, Chan ST, Huang TS. Brain abscess: with special reference to otolaryngologic sources of infection. Otolaryngol Head Neck Surg 1995;113:15.
44. Grigoriadis E, Gold WL. Pyogenic brain abscess caused by *Streptococcus pneumoniae*: case report and review. Clin Infect Dis 1997;25:1108.
45. Yang SY, Zhao CS. Review of 140 patients with brain abscess. Surg Neurol 1993;39:290.
46. Miller ES, Dias PS, Uttley D. CT scanning in the management of intracranial abscess: a review of 100 cases. Br J Neurosurg 1988;2:439.
47. Smith RR, Caldemeyer KS. Neuroradiologic review of intracranial infection. Curr Probl Diagn Radiol 1999;28:1.
48. Kim SH, Chang KH, Song IC, et al. Brain abscess and brain tumor: discrimination with in vivo H-1 MR spectroscopy. Radiology 1997;204:239.
49. Martinez-Perez I, Moreno A, Alonso J, et al. Diagnosis of brain abscess by magnetic resonance spectroscopy. Report of two cases. J Neurosurg 1997;86:708.
50. Zeidman SM, Geisler FH, Olivi A. Intraventricular rupture of a purulent brain abscess: case report. Neurosurgery 1995;36:189.
51. Seydoux C, Francioli P. Bacterial brain abscesses: factors influencing mortality and sequelae. Clin Infect Dis 1992;15:394.

Chapter 10
Acute Encephalitis

Clinical findings that are often diagnostic of acute encephalitis are fever, agitation, localizing neurologic signs, and changes in personal behavior. Progression to coma is expected in fulminant variants, and attending physicians may feel pressured because little in the presentation discriminates among the possible triggering agents.

There are a bewildering number of causes of encephalitis, but this chapter concentrates on those with more defined management and diagnostic tests. Viral infection remains most common, but other infectious disorders mimicking viral encephalitis may become more obvious after careful probing during history taking (Table 10.1). Noninfectious causes should be considered in appropriate circumstances, and the diagnostic considerations of major importance are listed in Table 10.2. This chapter discusses the confused, febrile patient with a deteriorating level of consciousness in whom acute encephalitis is suspected. It points out a practical approach to evaluation and triage.

Herpes Simplex Encephalitis

Epidemiologic registries have demonstrated that herpes simplex encephalitis is uncommon (2 cases per 1 million population annually) and can be implicated in less than 10% of all reported encephalitides in middle-aged and elderly adults.[1] Untreated, it frequently leads to further deterioration of consciousness, permanent morbidity, and brain death. The primary concern is to treat early and preempt further progression. Prompt treatment with acyclovir has considerably improved the neurologic outcome. But even so, there may be ravaging consequences despite early treatment.

Clinical Presentation

The clinical diagnosis of herpes simplex encephalitis should be urgently considered in patients with abrupt onset of a triad of fever (up to 39°C to 40°C), change in personality, and localizing neurologic findings (such as aphasia, hemiparesis, and apraxia).[2,3] Seizures, often focal and transient, are present in one-third of the patients. As the disorder progresses, epilepsia partialis continua and temporal lobe seizures may reflect frontal or temporal lobe involvement. Auras of temporal lobe seizures may consist of hallucinations and dysgeusia. Progression to coma may take days but can be rapid, and even the interval between the development of febrile illness and the late stages of coma with extensor responses may be surprisingly short. Some patients may be healthy in the morning and fulfill the criteria for brain death at night. Unusual features are visual field defects, papilledema (only in moribund patients), and memory loss (more commonly apparent in late survivors). Autonomic dysfunction with profound instability in blood pressure, tachypnea, and sweating may occur

Table 10.1. Infectious Diseases That Can Masquerade as Viral Central Nervous System Infections

Bacteria
Spirochetes
Syphilis (secondary or meningovascular)
Leptospirosis
Borrelia burgdorferi infection (Lyme disease)
Mycoplasma pneumoniae infection
Cat-scratch fever
Listeriosis
Brucellosis (particularly due to *Brucella melitensis*)
Tuberculosis
Typhoid fever
Parameningeal infections (epidural infection, petrositis)
Partially treated bacterial meningitis
Brain abscesses
Whipple's disease
Fungi
Cryptococcosis
Coccidioidomycosis
Histoplasmosis
North American blastomycosis
Candidiasis
Parasites
Toxoplasmosis
Cysticercosis
Echinococcosis
Trichinosis
Trypanosomiasis
Plasmodium falciparum infection
Amebiasis (due to *Naegleria* and *Acanthamoeba*)

Modified from Johnson RT. Acute encephalitis. Clin Infect Dis 1996;23:219. By permission of The University of Chicago.

(60% of biopsy-proven cases) and in exceptional cases may further deteriorate into a sympathetic overdrive with catatonia and extensive rigidity. For unclear reasons, herpes simplex encephalitis in immunocompromised patients seems to occur more often as a brain stem encephalitis with diplopia, dysarthria, and ataxia.[4,5]

Recently, an anterior operculum syndrome was reported,[6] and failure to recognize its distinguishing features may potentially delay therapy. Involvement of the anterior operculum (the operculum is the cortex and white matter tissue overlying the insula) results in difficulty chewing, a tendency for the mouth to be half open, bifacial palsy, dysphagia, drooling, anarthria, and trismus. Automatic facial movements, such as yawning, are preserved.[6,7] Manic behavior (hallucinations, elevated mood, decreased need for sleep, increased sexual desire, flirtations) has been pointed out (patients feel "absolutely marvelous, relaxed and happy") but is uncommon.[8] These complex presentations should alert the neurologist to herpes simplex encephalitis, but the very untraditional presentation may not be associated with this encephalitis.

Table 10.2. Noninfectious Diseases Mimicking Encephalitis

CNS vasculitis
Fulminant bacterial meningitis
ADEM
Thrombotic thrombocytopenic purpura
Fulminant hepatic failure, Reye's syndrome
Endocrine crisis (myxedema, Addison's disease)
Toxic encephalopathy (cyclosporine, tacrolimus, MTX, 5-FU, illicit drugs)

(ADEM = allergic demyelinating encephalomyelitis; CNS = central nervous system; 5-FU = 5-fluorouracil; MTX = methotrexate.)

Interpretation of Diagnostic Tests

Time is needed to document the source and nature of any infection, whether for careful preparation of cerebrospinal fluid (CSF) for cultures, priming of a polymerase chain reaction (PCR), or awaiting the results of blood cultures. Certain laboratory tests are helpful in the emergency department and can be used in early assessment of prognosis.

Cerebrospinal Fluid

Pleocytosis with lymphocytes (50 to 2,000/mm^3) and a fivefold increase in protein are common. CSF glucose may be decreased. CSF is normal only exceptionally, mostly in patients examined very early in the course of the illness. CSF PCR has a sensitivity of 98% and a specificity of 94% (Capsule 10.1 and Table 10.3). Acyclovir may reduce PCR sensitivity, but herpes simplex DNA can still be detected in one-third of cases long after acyclovir treatment.[1]

Capsule 10.1. Polymerase Chain Reaction Technology for Fulminant Encephalitis

Polymerase chain reaction (PCR) has revolutionized the diagnosis of herpes simplex, cytomegalovirus, and toxoplasmic encephalitides. Small quantities of viral DNA or RNA in cerebrospinal fluid can be selectively amplified. Target sequences of DNA are amplified by DNA polymerase, and with multiple repeating of cycles, large copies can be obtained. This amplified DNA is visualized on gel stained by ethidium bromide. PCR is the method of choice for diagnosis but not useful to monitor treatment efficacy. In addition, persistent viral load DNA does not correlate with outcome.[9] False-negative PCR may result from antiviral treatment or, more commonly, technical difficulty with primers.[10–12]

Table 10.3. Sensitivity and Specificity of Polymerase Chain Reaction in Cerebrospinal Fluid

Agent	Sensitivity (%)	Specificity (%)
Herpes simplex[11]	98	94
Cytomegalovirus[13]	79	95
Toxoplasma[14]	42	100

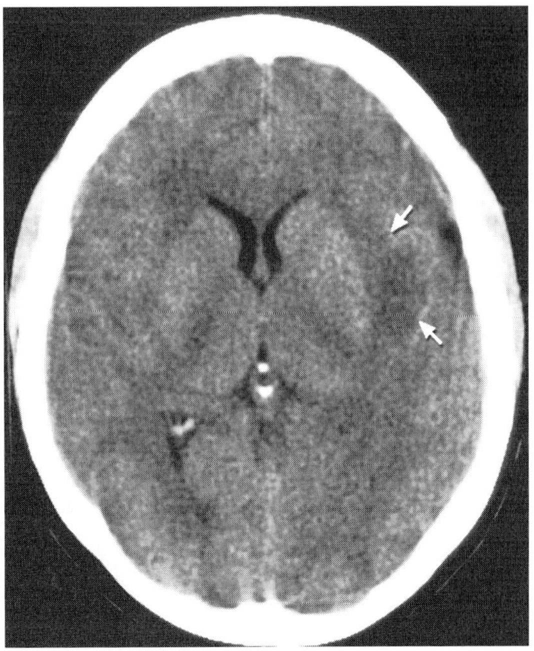

Figure 10.1. Computed tomography scan findings of early herpes encephalitis with subinsular hypodensity.

Electroencephalography

In the electroencephalogram (EEG), typical but not-to-be-mistaken nonspecific abnormalities over the temporal regions are spike-and-slow-wave activity, delta waves, or triphasic waves evolving into unilateral periodic lateralized epileptiform discharges, which rapidly spread to both temporal hemispheres.[15] This pattern is seen in 84% of typical cases of herpes simplex encephalitis but with a specificity of only 30%.[15]

Computed Tomography and Magnetic Resonance Imaging

Computed tomography (CT) scanning is generally not useful in herpes simplex encephalitis, and the findings become abnormal only after days and predominantly in advanced cases evolving into coma. Abnormal CT scan findings in the temporal and insular regions (Figure 10.1) develop in approximately 50% of patients, but the reported radiologic series are certainly skewed toward the more severe cases. Hypodensity and swelling in the temporal lobe may become prominent and hemorrhagic and be initially misinterpreted as a lobar hematoma or hemorrhagic infarct (Figure 10.2). Unilateral swelling may suggest a glioma or an abscess (and sometimes it is).

Magnetic resonance imaging (MRI) is the definitive diagnostic test, with a high sensitivity and specificity for early T2 changes in the temporal lobe and, to a lesser extent, in the frontobasal or cingulate gyrus of the frontal lobe, in the insular cortex, and across the splenium (Figure 10.3). Fluid-attenuated inversion recovery is more sensitive and may clearly show abnormal images not evident on routine T2-weighted sequences.[16] The MRI abnormalities may appear within 1 day of herpes simplex

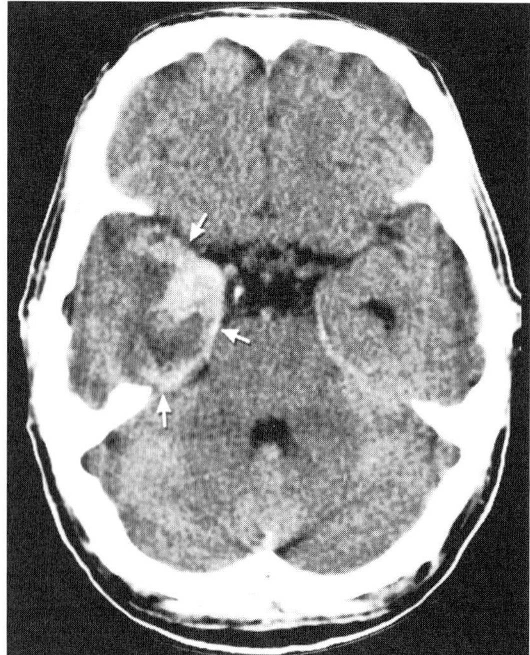

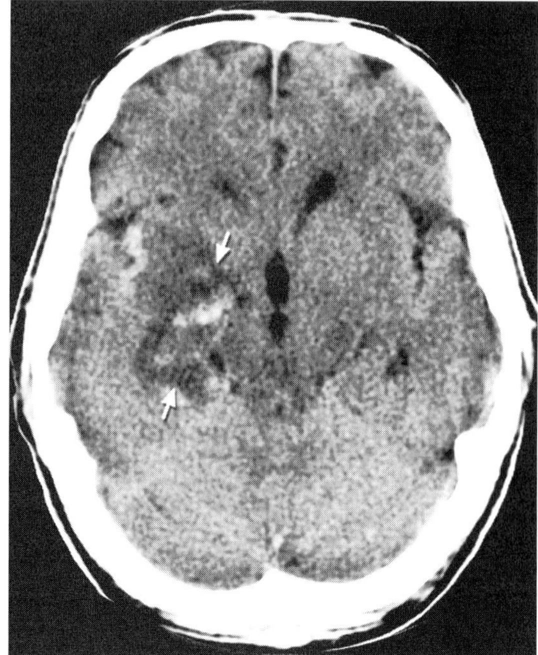

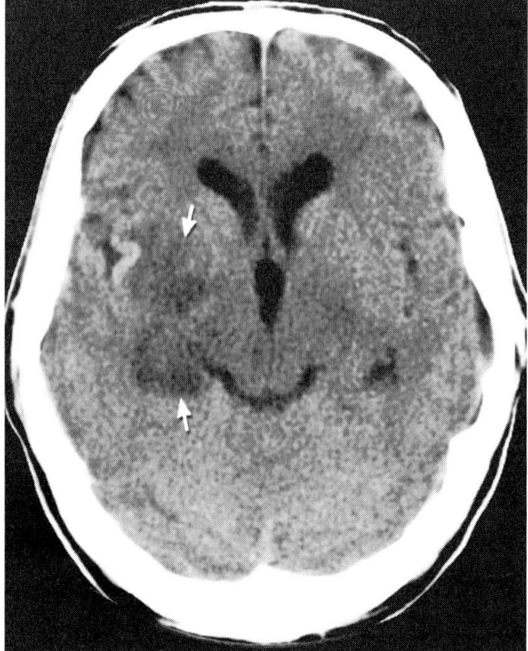

Figure 10.2. Computed tomography scans showing unilateral swollen, hypodense, and mixed hemorrhagic temporal lobe lesion from herpes simplex encephalitis.

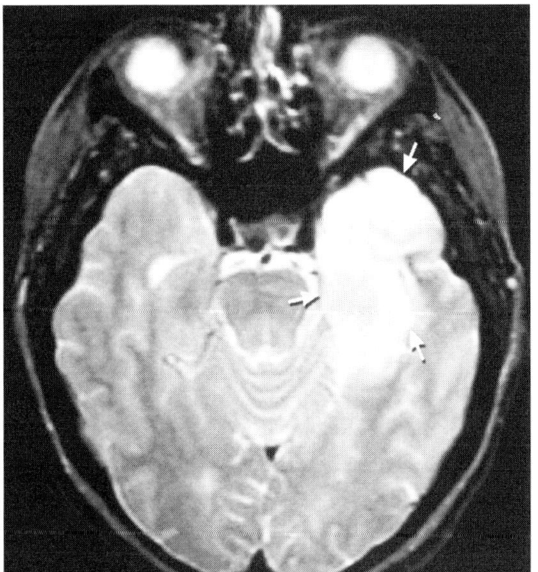

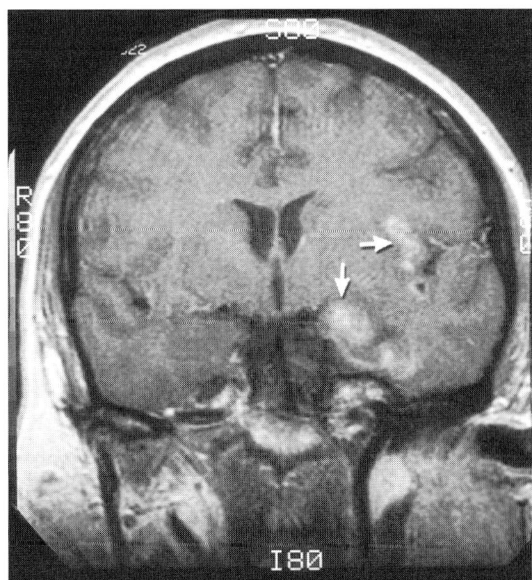

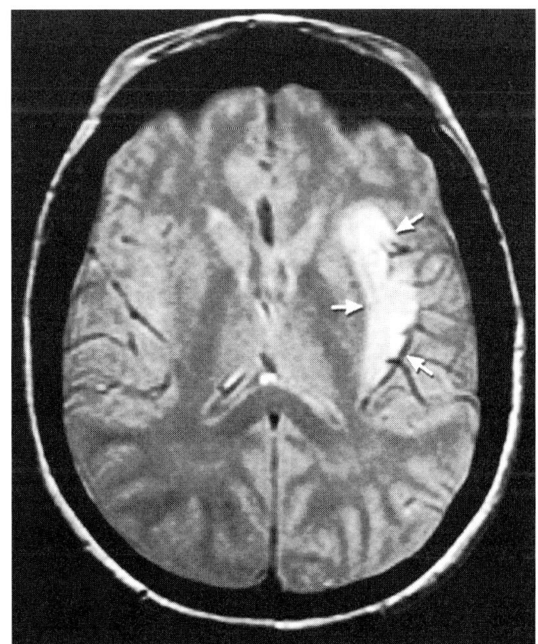

Figure 10.3. Magnetic resonance images with typical hyperintensities (T2-weighted [left], T1-weighted [upper right], fluid attenuated inversion recovery [lower right]) in temporal, frontal lobe, and insular regions from herpes simplex encephalitis.

encephalitis. Conversely, normal MRI findings in a comatose patient virtually exclude herpes simplex encephalitis.

Single-Photon Emission Computed Tomography

With single-photon emission computed tomography (SPECT) in which technetium Tc 99m hexamethylpropyleneamine oxime is the radiopharmaceutical, unilateral hyperfusion is a common finding, and, as expected, the tracer preferentially lodges in the temporal lobe and adjacent frontal lobe. This phenomenon of increased uptake is not specific for herpes simplex encephalitis and indicates only inflammation and early neuronal injury.

Approximately half of the SPECT scans performed within days of symptoms yield normal results. It may become a preferred test in patients seen in the emergency department because data are rapidly acquired, and despite moderate sensitivity, it may be more helpful than EEG or MRI in the first days after presentation.

First Priority in Management

An immediate intravenous dose of acyclovir, 10 mg/kg, is needed, followed by maintenance with 10 mg/kg every 8 hours for 10 days. Intravenous loading with fosphenytoin, 18 to 20 mg/kg, is needed after presentation with seizures, but its use as prophylaxis is not established. Midazolam infusion, 0.4 mg/kg per minute, may be useful to control extreme agitation. With the introduction of PCR and MRI, earlier dilemmas about the need for brain biopsy have almost been resolved.[17,18] Biopsy should be considered if the PCR result is negative, if CSF pleocytosis is absent, and when, primarily to exclude a glioma, only unilateral temporal lobe swelling is present. In patients with a markedly swollen temporal lobe and shift and impending herniation, craniotomy with dural grafting is indicated. Some of the necrotic tissue may need to be removed to decompress the supratentorial compartment.

Predictors of Outcome

Treatment with acyclovir within 5 days of onset of the first symptoms remains associated with a 25% incidence of fatal outcome. Fatal outcome is associated with brain edema but more commonly with persistent vegetative state and terminal systemic infection. Good recovery with return to a similar productive life is possible in 50% of patients.[19] MRI abnormalities[20] and bilateral EEG abnormalities predict poor outcome, with memory deficits[21] and inability to function at a similar intellectual level.

SPECT may have a good predictive value: A close association between focal hyperfusion on SPECT and poor outcome was emphasized in a large study of patients with acute encephalitis.[22]

Triage

- Monitor and manage increased intracranial pressure in the neurologic intensive care unit.
- Consider EEG or video monitoring in the intensive care unit if the patient had seizures and impaired consciousness.

Arthropod-Borne Viral Encephalitis

These encephalitides are widespread geographically and commonly endemic, sporadic cases are seasonal during the summer months, and cluster cases may signal an outbreak. Fatality depends on the type of virus and amplifying host. The virus is transmitted through ticks and mosquitoes after replication in wild animals. The most common viruses are Bunyavirus (La Crosse, California), Alphavirus (eastern and western equine), and Flavivirus (St. Louis).[23,24]

Clinical Presentation

Differences in presentation are apparent. La Crosse (California) encephalitis is most commonly reported to the Centers for Disease Control and predominates in children younger than 15 years. The hosts for the mosquito are chipmunks and squirrels, and the mosquito breeds in rainwater-filled tires and birdhouses. In California encephalitis, seizures are common (50%), and seizure disorder develops later in many patients. Within 2 weeks after prodromal fever, the patient may experience malaise, very severe headaches, confusion, drowsiness, and coma—in roughly that order.

The equine encephalitides (western and eastern) differ substantially in mortality.[25] The mosquito breeds in freshwater swamps, and birds (sparrows, ducks, and pheasants) are the hosts. It is prevalent along the Atlantic and Gulf coasts, but eastern encephalitis is infrequent. Evolution to coma from massive cerebral edema is rapid, usually within 1 week.[25,26] The virus causes an acute encephalitis in horses, and it can be isolated from brain tissue specimens.[26] Western equine encephalitis peaks in August and September, and outbreaks have been reported from the Midwest United States. Improved vector control has reduced the incidence of both types of encephalitis.

St. Louis encephalitis occurs commonly in the United States. Its manifestations appear to be milder in children than in adults. The susceptible populations are persons living in public housing projects and, possibly, patients infected with human immunodeficiency virus (HIV).

In the tropics, Venezuelan equine encephalitis is most common, particularly in Central and South America, and is very comparable to western equine encephalitis in prevalence, clinical presentation, morbidity, and mortality. Japanese encephalitis is endemic in Southeast Asia and India. Vaccination of children has markedly decreased its prevalence in Japan, but vaccination for travelers to endemic areas is recommended. Most cases occur in China, India, and Thailand.[27] Japanese encephalitis peaks during the rainy season. It may occur during only brief stays, such as a vacation,[28] although the risk of exposure increases with a longer stay.

The clinical features of Japanese encephalitis are nonspecific, with elements of diffuse involvement of both hemispheres, but spinal cord involvement (often leading to the incorrect diagnosis of fulminant multiple sclerosis) has been noted.[27,29]

Recently, tick-borne encephalitis became a serious health problem in forested areas of Europe and Russia.[30–33] Flaviviruses are transmitted by tick bites. Encephalitis develops in only 1 of 10 infected persons, usually after a flulike illness.

Interpretation of Diagnostic Tests

Diagnosis of arthropod-borne viral encephalitis is often delayed, and no specific neuroimaging finding has been reported in certain types of encephalitides.

Computed Tomography and Magnetic Resonance Imaging

CT scans are normal or may show diffuse edema (see Chapter 2). Abnormal MRI findings have been described in a large series of patients with a predilection for basal ganglionic and thalamic lesions in all types of arbovirus encephalitis. The midbrain and cortex may be involved in some. In one study, MRI findings were abnormal in 11 comatose patients, but other arboviruses can produce coma without MRI abnormalities in the earlier diagnostic phase.[25] MRI abnormalities, however, can be present soon after the onset of neurologic symptoms. Diffuse cerebral edema appears after several days of coma. Similar MRI findings have been reported in Japanese encephalitis[34–36] and European tick-borne encephalitis. The sensitivity of MRI in these types of encephalitis is not known.

Cerebrospinal Fluid and Serology

As expected, pleocytosis with lymphocytosis is found along with increased protein. A CSF profile mimicking bacterial meningitis has been described in eastern equine encephalitis. The diagnosis of arbovirus encephalitis is based on determination of IgM antibodies by an enzyme-linked immunosorbent assay, which has a high sensitivity but is time-consuming. Isolation of the virus from blood or CSF is unrewarding. A recent study documented positive findings in 10% of tested specimens of CSF.[37] PCR detection is currently under investigation.

First Priority in Management

No specific antiviral therapy is available, but acyclovir (10 mg/kg intravenously every 3 hours) should be administered until PCR results are confirmed negative. Supportive therapy consists of antiepileptic drugs, mechanical ventilation, and prevention of medical complications in the more severe cases. Corticosteroids are not effective.[38]

Predictors of Outcome

Mortality in La Crosse and California encephalitides is fortunately low, but neurologic sequelae with hemiparesis or aphasia are possible in 15% of patients. Eastern equine encephalitis may cause numerous deaths, and up to 70% of patients have severe neurologic disability. In western equine encephalitis, in contrast, full recovery occurs, although elderly patients may die. The death rate in St. Louis encephalitis is approximately one in four for elderly patients. Neuropsychologic sequelae seem more common than overt localizing neurologic signs in tick-borne encephalitis.

Triage

- Neurologic intensive care unit for supportive care.
- Early administration of mannitol, 1 g/kg, in rapidly developing coma from brain edema.

Cytomegalovirus and Varicella-Zoster Virus Encephalitis

Cytomegalovirus (CMV) is an opportunistic infectious agent. In a review of 676 patients, 85% of the patients with CMV encephalitis were infected with the acquired immunodeficiency syndrome (AIDS) virus.[13,39] CMV ventriculoencephalitis is the hallmark of the infection and the cause of death.

The patterns of varicella-zoster virus (VZV) encephalitis have recently been classified by Amlie-Lefond et al.[9] and Kleinschmidt-DeMasters et al.[40] into three major categories. These are (1) large- or medium-vessel vasculopathy involving large vessels at the base of the brain or convexity; the infection may affect large territories and cause hemorrhagic infarctions (arteritis and the virus inside the artery have been well documented); (2) small-vessel vasculopathy producing demyelinating ischemic lesions with a more subacute clinical course; and (3) ventriculitis. VZV encephalitis has been associated with hematologic-oncologic malignant disease, sarcoidosis, rheumatoid arthritis, tuberculosis, transplantation, and AIDS.

Clinical Presentation

Confusion and lethargy in a patient with a history of CMV retinitis or pneumonitis should suggest the diagnosis. The clinical features include confusion (60% of patients), coma (45%), cranial nerve palsy (40%), and seizures (25%).[39] Ventriculitis and hydrocephalus may be the cause of reduced consciousness. Hyponatremia from CMV adrenalitis is common and an important laboratory indicator in patients with AIDS and rapidly developing encephalitis.

VZV encephalitis should be the first consideration in immunosuppressed (e.g., HIV-infected) patients with recent shingles.[41] In most reported cases, however, a rash developed days to months before the onset but was not always remembered by the patients. In several reports, VZV encephalitis actually occurred without a skin eruption.

Progressive multifocal neurologic deficits occur, often leading to visual field defects, aphasia, apraxia, hemiparesis, and more specific neurocognitive syndromes, such as Gerstmann's syndrome (acalculia, finger agnosia, right-left confusion, and agraphia) and Anton's syndrome (cortical blindness). Progressive mental impairment with frontal release signs and spastic paraparesis has been observed in patients with a type of small-vessel vasculopathy causing widespread white matter demyelination without cortical involvement.

Interpretation of Diagnostic Tests

Computed Tomography and Magnetic Resonance Imaging

MRI in CMV encephalitis may show nonspecific brain atrophy and enlarged ventricles with typical ependymal signal enhancement.[39] Brain stem and cerebellar abnormalities after gadolinium have been reported in isolated cases.

In patients with VZV encephalitis, both neuroimaging studies show multiple T1-weighted hypointensity and T2-weighted hyperintensity involving the white and gray matter. Subcortical enhancing, coalescing lesions followed by gray matter involvement are characteristic.[42] Involvement of multiple territories is compatible with several large intracranial vasculitides representing infarction (Figure 10.4).

Cerebrospinal Fluid

The CSF formula is normal in many instances, complicating detection. PCR of CMV has significantly increased the ability to make the diagnosis (sensitivity, 79%; specificity, 95%).

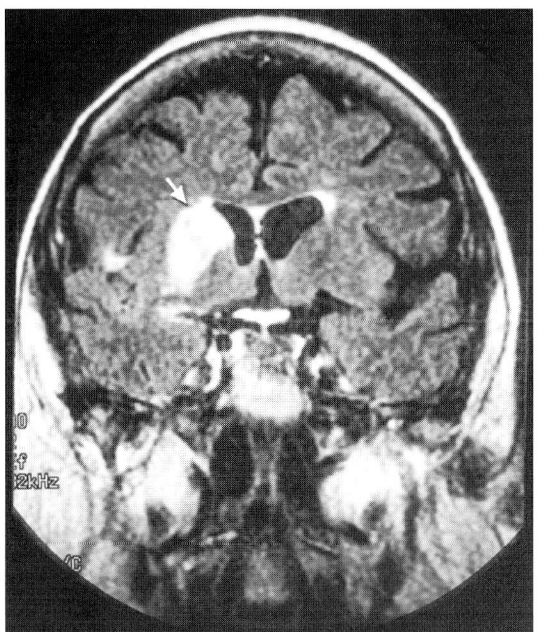

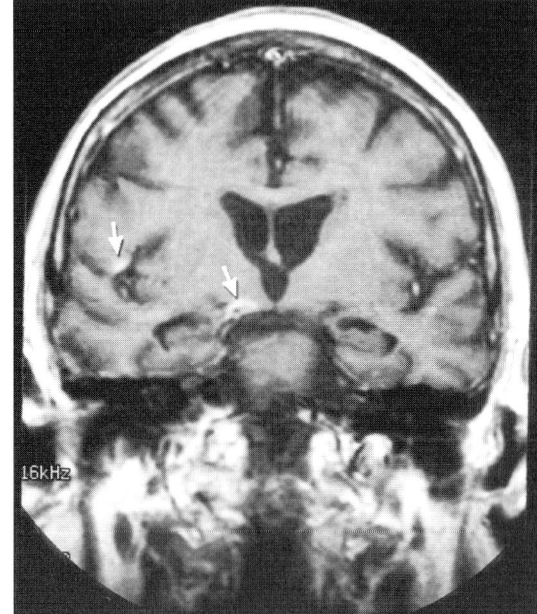

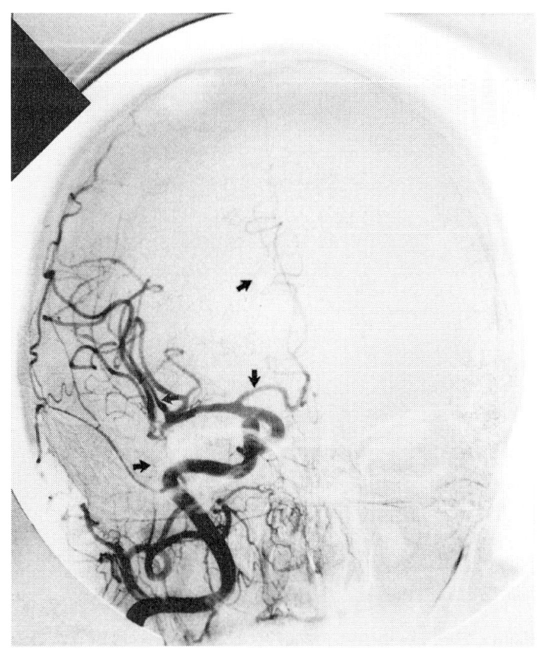

Figure 10.4. Varicella-zoster virus encephalitis with multiple infarcts (*large arrows*) and vasculitis (*small arrows*) on carotid angiogram.

In VZV encephalitis, a marked variation in inflammatory response is known, from only a few to several hundred cells, with accompanying increase in protein. Glucose concentration is normal. PCR has become available for VZV encephalitis, but the diagnostic validity is not yet known.[43]

First Priority in Management

Ganciclovir is the preferred agent (10 mg/kg), with maintenance of 10 mg/kg twice a day for 14 days. Patients previously receiving a maintenance dose of ganciclovir need the addition of foscarnet, 180 mg/kg every 8 hours.

Predictors of Outcome

The outcome in CMV-associated encephalitis is poor because of underlying HIV infection and, commonly, concomitant opportunistic infection. The outcome in VZV encephalitis is entirely determined by associated vasculitis; without it, full recovery is possible.

Triage

- Neurologic intensive care unit.
- Consider ventriculostomy in patients with hydrocephalus.

Encephalitis from Rickettsiae

Rickettsial diseases are transmitted through ticks, mites, lice, and fleas. The stings are often not remembered because they are painless and may not be followed by a rash at the injection site. The most important and potentially fatal disorder is Rocky Mountain spotted fever, which causes a generalized vasculitis and meningoencephalitis. It emerges in late spring and summer, predominantly in the Southeast region of the United States.[44]

Other rickettsial infections that may involve the central nervous system are encephalitides from the typhus group. The typhus group includes Q fever, epidemic typhus, murine typhus, and scrub typhus. The epidemic can be worldwide and produce similar neurologic manifestations, with typical maculopapular rash and multifocal central nervous system manifestations.[44]

Clinical Presentation

Rocky Mountain spotted fever is evident in patients with fever who have a marked purpuric rash involving the palms and soles. The flexor surfaces of the hands and feet are involved first before the rash spreads over the body. The purpuric lesions are a consequence of rickettsiae invading small blood vessels and causing occlusion and necrosis. This rash (Color Plate 20) may be absent early in the disease.[45]

Neurologic manifestations are protean, but severe headache, profound neck stiffness, and clouding of consciousness are common, with progression to stupor in more than one-fourth of affected patients.[46,47]

Q fever occurs as a result of exposure to farm animals, rabbits, or deer and may result in fever, pneumonia, myocarditis, endocarditis, and a meningoencephalitis. The involvement of the central nervous system is less common in Q fever but may mimic herpes simplex encephalitis.[48] Neurologic involvement from the responsible agent, *Coxiella burnetii*, is uncommon but can be dramatic. Severe headache and myalgias are common.[49] Neurologic manifestations that may precede stupor are cranial nerve involvement and cerebellar signs.[48] Acute confusion evolving into acute manic behavior has been reported as well. Epidemic, murine, and scrub types, which occur widely in Southeast Asia, the Pacific Islands, India, and Nepal, are not further considered here.

Interpretation of Diagnostic Tests

Computed Tomography and Magnetic Resonance Imaging

The findings in Rocky Mountain spotted fever are multiple small subcortical infarcts (often in the basal ganglia), development of cerebral edema with loss of gray-white matter differentiation, and sulci effacement.[2] A survivor in one report had multiple punctate areas of increased intensity throughout the white matter in the distribution of the perivascular (Virchow-Robin) spaces, possibly representing a perivascular inflammatory response.[50,51] Meningeal enhancement after gadolinium is typical.

Cerebrospinal Fluid and Serum

Increased protein occurred in only one-third of the patients, with only a mild pleocytosis (<50 mm^3) in most cases. PCR detection in blood samples from infected patients has been successful, even in those obtained on the day of onset.[52]

Predictors of Outcome

These types of encephalitides are typically diagnosed at autopsy, because patients deteriorate rapidly from brain edema.

No early clinical predictors are known other than brain edema, which may be difficult to control. Increased intracranial pressure (>40 mm Hg) despite aggressive mannitol therapy predicts poor outcome.

First Priority in Early Management

Early treatment of rickettsial or tick-borne encephalitis with oral tetracycline is needed (25 to 50 mg/kg per day in two or four divided doses). A relapse can be treated with chloramphenicol, but tetracycline remains the agent for first-line therapy.[53]

Triage

- Neurologic intensive care unit for monitoring of intracranial pressure.
- Cardiac consultation in Q fever for possible myocarditis.

Toxoplasmic Encephalitis

Normal host immunity contains an infection with *Toxoplasma gondii*. Therefore, toxoplasmic encephalitis is a leading cause of acute encephalitis in patients with AIDS or in immunosuppressed patients.[54] HIV encephalitis has a more protracted course. *Toxoplasma* infestation can be a defining illness in previously HIV-positive patients. It is much less common in transplant recipients, patients with Hodgkin's disease, or patients with systemic lupus erythematosus.[55] Its incidence may be lower in patients with AIDS receiving trimethoprim-sulfamethoxazole prophylaxis for *Pneumocystis carinii*.

Clinical Presentation

Toxoplasma infection may result in a single mass effect, multiple abscesses, or multiple hemorrhages in abscesses mimicking coagulopathy-associated hemorrhages. The total parasite burden to the brain determines the clinical manifestations, but many of these abscesses do not produce clinical signs other than headache and lethargy. Progression may be in days or protracted over months. Decreasing alertness, onset of seizures, and persisting headache should alert one to the diagnosis.[56] *Toxoplasma* has a predilection for the basal ganglia and cerebellum, but hemichorea, hemiballismus, and ataxia are uncommon manifestations.

Interpretation of Diagnostic Tests

The diagnosis is confirmed by CSF PCR, MRI of the brain, or biopsy of the brain in selected cases.

Computed Tomography and Magnetic Resonance Imaging

CT scanning underestimates the number of abscesses, even when contrast material is administered in double doses; therefore, its use is limited to initial screening.[57] Acute hydrocephalus without defined abscesses may point to the diagnosis in the proper clinical situation. Multiple intracerebral hemorrhages in patients with AIDS often indicate *Toxoplasma* (or *Aspergillus*) rather than a coagulopathy.[58,59]

MRI of toxoplasmic encephalitis, which displays multiple abscesses, is nonspecific, because very similar signal abnormalities and ring enhancement can be seen with lymphoma, tuberculous abscesses, nocardiosis, cryptococcosis, and, less commonly, syphilitic gummas.[57,59]

Hyperintensity on T2-weighted images is common, but after treatment, it evolves into T2-weighted isointensity comparable with that of necrotizing abscesses[61] (Figure 10.5). Marked perilesional edema is typical.

Cerebrospinal Fluid

An inflammatory profile is present in the CSF, with increased protein concentration and, rarely, marked mononuclear pleocytosis (<100 cells). The sensitivity of PCR for *Toxoplasma* is 42%, but the specificity is 100%.[14,62] The comparatively low sensitivity is determined by intraparenchymal localization of *Toxoplasma*, so that it is more likely that CSF does not contain *Toxoplasma* DNA. Its diagnostic value, therefore, is limited, but PCR technology has reduced the number of brain biopsies for confirmation.

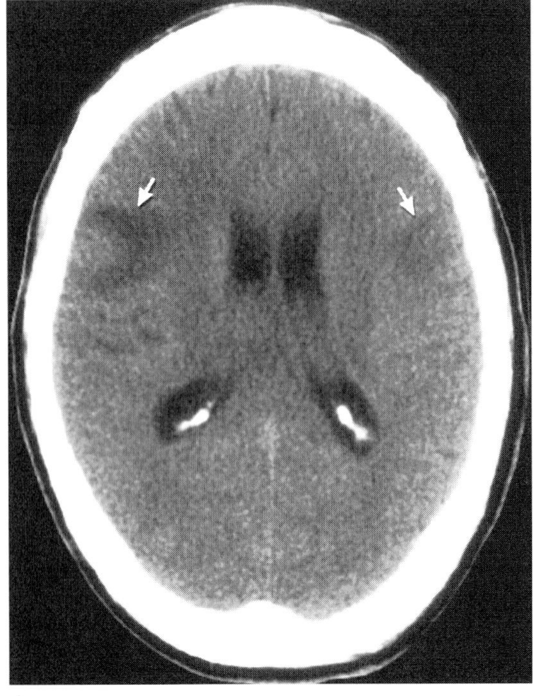

A

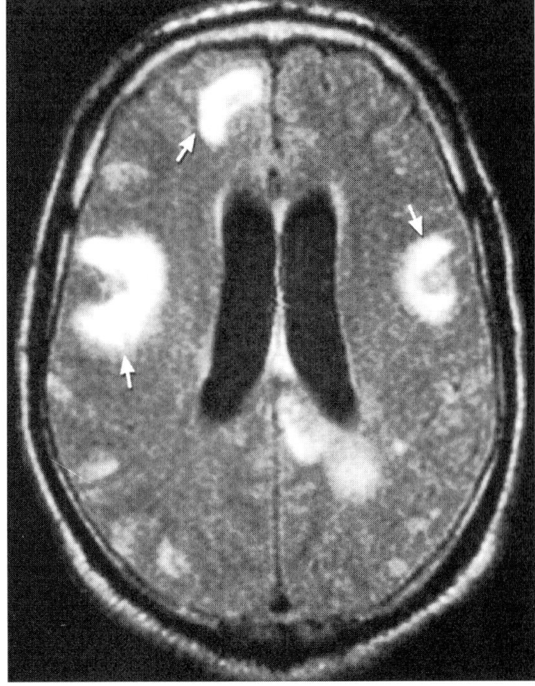

B

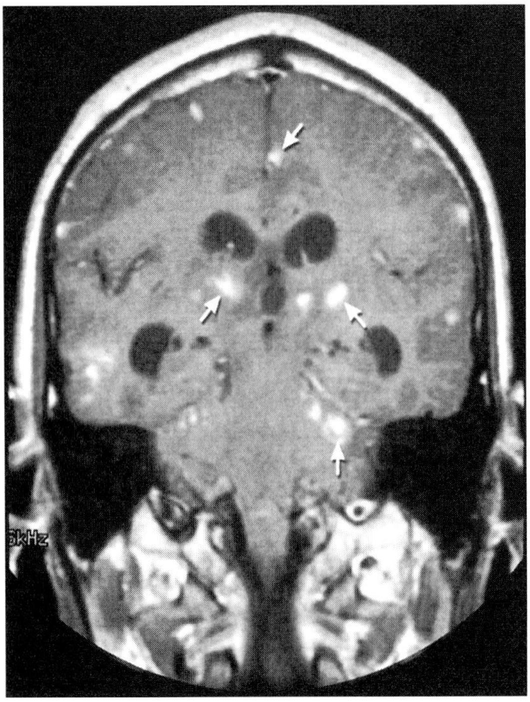

C

Figure 10.5. Toxoplasmic encephalitis with multiple abscesses (*arrows*). The abcesses are poorly defined by computed tomography scan **(A)** and more evident by magnetic resonance imaging fluid-attenuated inversion recovery **(B)** and postcontrast T1-weighted scan **(C)**.

Single-Photon Emission Computed Tomography

SPECT of the brain with thallium 201 may differentiate lymphoma from toxoplasmic encephalitis. The high mitotic activity of the lymphoma increases uptake, causing a "hot" region. Its accuracy in predicting lymphoma is questioned despite impressive predictive value in a first series of patients.[63–65]

Serum Serology

Low or absent antitoxoplasmic antibody titers (IgG) are common in immunosuppressed patients, and IgM titers are negative. Variation is great—from 1:8 to titers exceeding 1:1,024. A significant increase in serum titer over time has no significance, because it may occur in immunocompromised patients without active *Toxoplasma* infection.

First Priority in Management

The standard therapeutic agents in toxoplasmic encephalitis are pyrimethamine, 50 to 100 mg, and sulfadiazine, 4 to 8 g, daily, combined with folinic acid, 10 mg/day, to reduce bone marrow depression.[66]

Adverse reactions are a rash and anemia, leukopenia, or thrombocytopenia, occurring in 20% of patients. Any allergic reaction should result in replacement of sulfadiazine by clindamycin (600 to 900 mg every 8 hours).[67] When *Toxoplasma* is the culprit, within 3 weeks radiologic improvement (defined as less edema and isointense signals rather than hyperintense signals on MRI) or complete resolution should be expected in 70% of patients.

Predictors of Outcome

Fatal outcome occurs in patients with multiple hemorrhagic abscesses. The response to therapy determines outcome.[66,68] Often, underlying central nervous system lymphoma (together with toxoplasmic encephalitis) reduces prospects of full recovery.

Triage

- Most patients can be initially managed on wards rather than in an intensive care unit.
- Surgical drainage of a large abscess should be considered if a mass effect is present.
- Biopsy should be strongly considered when PCR is negative, primarily to exclude lymphoma. Immunofluorescence techniques can confirm *Toxoplasma* in brain tissue with the use of monoclonal antibodies in the tissue samples.

Fungal Encephalitis

Viral meningoencephalitis is the most common cause in patients with progressive headache, nuchal rigidity, confusion, and lymphocytic predominance, but a fungal cause should always be considered.[69] One should be especially alert if an acute presentation is followed by an insidious course, particularly in endemic regions. Prompt diagnosis and therapy with amphotericin B result in survival and reduced morbidity.

Clinical Presentation

The lung is the port of entry of the fungus and generally the primary site of infection. Evidence of infection in organ systems outside the central nervous system, such as skin, bone, and prostate, is commonly needed to implicate fungal infection. Typical clinical features are headaches, myalgia, fever, intermittent nausea, and photophobia. Cognition may rapidly become impaired, and patients may have marked abulia and lethargy due to irreversible, devastating brain damage. The presentation often is nonspecific and atypical, making the diagnosis very difficult.

Coccidioides immitis is endemic to the southwestern United States and the central valley of California. Dissemination is usually seen only in immunosuppressed patients but occurs in 1% of infected patients. Central nervous system involvement is typically severe and is fatal if untreated.

Other fungal causes must be considered in the differential diagnosis. Organisms include *Cryptococcus neoformans, Blastomyces dermatitidis, Histoplasma capsulatum, Aspergillus* species, and a number of uncommon pathogens, all with possibly similar presentations and CSF formulae. Meningitis is the most common manifestation of infection by *Cryptococcus neoformans* and is generally found in immunocompromised patients. It is ubiquitous and protean in its presentation, ranging from indolent changes in cognitive function to florid meningoencephalitis.[70,71] *Histoplasma capsulatum* is found in the Ohio and Mississippi river valleys, and most persons in endemic areas have positive skin tests for previous infection. Active disease is rare and, again, is seen most commonly in immunocompromised hosts. *Aspergillus* is a common fungal pathogen with a predilection for the brain parenchyma over the meninges. Abscess formation is common, as is central nervous system vasculitis.

Case reports of blastomycotic meningitis are noteworthy for the frequent misdiagnosis of tuberculous meningitis[72,73] (see Chapter 9). The similar clinical characteristics and the nodular appearance of meningeal enhancement on MRI in both diseases make distinction between the two difficult. Many patients have been treated with antituberculous agents before the accurate diagnosis of blastomycotic meningitis. This can further confuse the diagnosis, because rifampin has some therapeutic benefit in treating blastomycosis and incomplete treatment with that drug may lead to reactivation of disease.

Interpretation of Diagnostic Tests

Magnetic Resonance Imaging

Prominent enhancement of the basilar meninges can be found. A nodular character may suggest a fungal cause. Scattered hyperintensities in the basal ganglia may represent extension of infection along perforating arteries[74] (Figure 10.6).

Cerebrospinal Fluid

Typical findings are lymphocytic pleocytosis, borderline decreased glucose concentration, and mildly increased protein level. CSF serology for *Cryptococcus neoformans, Coccidioides immitis, Histoplasma capsulatum,* and *Blastomyces dermatitidis* should be done, but the results may be negative.

Brain Biopsy

Brain biopsy should be considered early, but the poor sensitivity of microscopy in identifying the organism in biopsied specimens is often remarkable. Culture of CSF and brain tissue obtained at operation remains the prime diagnostic test.

First Priority in Management

Ketoconazole or, more recently, itraconazole is the first-line agent for pulmonary blastomycosis.[75] Amphotericin B is usually reserved for more serious clinical situations or refractory disease, but many experts believe that it is the drug of choice in patients with meningeal involvement. Most authorities recommend a total dose of amphotericin B of 2 to 3 g. Hydrocephalus may become considerable, and ventriculostomy is needed. This provides the opportunity to culture CSF, but brain biopsy may be needed to unveil the fungus.[76]

Predictors of Outcome

These disorders are rare, but morbidity is substantial. Amphotericin therapy may be successful in arresting progression of neurologic manifestations. Despite early initiation of empirical treatment with amphotericin, death has been reported.

Triage

- Brain biopsy to confirm the diagnosis, and surgery may be indicated if a single abscess has formed.
- Ventriculostomy may be needed to relieve hydrocephalus.
- Ward for intravenous amphotericin B therapy.

Paraneoplastic Limbic Encephalitis

This rare disorder should be considered when infectious agents seem highly unlikely. A history of depression, agitation, paranoia, and feelings of depersonalization and memory loss may be obtained.[77] The pathologic substrate can be extensive, with neuronal loss, perivascular monocytic infiltrates, and microglial nodules, predominantly in the limbic and insular cortices but also located in the brain stem, spinal cord, and dorsal root gan-

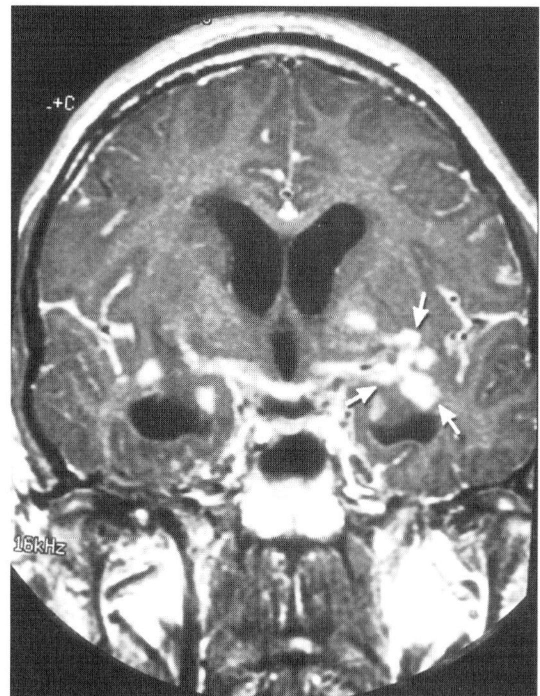

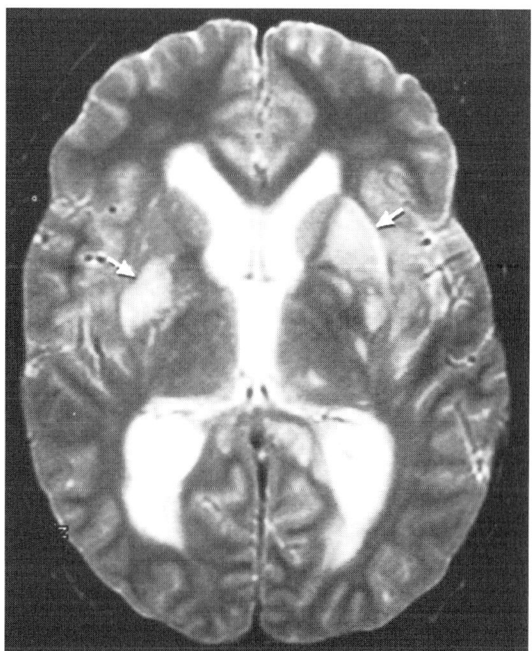

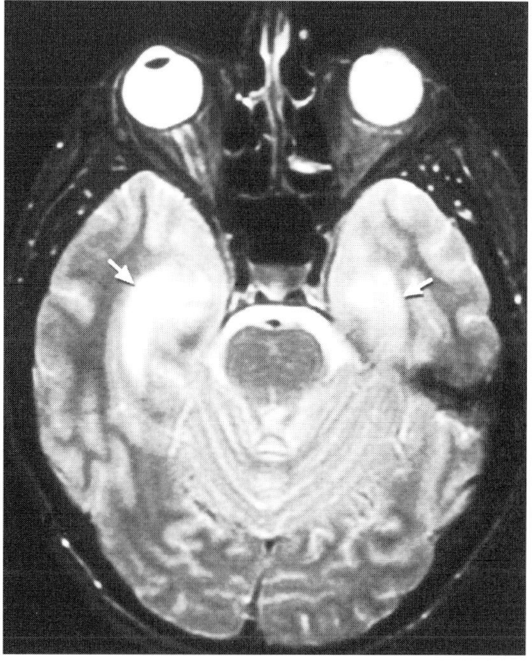

Figure 10.6. Magnetic resonance images showing diffuse nodular enhancement of basal meninges, with abnormal T2 signal in the basal ganglia bilaterally and bitemporal lesions representing encephalitis (*arrows*). The fungus isolated from brain biopsy culture was *Blastomyces*.

glia.[78] It is uncommon to find a neoplasm during life, but the condition can be the first manifestation or appear in a patient with a previous diagnosis of small cell (oat cell) carcinoma, Hodgkin's disease, or testicular seminoma.[79–82]

Clinical Presentation

Rapid onset of mood changes, usually sadness, detachment, and loss of recent memory, is the characteristic presentation, but more fulminant forms are manifested

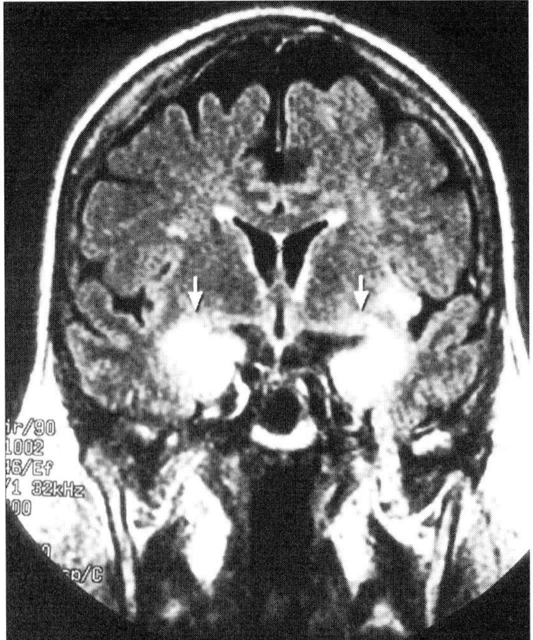

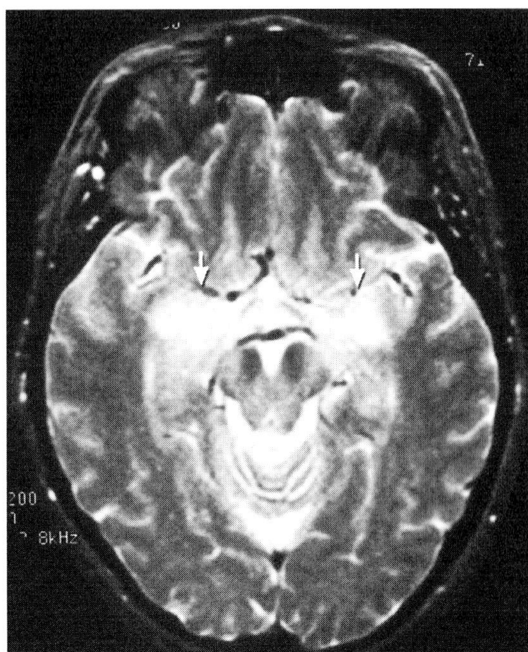

Figure 10.7. Magnetic resonance images of limbic paraneoplastic encephalitis, showing symmetrical T2 signal in mesial temporal lobe (*arrows*).

by agitation, hallucinations, and bizarre behavior preceding a decrease in alertness. (The diagnosis is often suggested when the psychiatric symptoms progress despite psychotropic drugs.) Coma is uncommon and, if present, mostly from secondary causes, such as infections, sepsis, and acute metabolic derangements.

Neurologic examination clearly demonstrates only poor recall and clinical signs of major depression and, if the patient is specifically asked, behavioral abnormalities and hallucinations. Subtle brain stem or cerebellar abnormalities may be evident in some patients.

Interpretation of Diagnostic Tests

Full evaluation for a possible malignancy workup is therefore needed and should include CT scan of the chest and lymph node biopsy in patients with lymphadenopathy because of the common association with Hodgkin's disease and lung cancer. However, diagnostic evaluation may be extended to exclude gastrointestinal, kidney, and gynecologic malignant diseases and thus should include mammogram, pelvic examination, testicular ultrasonography, serum cancer markers, and antineuronal nuclei antibodies.[80,81,83,84]

Electroencephalography

The EEG may be normal early in the course but will show progressive nonspecific slowing of the background rhythm with sparing of temporal slow waves and spike foci. Epileptiform activity is uncommon.

Computed Tomography and Magnetic Resonance Imaging

Normal findings are typical and often suggest the diagnosis in the proper situation. However, in an anecdotal report, T2-weighted hyperintensity changes in the medial temporal lobes appeared with contrast enhancement in the temporal lobes, amygdala, and hippocampus[82] (Figure 10.7).

Cerebrospinal Fluid and Serum

CSF is under normal opening pressures, but an increased protein and mononuclear pleocytosis varied from 30 to 150 total cells in more than 50% of the reported cases. Normal CSF or only mildly increased protein is less common.

Anti-HU (term derived from a patient's initials) denotes an autoantibody in patients with cancer, predominantly small cell lung cancer. It is found mostly in patients with subacute sensory neuropathy leading to severe ataxia but can be found in paraneoplastic limbic encephalitis.[83] Anti-HU is a polyclonal IgG antibody reacting with neuron nuclei in vitro. The HU antigen has been cloned, and recently a cell-mediated response toward one of the HU antigens (HUD) was documented.[84] The specificity and sensitivity for the anti-HU test are not exactly known, but low titers can be found in patients with cancer and no neurologic involvement.

Brain Biopsy

Stereotactic brain biopsy may show perivascular infiltrates with predominantly B cells, and microglial-like cells may be observed surrounding neurons.[85]

Predictors of Outcome

The clinical course is progressive, but fluctuations may occur. The interval from initial psychiatric signs to death due to infections varies greatly, from 1 month to 2 years. Treatment of underlying cancer has resulted in substantial improvement in only some of the patients.

Triage

- Supportive measures and hospital admission for full medical evaluation and a search for the underlying cancer are needed.
- Management of respiratory complications from aspiration or sepsis and brain biopsy to exclude other treatable disorders may justify brief intensive care admission.

References

1. Koskiniemi M, Piiparinen H, Mannonen L, et al. Herpes encephalitis is a disease of middle aged and elderly people: polymerase chain reaction for detection of herpes simplex virus in the CSF of 516 patients with encephalitis. J Neurol Neurosurg Psychiatry 1996;60:174.
2. Bonawitz C, Castillo M, Mukherji SK. Comparison of CT and MR features with clinical outcome in patients with Rocky Mountain spotted fever. AJNR Am J Neuroradiol 1997;18:459.
3. Sköldenberg B. Herpes simplex encephalitis. Scand J Infect Dis Suppl 1996;100:8.
4. Chretien F, Belec L, Hilton DA, et al. Herpes simplex virus type 1 encephalitis in acquired immunodeficiency syndrome. Neuropathol Appl Neurobiol 1996;22:394.
5. Hamilton RL, Achim C, Grafe MR, et al. Herpes simples virus brainstem encephalitis in an AIDS patient. Clin Neuropathol 1995;14:45.
6. McGrath NM, Anderson NE, Hope JK, et al. Anterior opercular syndrome, caused by herpes simplex encephalitis. Neurology 1997;49:494.
7. van der Poel JC, Haenggeli CA, Overweg-Plandsoen WC. Operculum syndrome: unusual feature of herpes simplex encephalitis. Pediatr Neurol 1995;12:246.
8. Fisher CM. Hypomanic symptoms caused by herpes simplex encephalitis. Neurology 1996;47:1374.
9. Amlie-Lefond C, Kleinschmidt-DeMasters BK, Mahalingam R, et al. The vasculopathy of varicella-zoster virus encephalitis. Ann Neurol 1995;37:784.
10. Jeffery KJ, Read SJ, Peto TE, et al. Diagnosis of viral infections of the central nervous system: clinical interpretation of PCR results. Lancet 1997;349:313.
11. Lakeman FD, Whitley RJ. Diagnosis of herpes simplex encephalitis: application of polymerase chain reaction to cerebrospinal fluid from brain-biopsied patients and correlation with disease. J Infect Dis 1995;171:857.
12. Wildemann B, Ehrhart K, Storch-Hagenlocher B, et al. Quantitation of herpes simplex virus type 1 DNA in cells of cerebrospinal fluid of patients with herpes simplex virus encephalitis. Neurology 1997;48:1341.
13. Arribas JR, Storch GA, Clifford DB, Tselis AC. Cytomegalovirus encephalitis. Ann Intern Med 1996;125:577.
14. Novati R, Castagna A, Morsica G, et al. Polymerase chain reaction for *Toxoplasma gondii* DNA in the cerebrospinal fluid of AIDS patients with focal brain lesions. AIDS 1994;8:1691.
15. Smith JB, Westmoreland BF, Reagan TJ, Sandok BA. A distinctive clinical EEG profile in herpes simplex encephalitis. Mayo Clin Proc 1975;50:469.
16. White ML, Edwards-Brown MK. Fluid attenuated inversion recovery (FLAIR) MRI of herpes encephalitis. J Comput Assist Tomogr 1995;19:501.
17. Revello MG, Manservigi R. Molecular diagnosis of herpes simplex encephalitis. Intervirology 1996;39:185.
18. Tebas P, Nease RF, Storch GA. Use of the polymerase chain reaction in the diagnosis of herpes simplex encephalitis: a decision analysis model. Am J Med 1998;105:287.
19. Preiser W, Weber B, Klos G, et al. Unusual course of herpes simplex virus encephalitis after acyclovir therapy. Infection 1996;24:384.
20. Takanashi J, Sugita K, Ishii M, et al. Longitudinal MR imaging and proton MR spectroscopy in herpes simplex encephalitis. J Neurol Sci 1997;149:99.
21. Hokkanen L, Salonen O, Launes J. Amnesia in acute

herpetic and nonherpetic encephalitis. Arch Neurol 1996;53:972.
22. Launes J, Siren J, Valanne L, et al. Unilateral hyperfusion in brain-perfusion SPECT predicts poor prognosis in acute encephalitis. Neurology 1997;48:1347.
23. Lowry PW. Arbovirus encephalitis in the United States and Asia. J Lab Clin Med 1997;129:405.
24. Mancao MY, Law IM, Roberson-Trammell K. California encephalitis in Alabama. South Med J 1996;89:992.
25. Deresiewicz RL, Thaler SJ, Hsu L, Zamani AA. Clinical and neuroradiographic manifestations of eastern equine encephalitis. N Engl J Med 1997;336:1867.
26. Komar N, Spielman A. Emergence of eastern encephalitis in Massachusetts. Ann N Y Acad Sci 1994;740:157.
27. Igarashi A. Epidemiology and control of Japanese encephalitis. World Health Stat Q 1992;45:299.
28. Wittesjö B, Eitrem R, Niklasson B, et al. Japanese encephalitis after a 10-day holiday in Bali (letter to the editor). Lancet 1995;345:856.
29. Jelinek T, Nothdurft HD. Japanese encephalitis vaccine in travellers. Is wider use prudent? Drug Safety 1997;16:153.
30. Haglund M, Forsgren M, Lindh G, Lindquist L. A 10-year follow-up study of tick-borne encephalitis in the Stockholm area and a review of the literature: need for a vaccination strategy. Scand J Infect Dis 1996;28:217.
31. Prokopowicz D, Bobrowska E, Bobrowski M, Grzeszczuk A. Prevalence of antibodies against tick-borne encephalitis among residents of north-eastern Poland. Scand J Infect Dis 1995;27:15.
32. Roggendorf M. Epidemiology of tick-borne encephalitis virus in Germany. Infection 1996;24:465.
33. Treib J, Haass A, Mueller-Lantzsch N, et al. Tick-borne encephalitis in the Saarland and the Rhineland-Palatinate. Infection 1996;24:242.
34. Kumar S, Misra UK, Kalita J, et al. MRI in Japanese encephalitis. Neuroradiology 1997;39:180.
35. Misra UK, Kalita J, Jain SK, Mathur A. Radiological and neurophysiological changes in Japanese encephalitis. J Neurol Neurosurg Psychiatry 1994;57:1484.
36. Shoji H, Murakami T, Murai I, et al. A follow-up study by CT and MRI in 3 cases of Japanese encephalitis. Neuroradiology 1990;32:215.
37. Huang C, Chatterjee NK, Grady LJ. Diagnosis of viral infections of the central nervous system (letter to the editor). N Engl J Med 1999;340:483.
38. Hoke CH Jr, Vaughn DW, Nisalak A, et al. Effect of high-dose dexamethasone on the outcome of acute encephalitis due to Japanese encephalitis virus. J Infect Dis 1992;165:631.
39. Pierelli F, Tilia G, Damiani A, et al. Brainstem CMV encephalitis in AIDS: clinical case and MRI features. Neurology 1997;48:529.
40. Kleinschmidt-DeMasters BK, Amlie-Lefond C, Gilden DH. The patterns of varicella zoster virus encephalitis. Hum Pathol 1996;27:927.
41. Case records of the Massachusetts General Hospital. N Engl J Med 1996;335:1587.
42. Weaver S, Rosenblum MK, DeAngelis LM. Herpes varicella zoster encephalitis in immunocompromised patients. Neurology 1999;52:193.
43. Bergstrom T. Polymerase chain reaction for diagnosis of varicella zoster virus central nervous system infections without skin manifestations. Scand J Infect Dis Suppl 1996;100:41.
44. Marrie TJ, Raoult D. Rickettsial infections of the central nervous system. Semin Neurol 1992;12:213.
45. Horney LF, Walker DH. Meningoencephalitis as a major manifestation of Rocky Mountain spotted fever. South Med J 1988;81:915.
46. Katz DA, Dworzack DL, Horowitz EA, Bogard PJ. Encephalitis associated with Rocky Mountain spotted fever. Arch Pathol Lab Med 1985;109:771.
47. Kirk JL, Fine DP, Sexton DJ, Muchmore HG. Rocky Mountain spotted fever. A clinical review based on 48 confirmed cases, 1943-1986. Medicine (Baltimore) 1990;69:35.
48. Sempere AP, Elizaga J, Duarte J, et al. Q fever mimicking herpetic encephalitis. Neurology 1993;43:2713.
49. Silpapojakul K, Ukkachoke C, Krisanapan S, Silpapojakul K. Rickettsial meningitis and encephalitis. Arch Intern Med 1991;151:1753.
50. Baganz MD, Dross PE, Reinhardt JA. Rocky Mountain spotted fever encephalitis: MR findings. AJNR Am J Neuroradiol 1995;16(Suppl 4):919.
51. Lorenzl S, Pfister HW, Padovan C, Yousry T. MRI abnormalities in tick-borne encephalitis (letter to the editor). Lancet 1996;347:698.
52. Tzianabos T, Anderson BE, McDade JE. Detection of *Rickettsia rickettsii* DNA in clinical specimens by using polymerase chain reaction technology. J Clin Microbiol 1989;27:2866.
53. Shaked Y. Rickettsial infection of the central nervous system: the role of prompt antimicrobial therapy. Q J Med 1991;79:301.
54. Peacock JE Jr, Folds J, Orringer E, et al. *Toxoplasma gondii* and the compromised host. Antibody response in the absence of clinical manifestations of disease. Arch Intern Med 1983;143:1235.
55. Deleze M, Mintz G, del Carmen Mejia M. *Toxoplasma gondii* encephalitis in systemic lupus erythematosus. A neglected cause of treatable nervous system infection. J Rheumatol 1985;12:994.
56. Porter SB, Sande MA. Toxoplasmosis of the central nervous system in the acquired immunodeficiency syndrome. N Engl J Med 1992;327:1643.
57. Knobel H, Guelar A, Graus F, et al. Toxoplasmic encephalitis with normal CT scan and pathologic MRI. Am J Med 1995;99:220.
58. Casado-Naranjo I, Lopez-Trigo J, Ferrandiz A, et al. Hemorrhagic abscess in a patient with the acquired immunodeficiency syndrome. Neuroradiology 1989;31:289.
59. Wijdicks EFM, Borleffs JC, Hoepelman AI, Jansen GH. Fatal disseminated hemorrhagic toxoplasmic encephali-

tis as the initial manifestation of AIDS. Ann Neurol 1991;29:683.

60. Levy RM, Rosenbloom S, Perrett LV. Neuroradiologic findings in AIDS: a review of 200 cases. AJNR Am J Neuroradiol 1988;7:833.
61. Brightbill TC, Post MJ, Hensley GT, Ruiz A. MR of toxoplasma encephalitis: signal characteristics on T2-weighted images and pathologic correlation. J Comput Assist Tomogr 1996;20:417.
62. Roberts TC, Storch GA. Multiplex PCR for diagnosis of AIDS-related central nervous system lymphoma and toxoplasmosis. J Clin Microbiol 1997;35:268.
63. Campbell BG, Hurley J, Zimmerman RD. False-negative single-photon emission CT in AIDS lymphoma: lack of effect of steroids (letter to the editor). Am J Neuroradiol 1996;17:1000.
64. O'Malley JP, Ziessman HA, Kumar PN, et al. Diagnosis of intracranial lymphoma in patients with AIDS: value of ^{201}TI single photon emission computed tomography. AJR Am J Roentgenol 1994;163:417.
65. Ruiz A, Ganz WI, Post MJ, et al. Use of thallium-201 brain SPECT to differentiate cerebral lymphoma from toxoplasma encephalitis in AIDS patients. AJNR Am J Neuroradiol 1994;15:1885.
66. Fung HB, Kirschenbaum HL. Treatment regimens for patients with toxoplasmic encephalitis. Clin Ther 1996;18:1037.
67. Dannemann BR, Israelski DM, Remington JS. Treatment of toxoplasmic encephalitis with intravenous clindamycin. Arch Intern Med 1988;148:2477.
68. Green JA, Spruance SL, Cheson BD. Favorable outcome of central nervous system toxoplasmosis occurring in a patient with untreated Hodgkin's disease. Cancer 1980;45:808.
69. Treseler CB, Sugar AM. Fungal meningitis. Infect Dis Clin North Am 1990;4:789.
70. Minamoto GY, Rosenberg AS. Fungal infections in patients with acquired immunodeficiency syndrome. Med Clin North Am 1997;81:381.
71. Lyons RW, Andriole VT. Fungal infections of the CNS. Neurol Clin 1986;4:159.
72. Gonyea EF. The spectrum of primary blastomycotic meningitis: a review of central nervous system blastomycosis. Ann Neurol 1978;3:26.
73. Harley WB, Lomis M, Haas DW. Marked polymorphonuclear pleocytosis due to blastomycotic meningitis: case report and review. Clin Infect Dis 1994;18:816.
74. Friedman J, Wijdicks EFM, Fulgham J, Wright A. Meningoencephalitis from blastomycosis (submitted for publication).
75. Sarosi GA, Davies SF. Therapy for fungal infections. Mayo Clin Proc 1994;69:1111.
76. Ward BA, Parent AD, Raila F. Indications for the surgical management of central nervous system blastomycosis. Surg Neurol 1995;43:379.
77. Newman NJ, Bell IR, McKee AC. Paraneoplastic limbic encephalitis: neuropsychiatric presentation. Biol Psychiatry 1990;27:529.
78. Camara EG, Chelune GJ. Paraneoplastic limbic encephalopathy. Brain Behav Immun 1987;1:349.
79. Corsellis JA, Goldberg GJ, Norton AR. "Limbic encephalitis" and its association with carcinoma. Brain 1968;91:481.
80. Deodhare S, O'Connor P, Ghazarian D, Bilbao JM. Paraneoplastic limbic encephalitis in Hodgkin's disease. Can J Neurol Sci 1996;23:138.
81. Wingerchuk DM, Noseworthy JH, Kimmel DW. Paraneoplastic encephalomyelitis and seminoma: importance of testicular ultrasonography. Neurology 1998; 51:1504.
82. Kodama T, Numaguchi Y, Gellad FE, et al. Magnetic resonance imaging of limbic encephalitis. Neuroradiology 1991;33:520.
83. Greenlee JE, Lipton HL. Anticerebellar antibodies in serum and cerebrospinal fluid of a patient with oat cell carcinoma of the lung and paraneoplastic cerebellar degeneration. Ann Neurol 1986;19:82.
84. Benyahia B, Liblau R, Merle-Beral H, et al. Cell-mediated autoimmunity in paraneoplastic neurological syndromes with anti-Hu antibodies. Ann Neurol 1999;45:162.
85. Jean WC, Dalmau J, Ho A, Posner JB. Analysis of the IgG subclass distribution and inflammatory infiltrates in patients with anti-Hu-associated paraneoplastic encephalomyelitis. Neurology 1994;44:140.

Chapter 11
Acute White Matter Diseases

Devastating white matter disorders are fulminant multiple sclerosis (MS), transverse myelitis, and disseminated encephalomyelitis. Even in academic institutions, they are sporadically seen. They are included in this monograph because it is important to diagnose and manage these disorders quickly.

Acute demyelination of the neuraxis may turn out catastrophic, and treatment in the acute phase remains problematic. Rapid cures remain few and far between. For one thing, aggressive immunosuppression may shorten the relapse or resolve some or virtually all of its manifestations.

A related disorder, often with an acute onset, is acute leukoencephalopathy occurring in a diverse group of patients. In this entity, demyelination is part of a more global involvement of white matter structures, including axis cylinders. Toxins, illicit drug abuse, toxicity from immunosuppressive agents, and hypertensive crises are common. These disorders may resolve quickly after elimination of the trigger alone.

Acute Disseminated Encephalomyelitis

Acute disseminated encephalomyelitis (ADEM) is a dramatic monophasic illness from an autoimmune response activated by a viral infection or vaccination. ADEM occurs more often in children and young adults, and most infections are mundane viral respiratory episodes. ADEM may follow any well-defined illness (e.g., rubeola, varicella, mycoplasmal pneumonia,[1,2] and infectious mononucleosis) or may occur without an identifiable antecedent event.

Pathologic features of ADEM include multifocal patchy perivenous demyelination. Even in the most severe cases, use of polymerase chain reaction analysis to recover a virus (e.g., enterovirus, adenovirus, herpesvirus, and respiratory syncytial virus) from the brain during autopsy has not been successful. Human herpesvirus 6 has recently been associated with ADEM.[3] However, no virus has yet been isolated from cerebrospinal fluid (CSF). Recognition of human herpesvirus 6 (polymerase chain reaction is currently in development) may be clinically pertinent, because this virus can potentially be treated with acyclovir.

Clinical Presentation

Patients and their consulted family members recall a flulike illness with a variable combination of fever, aching joints, swollen lymph nodes, and fatigue. Some of these constitutional symptoms may still be present at onset.

Neurologic manifestation occurs after an "incubation" of 1 to 3 weeks but progresses rapidly to a maximum within days. Widespread involvement of the central nervous system may affect many eloquent areas of the brain and cord. White matter destruction involving the optic tract, brain stem, and spinal cord that resembles acute transverse myelitis is a classic

Table 11.1. Disorders Mimicking Acute Disseminated Encephalomyelitis

Acute viral encephalitis (arboviruses)
Herpes simplex encephalitis
Central nervous system vasculitis
Intravascular lymphoma
Progressive multifocal leukoencephalopathy
Neurosarcoidosis
Systemic lupus erythematosus

finding if the disorder progresses. Initially, headaches with transient focal neurologic signs may be prominent and fluctuating. Neurologic findings further reflect acute myelin destruction and may consist of any degree of impairment of consciousness with several prompts needed to alert patients to their surroundings, ophthalmoplegia, cerebellar ataxia, and, in many patients, evolution to muteness.

Spinal cord involvement may be the first presenting symptom or quickly merge into a more diffuse or multifocal neurologic symptom complex. Progressive quadriparesis may result in early inability to walk, but level of consciousness should also become involved at this time.

Progression is within days, but a clinical course with up to 2 months of gradual, protracted change has been documented. ADEM can be mistaken for central nervous system lymphoma, vasculitis, and viral encephalitis (Table 11.1).

Interpretation of Diagnostic Tests

Computed Tomography and Magnetic Resonance Imaging

Computed tomography (CT) and magnetic resonance imaging (MRI) findings are fairly typical but may be rather subtle in earlier stages. The typical appearance in ADEM is multiple discrete lesions in the cerebral white matter and rarely in periventricular areas, a location much more typical for fulminant MS. The lesions predominate in occipital-parietal white matter (Figure 11.1, A and B) but may involve the basal ganglia, hypothalamus, and brain stem.[4,5] Symmetrical cerebellar white matter and basal ganglia involvement may differentiate it from MS.[6,7] All these abnormalities may hardly be detected by CT, and only some decreased attenuation in the white matter of the centrum semiovale is seen, even at the stage of prominent neurologic manifestations. MRI remains a crucial determinant for its diagnosis. Gadolinium enhancement is a reflection of the blood-brain barrier breakdown in the earlier stages of demyelination. Enhancement may appear in some lesions on MRI and not in others, suggesting different stages in demyelination.[8,9] Enhancement may be marginal because of corticosteroid treatment that reduces the blood-brain barrier permeability.[10] If enhancement is found, abnormal signal intensity bilaterally in the optic neuritis is more common (as opposed to the more common unilateral optic neuritis in MS). Generally, these MRI features cannot be easily differentiated from those of MS, and a more distinct histologic feature of brain tissue has not been identified in tissue specimens.

Hemorrhagic changes (Figure 11.1, C and D) suggest an acute hemorrhagic leukoencephalitis (or Weston Hurst disease), and this disorder, noted after similar triggering circumstances, may primarily be an aggressive variant of ADEM, commonly with massive brain edema.[11] Hyperintense lesions on T2-weighted images, with ringlike solid enhancing lesions and perifocal edema, have been reported as well. Cortical involvement is compatible with the diagnosis albeit less extensively distributed.

Cerebrospinal Fluid

CSF may show moderate pleocytosis (up to 200 cells/mm^3). In ADEM, the CSF contains lymphocytes; in Weston Hurst disease, polymorphonuclear leukocytes are prominent.[11] The pleocytosis is usually out of proportion to what is expected during a flare-up of MS. Oligoclonal bands can be found and may disappear after treatment (oligoclonal bands commonly persist in MS).

First Priority in Management

High-dose methyl prednisolone (1,000 mg intravenously daily) remains the first therapy of choice. Excellent recovery has also been observed with plasma exchange, but failure to improve rapidly with corticosteroids should prompt its use. The exact number of plasma exchanges is unknown, although exchanges for up to 10 days (or until improvement) have been pro-

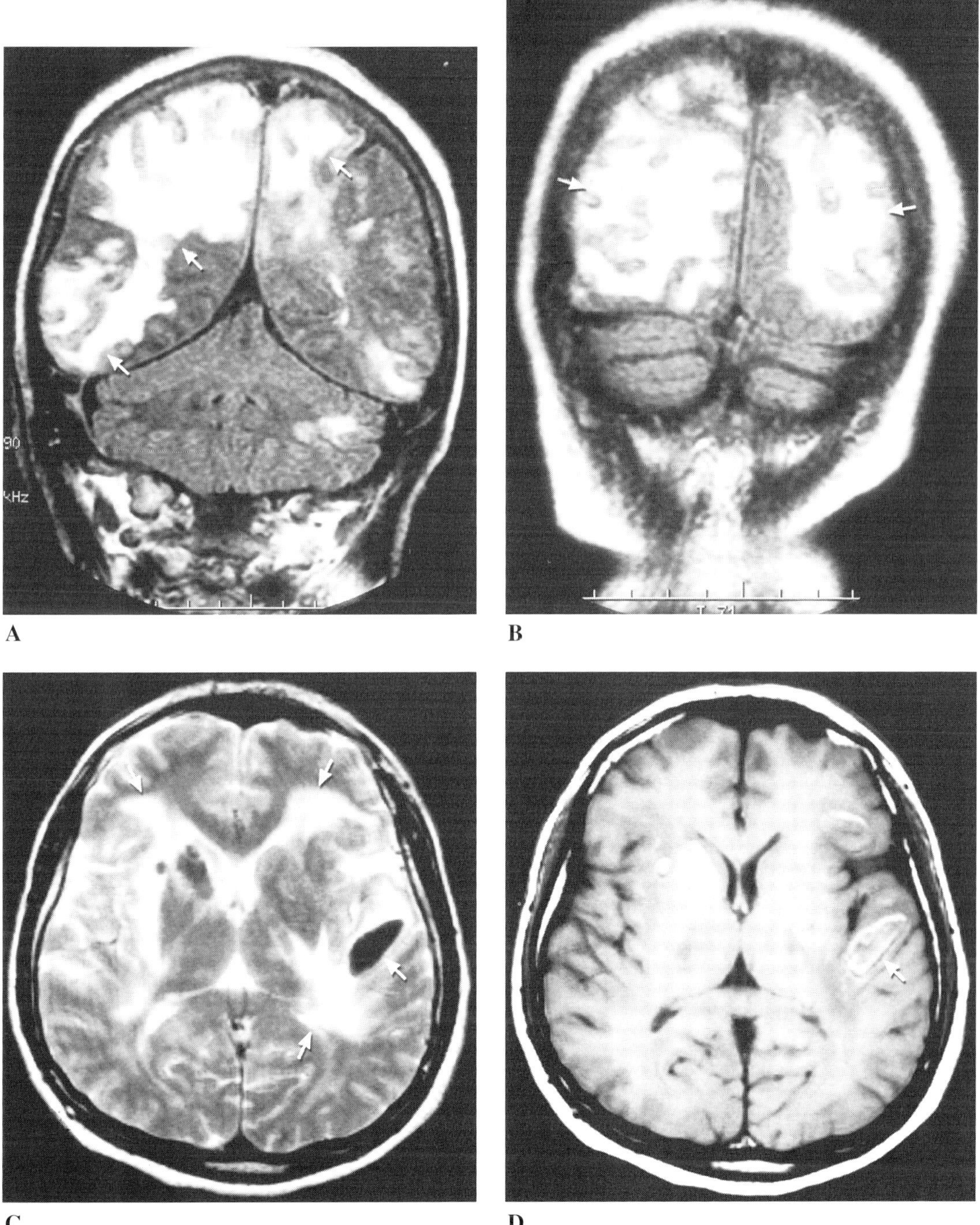

Figure 11.1. Magnetic resonance imaging with coronal views of acute disseminated encephalomyelitis (see text).

posed.[12–14] Alternatively, intravenous immunoglobulin, 0.4 g/kg for 3 to 5 days, can be used.[15,16]

Predictors of Outcome

Improvement can be rather rapid with specific measures, such as corticosteroid treatment. Awakening is followed by reduction in diplopia and bulbar abnormalities and more gradually by improved ambulation. MRI findings should closely parallel clinical improvement. Full recovery after Weston Hurst disease has been described in several cases.

Triage

- A brief period of observation in the intensive care unit and support with mechanical ventilation may be needed, but many patients are soon able to protect their airway.
- Brain biopsy should be deferred until the effect of specific therapy has been evaluated.

Fulminant Multiple Sclerosis

Patients with clinically or laboratory-supported definitive MS may have fulminant exacerbations. Progression into a devastating condition or death rarely is the first presentation. The designation "fulminant" in this condition is usually defined by days rather than weeks and presupposes involvement of multiple areas in the cerebral white matter and often the brain stem. Demyelination, which leads to loss of ambulation from weakness or ataxia, may involve the bulbar function and respiratory centers. A brain biopsy performed for diagnosis shows fairly typical neuropathologic features of marked inflammatory perivascular infiltrates, extensive myelin breakdown that spares the nerve cell bodies and axis cylinders, and diffuse macrophage infiltration.

Clinical Presentation

Earlier descriptions of this fulminant variant emphasized an accelerated development of ataxia, hemiparesis, or paraparesis; blindness or progressive ophthalmoplegia; and a notable bulbar involvement leading to dysphagia and aspiration. Brain stem involvement is a common feature in acute fulminant MS. Quadriparalysis and involvement of the lower cranial nerves with sparing of only the oculomotor nerves closely resemble a locked-in syndrome and often is linked to a fatal outcome.[17,18]

The most dramatic variant, one with high mortality, is the Marburg variant.[19] Within days, progressive ophthalmoplegia, dysarthria, dysphagia, and blindness may develop and the patient becomes comatose. An uncal herniation pattern appears when a large inflammatory demyelinating mass shifts brain tissue.

Mechanical ventilation is often instituted in patients whose condition deteriorates to coma and in patients with bulbar signs. Pulmonary edema as a result of sympathetic disinhibition may accompany the fulminant form.[20] In most patients, marked bulbar failure and inability to swallow secretions lead to aspiration pneumonitis rather than true neurogenic pulmonary edema.

Interpretation of Diagnostic Tests

The diagnostic criteria of MS, including laboratory abnormalities, have recently been expertly outlined. A modification of the Poser criteria is shown in Capsule 11.1.

Computed Tomography and Magnetic Resonance Imaging

MRI assists in the diagnosis, but findings are nonspecific. MRI shows demyelination, which is hypointense or isointense on T1-weighted images, occasionally with hyperintense edges; lesions are small, irregular, or confluent. White matter lesions are invariably located in the pons, medulla, and additional hemispheric areas involving the junctions of gray and white matter and in the corpus callosum. Larger confluent areas of demyelination in periventricular white matter can be seen as well.[21,22] Ovoid lesions at right angles to the ventricular surface are characteristic (Figure 11.2). Unilateral mass effect with developing edema may occur. Mass effect may be the most prominent CT scan manifestation (Figure 11.3). Ringlike structures may appear, corresponding to layers of macrophages, which generate

Capsule 11.1. Diagnostic Criteria for Multiple Sclerosis

Category	Subcategory	Number of clinical attacks	Number of clinically evident lesions	Paraclinical evidence*	CSF oligoclonal bands
CDMS	A1	2	2	N/A	N/A
	A2	2	1	and 1 (or more)	N/A
	A3	1	1	2†	N/A
LSDMS	B1	2	1	or 1 (or more)	+
	B2	1	2		+
	B3	1	1	and 1 (or more)	+

(CDMS = clinically definite multiple sclerosis; CSF = cerebrospinal fluid; LSDMS = laboratory-supported definite multiple sclerosis; N/A = not applicable; + = present.)
*Implies MRI, evoked potentials, or CSF.
†A diagnosis of CDMS A3 requires paraclinical evidence for dissemination in time as well as space.
From Paty DW, Noseworthy JH, Ebers GC. Diagnosis of Multiple Sclerosis. In DW Paty, GC Ebers (eds), Multiple Sclerosis (Contemporary Neurology Series). Philadelphia: FA Davis Company, 1998;48. By permission of Oxford University Press.

free radicals to produce this paramagnetic effect.[23] However, more recent magnetic resonance spectroscopy studies found that these rings represent central edema in the core of the ring plaque.[24]

Evoked Potentials

Evoked potential studies may detect asymptomatic lesions not apparent on MRI.[25,26] Pattern reversal visual evoked potential is sensitive for lesions in the optic nerve and chiasm, and findings are abnormal in 40% to 60% of patients with early MS.[22] The sensitivity in median nerve somatosensory evoked potentials is similar. Brain stem auditory evoked potentials are less sensitive and are positive in only 20% to 25% of patients with MS.[25]

Evoked potentials probably are most useful in providing supportive laboratory evidence of MS when results of two or more diagnostic tests are abnormal.[26]

Cerebrospinal Fluid

Cell count can vary from 10 to 50 lymphocytes/mm^3, with a mixture of monocytes, plasma cells, and macrophages. Total protein is mildly increased, and IgG is increased in 70% of clinically definite instances of MS. Two or more oligoclonal bands in the gamma field may be detected in only 40% of patients with first presentation of MS. Intrathecal immunoglobulin in the CSF is a result of increased plasma cell synthesis and leakage from the brain through a defective blood-brain barrier. Oligoclonal bands in the CSF (at least two different and distinct bands) but not in the serum are typical for MS but can occur in 8% of patients with other neurologic disease that may superficially mimic MS (viral meningoencephalitis, neurosyphilis, sarcoidosis, and fungal meningitis). The sensitivity of oligoclonal bands in CSF for MS is more than 90%.[27]

First Priority in Management

Intravenous administration of methylprednisolone, 1 g per day for 3 to 5 days, is followed by 60 mg of prednisone.[28] Tapering of oral prednisone should be completed in 14 days. Overall prognosis is not affected by corticosteroids. Azathioprine, methotrexate, cyclophosphamide, and cyclosporine have no demonstrated benefit in acute progressive MS.

High doses of corticosteroids may not be sufficient to counter the fulminant attack, and recent evidence in patients with fulminant MS suggests that plasma exchange may be useful.[29] Improvement begins within several days, reversing quadriplegia and dependency on a mechanical ventilator. Plasmapheresis has shown no effect in progressive MS, but

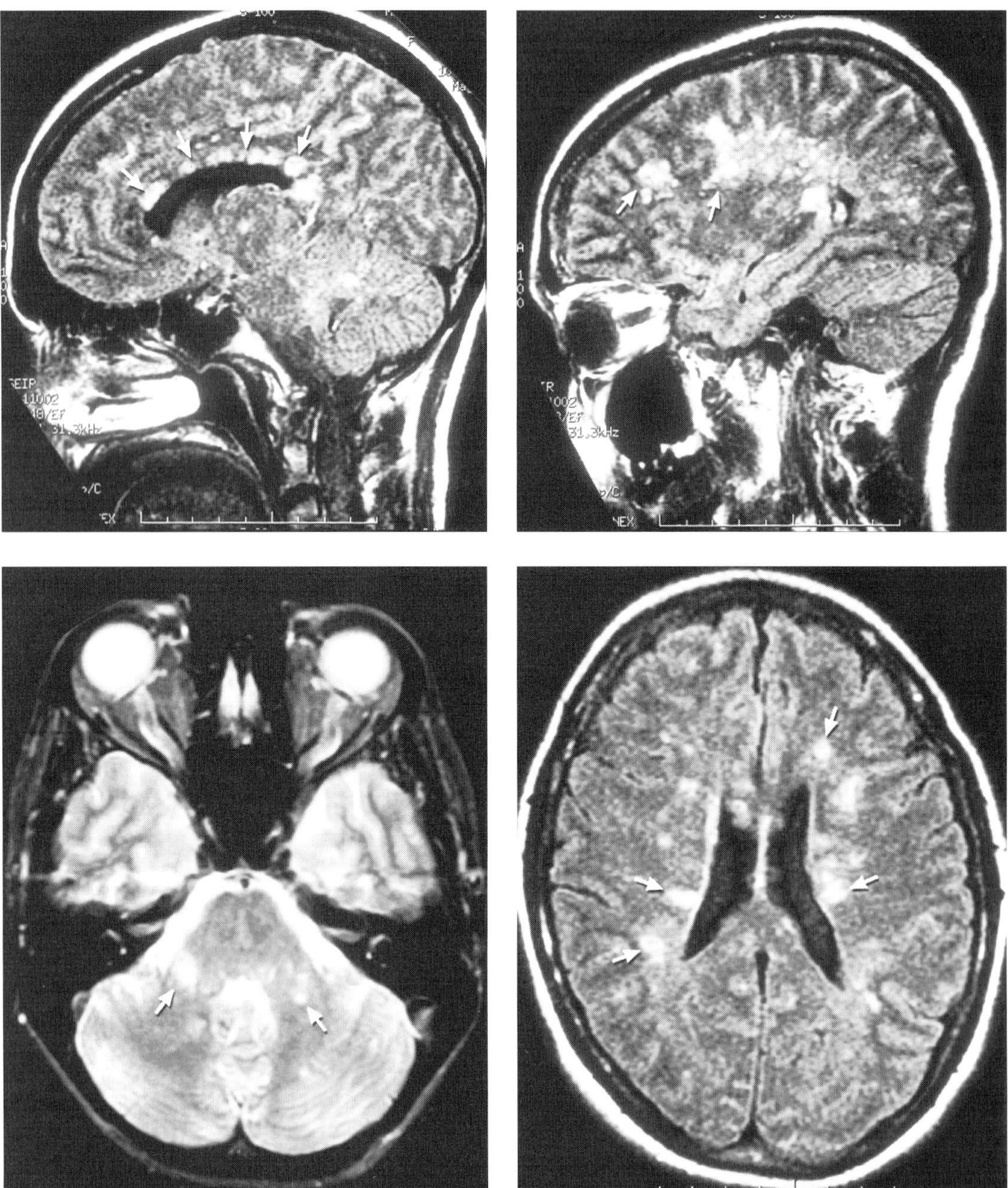

Figure 11.2. Fulminant multiple sclerosis with multiple periventricular white matter lesions and characteristic scattered lesions in the corpus callosum and brain stem.

it has been speculated that it may be beneficial in fulminant exacerbations by removing soluble factors involved in the process of demyelination. The number of plasma exchanges is unknown; six exchanges every other day were needed in one pilot study.[29]

Two forms of recombinant interferon beta should be considered. These agents decrease clinical relapses by 30%, halve the number of severe relapses, and lengthen time to first relapse. They are administered subcutaneously (interferon beta-1b, 8 million units every other day) or intramuscularly (interferon beta-1a, 6 million units weekly). The effects of a new agent, glatiramer acetate (20 mg subcutaneously daily), are similar.[30]

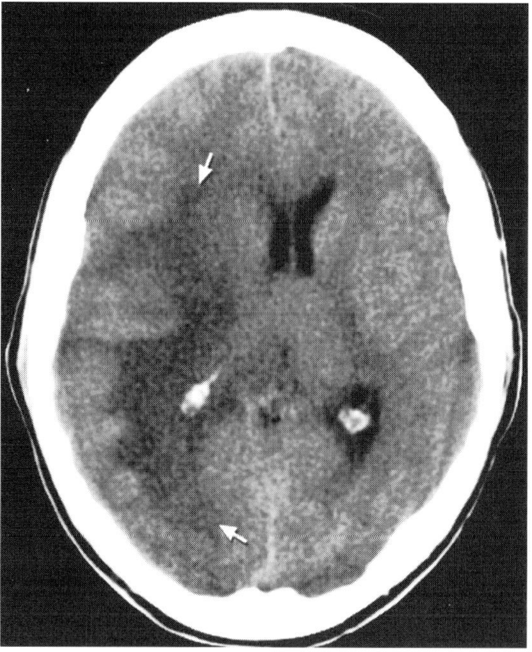
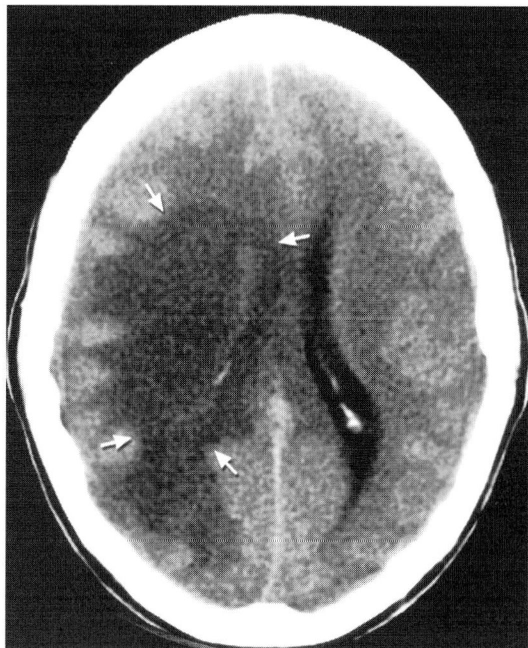

Figure 11.3. Marked mass effect and edema common in the Marburg variant of multiple sclerosis.

Predictors of Outcome

Fulminant MS is associated with a high probability of permanent disability and also with a somewhat shortened life span, strongly dependent on the degree of disability. Unfavorable prognostic factors are age over 40, male, and extensive MRI abnormalities (increased T2 lesion load and number of active enhancing lesions). The relapse rate varies after a first major attack but decreases over time. After the first attack, approximately 25% of patients have a relapse within 1 year and 50% within 3 years. The extent of disability 5 years after the diagnosis strongly determines the future clinical course.[31] Recovery may be protracted, lasting 3 to 4 weeks, and intercurrent infections may contribute to early mortality.

Triage

- Early aspiration, fever, or major bulbar involvement justifies admission to an intensive care unit.
- Placement of an intracranial pressure device is warranted in the Marburg variant to monitor progression and treat increased intracranial pressure.
- Neurosurgical consultation for craniotomy or biopsy may be needed to pathologically confirm the diagnosis.

Acute Transverse Myelitis

Acute transverse myelitis is an uncommon, potentially devastating disorder associated with many viral illnesses (Table 11.2). A vigorously mounted immune response is attributed to its pathogenesis. Demyelination and inflammation involve the spinal cord at any level, but often the effects are limited to a few segments. However, patients presenting with acute paraparesis and a distinct sensory level more commonly have extramedullary cord compression or another cause of myelitis. Chapter 5 presents the overall evaluation of acute spinal cord compression.

Clinical Presentation

Acute development of ascending sensory deficit and difficulty walking within days are hallmarks of the disorder.[32] Fever and nuchal rigidity may occur in 27% and 13% of the patients, respectively.[33] Pares-

Table 11.2. Causes of Acute Transverse Myelitis

Echovirus
Varicella
Herpes zoster
Influenza
Epstein-Barr virus
Cytomegalovirus
Mycoplasmal pneumonia
Parasite infection (e.g., schistosomiasis)
Vaccination
Multiple sclerosis
Lupus erythematosus

thesias may be widespread, but usually a sensory level below which sensation is abnormal is pointed out by the patient.

Motor weakness may vary substantially, with a maximum deficit usually within 1 to 2 days, although subacute progression up to 2 months is known. However, maximal motor deficit may be reached within several hours.

The neurologic findings are typical of a functional cord transection at one segment, with loss of motor and sensory function and areflexia. All spinal cord levels can become involved, but cervical localization is less prevalent. Partial variants have been described, with incomplete involvement, patchy and dissociated sensory symptoms, and sparing of the bladder.

Interpretation of Diagnostic Tests

Magnetic Resonance Imaging

MRI is preferred to exclude causes that are potentially reversible. The rarity of the disorder implies that other causes are more frequent in clinical practice. MRI should be performed at once, and if necessary, patients should be referred to a tertiary center.

MRI findings are swelling of the cord, increased T2-weighted signal, and, often, abnormal enhancement throughout the cord.[34–38]

More extensive involvement may be found on MRI than is clinically evident and vice versa (Figure 11.4). A swollen cord is difficult to differentiate from an intramedullary neoplasm or dural arteriovenous malformation causing venous hypertension (Chapter 5), but follow-up MRI, usually within weeks, should demonstrate complete resolution or substantial improvement. MRI of the brain is useful to demonstrate other demyelinating lesions that increase the probability of MS, with acute transverse myelitis as the first-defining illness.

Cerebrospinal Fluid

CSF examination may show pleocytosis of up to 10,000 cells (both lymphocytes and polymorphonuclear leukocytes), but findings can be normal. CSF protein is commonly increased (in more than three-fourths of patients) and may reach values as high as 500 mg/dL.

Miscellaneous

Vasculitis (e.g., systemic lupus erythematosus) and a vascular malformation are important considerations, and spinal angiography should be performed if involvement is at a high or middle thoracic level. This localization in a spinal watershed zone may suggest a vascular rather than an autoimmune mechanism.

Viral serology may be useful, because well-known viral agents may cause acute transverse myelitis,[39] but the effects of antiviral agents, even when administered early in the course, are not known.

First Priority in Management

Treatment with corticosteroids is controversial. No measurable effect has been reported, and with marked variability in recovery time, improvement cannot be attributed to this treatment without a formal clinical trial.

It is unknown whether specific antibiotic or antiviral therapy improves outcome. Experience with plasmapheresis and intravenous immunoglobulin is lacking. It is important to place an indwelling catheter in patients with minimal bladder reflex activity. Dysautonomia may occur from a distended bladder when the lesion is above the sympathetic outflow (T6), and any stimulus may produce severe hypertension. Prophylaxis for deep venous thrombosis (heparin subcutaneously or intermittent compression devices) should begin early.

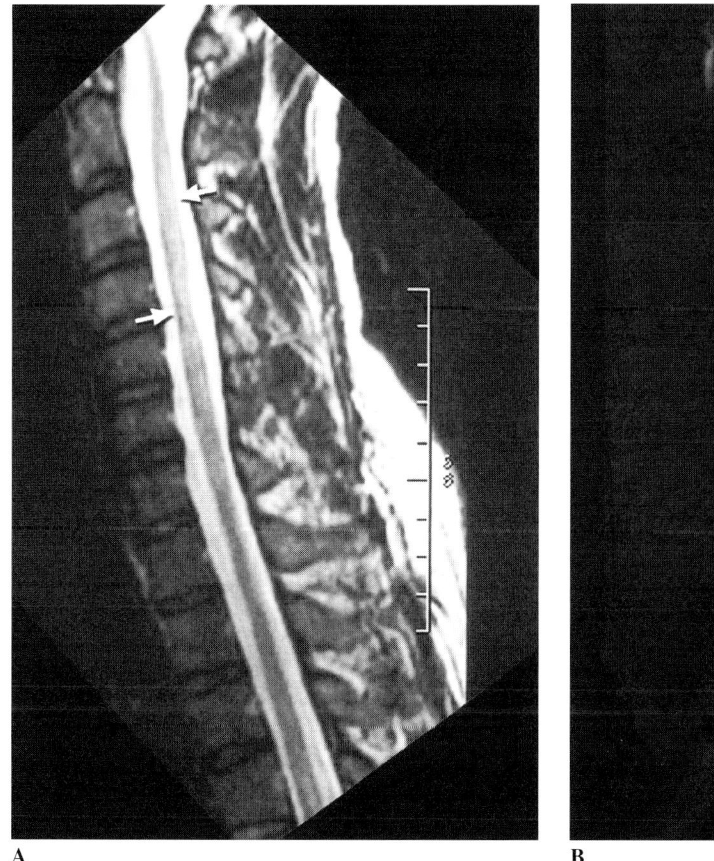

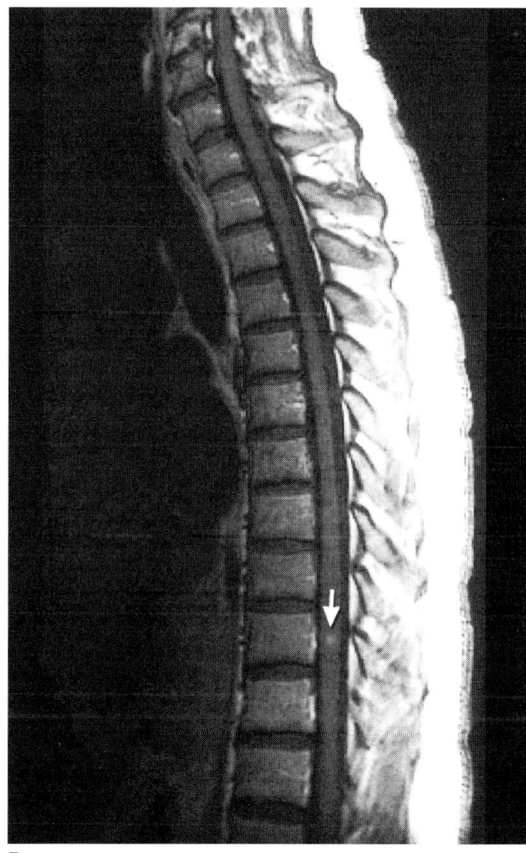

A B

Figure 11.4. Acute transverse myelitis (magnetic resonance images, sagittal view). **A.** Long segment of T2 signal in cervical cord. **B.** Subtle enhancing thoracic cord abnormality. Both patients had complete cord lesions on examination.

Predictors of Outcome

One-third of patients with acute transverse myelitis do not recover ambulation or bladder or bowel control. Partial recovery with a considerable handicap and good recovery each accounts for one-third of the patients.[40] Transverse myelitis has a much better prognosis if there is no progression to a complete cord syndrome and sensation remains preserved. MRI findings are not predictive of outcome. No correlation has been found with extent of the initial deficit, neurologic deficit and prognosis, and MRI findings.[41]

Triage

- ♦ MRI of the spine on an urgent basis.
- ♦ Neurology ward or rehabilitation unit.

Acute Leukoencephalopathy

Selective white matter damage has become more apparent with the introduction of immunosuppressive agents, street drugs, and chemotherapeutic agents. These lipophilic substances preferentially target myelin because of its high lipid content. MRI predominance in the bilateral parieto-occipital hemispheric regions justifies the term "posterior leukoencephalopathy."[42–46] This section describes acute leukoencephalopathy in adults. Causes are presented in Table 11.3. Chronic, protracted leukoencephalopathies consist of a very wide array of disorders, including aminoacidopa-

Table 11.3. Acute Leukoencephalopathy in Adults

Immunosuppressive agents (cyclosporine, tacrolimus)
Hypertensive crises
Eclampsia, HELLP syndrome
Chemotherapeutic agents (methotrexate, 5-fluorouracil, levamisole, intra-arterial nimustine [ACNU])
Fulminant multiple sclerosis
Postradiation period
Human immunodeficiency virus encephalopathy
Erythropoietin
Interferon-α
Heroin inhalation
Progressive multifocal leukoencephalopathy

(HELLP = hemolysis, elevated liver enzymes, and low platelet [count].)

thy, organic acid disorders, and lysosomal storage disease.

Clinical Presentation

Decrease in level of consciousness and marked cognitive decline, but also behavioral changes alone, may be presenting symptoms. Headache is prominent. Seizures are prevalent, mostly generalized tonic-clonic, but focal onset has been noted. The disorder may progress rapidly to cortical blindness, marked ataxia, and speech or language abnormalities. Akinetic mutism may occur if the disorder is not recognized in the earlier stages of presentation. Akinetic mutism (summarized by Cairns et al.[47] as "motionless, mindless wakefulness") can be explained by extensive involvement of the thalamofrontal fibers and isolation of the anterior cingulate cortex.

Immunosuppressive agents (cyclosporine and tacrolimus) in transplantation have been implicated in many well-documented cases of acute leukoencephalopathy. Breakdown of the blood-brain barrier or facilitated transport is required for these immunosuppressive drugs to enter the brain. Cyclosporine or tacrolimus may have a direct damaging effect on the vasculature, leading to microvascular damage and access to the brain.

Tremors, vivid visual hallucinations, and behavioral changes with paranoid behavior and wide mood swings are common and associated with a rambling, nonsensible speech. Commonly, the speech disorder is characterized by stuttering when words are spoken rapidly or even at a normal pace but normal output when the patient is instructed to speak slowly. Speech may be distorted, with similarity to a foreign accent, and a single generalized tonic-clonic seizure may be the only clue to toxicity. Less common presentations are blindness, cerebellar syndrome, orofacial dyskinesias, and mutism.[48] Presentation is similar in tacrolimus and cyclosporine neurotoxicity: signs and symptoms regress rapidly after discontinuation but may reoccur after a different immunosuppressive agent is substituted. With the oral microemulsion of cyclosporine (Neoral), neurotoxicity is less severe, mostly tremor and headache only.[49]

Another well-identified leukoencephalopathy has been associated with chemotherapeutic agents, predominantly 5-fluorouracil and levamisole. The estimated incidence of this toxic leukoencephalopathy is 2%.[50]

The lesions are more confluent and multifocal when tissue is examined. Perivascular lymphocytic inflammation is found next to demyelination. A more delayed manifestation, but often with seizures, has been reported with chemotherapeutic agents. In these patients, a history of insidious decline in intellectual function is obtained, together with clinical evidence of a progressive disorder characterized by spasticity and bulbar palsy. Its clinical presentation can be nothing more specific than depression and withdrawal, sometimes mistaken as a response to the diagnosis of cancer. Ataxia, impaired thinking, slurring of speech, and memory impairment follow, and profound stupor or coma may ensue. The predominant trigger of neurotoxicity is 5-fluorouracil,[50-52] but toxicity with levamisole alone has been reported as well.[53]

Methotrexate is used intravenously, intrathecally, and orally.[54] All these modes of administration may be associated with toxicity to the central nervous system white matter.[55,56] Methotrexate barely crosses the blood-brain barrier because it is an ionized and lipid-insoluble compound, but radiation-induced damage to the integrity of the blood-brain barrier may facilitate its transport. Intra-arterially administered nimustine (ACNU) has produced leukoencephalopathy in the treatment of glioma, but radiation may cause a similar clinical phenotype.[57] Combined use may complicate finding a precise cause-and-effect relationship.

In the management of leukemia, three recognized chemotherapy-associated leukoencephalopathy syndromes have been described: (1) an acute syndrome within 24 hours after intrathecal administration of methotrexate, cranial irradiation, or use of cytarabine, resulting in an acute confusional state and seizures resolving in 2 to 3 days; (2) subacute leukoencephalopathy 1 to 2 weeks after intravenous administration of methotrexate, with focal motor neurologic signs, behavioral changes, and seizures; and (3) insidious leukoencephalopathy progressing over months, with personality changes, marked intellectual decline, and spasticity.[58]

Leukoencephalopathy may occur after heroin abuse, particularly after inhalation of heroin ("Chinese blowing," or "Chinesing").[59,60] Progression from cerebellar symptoms to extrapyramidal involvement to spasticity to akinetic mutism is due to involvement of both cerebral hemispheres, the cerebellar peduncles, and the midbrain.

Anecdotal reports of acute leukoencephalopathy with erythropoietin,[61] amphotericin,[62] and interferon-α have appeared.[45] Hypertensive encephalopathy and eclampsia may cause headache, seizures, cortical blindness, and papilledema and may produce reversible posterior leukoencephalopathy.[63]

It remains important to exclude multifocal leukoencephalopathy associated with human immunodeficiency virus (HIV) and progressive multifocal leukoencephalopathy associated with JC virus by examination of CSF, polymerase chain reaction, or brain biopsy.[64–67]

Interpretation of Diagnostic Tests

Computed Tomography and Magnetic Resonance Imaging

CT scanning is not nearly as sensitive as MRI in leukoencephalopathy, and findings may be surprisingly normal. Any comatose patient with any of the toxins or triggers mentioned above should therefore undergo MRI.

Routine MRI sequences, gadolinium enhancement, and, if available, diffusion-weighted imaging may further delineate the white matter lesion. Increased diffusion on diffusion-weighted MRI may support vasogenic edema rather than cytotoxic edema, which indicates ischemia and is associated with decreased diffusion.[68]

The extensive lesions are nonspecific, but some MRI characteristics may point to a certain cause. These are sparing of the U fibers (cytomegalovirus and HIV encephalopathy); capping of the lateral ventricles, centrum semiovale, and corpus callosum (MS); additional gray matter involvement (central nervous system vasculitis, organic acidurias, postanoxic encephalopathies, including carbon monoxide and cyanide); enhancement with gadolinium (ADEM, MS, Alexander's disease, Schilder's diffuse sclerosis); and no involvement of the basal ganglia (lysosomal disorders, including sphingolipidosis). Several examples of acute leukoencephalopathies are shown in Figures 11.5, 11.6, and 11.7. Most patients with mild forms of cyclosporine or tacrolimus neurotoxicity do not have MRI abnormalities,[69,70] which are typically seen in the most severe instances,[71–73] often in patients with seizures at presentation. MRI abnormalities with immunosuppressive agents have largely been a consequence of inexperience with dosage in the early years of cyclosporine. Progressive multifocal leukoencephalopathy may mimic these disorders. Little or no mass effect or gadolinium enhancement is noted. The lesions are in focal areas of the gray-white junction (Figure 11.8).

Cerebrospinal Fluid and Serum

CSF examination is useful to obtain material for detecting the JC virus, and the test has 100% specificity in immunosuppressed patients after transplantation. Oligoclonal bands and IgG index are useful but not diagnostic and can be seen in many demyelinating disorders.

The correlation of cyclosporine and tacrolimus with blood or plasma levels is unreliable, and in some patients progression may occur despite declining blood levels. In 30% to 40% of the reported cases, trough plasma levels are increased or show a significant upward trend. Plasma levels of these immunosuppressive agents are more likely to be increased when leukoencephalopathy is demonstrated on MRI.

First Priority in Management

Discontinuation of therapy with the causative drug may resolve most of the symptoms within 2 days. Methylprednisolone has been administered intravenously in inflammatory leukoencephalopathies

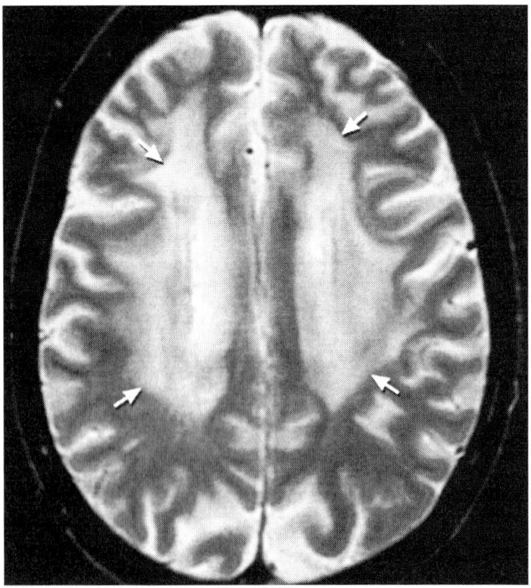

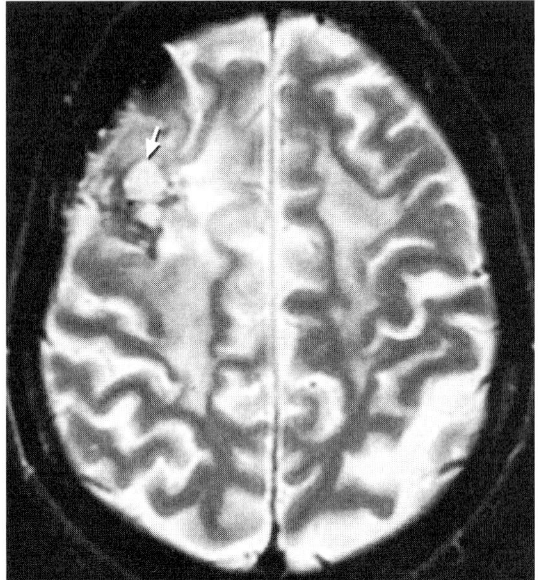

Figure 11.5. Magnetic resonance images demonstrate radiation leukoencephalopathy (radiation for glioma).

associated with chemotherapeutic agents, with a successful result but no proof of its effect.[53] The recommended dose is 1 g of methylprednisolone for 3 to 5 days. Suspicion of progressive multifocal leukoencephalopathy should be high in patients who have acquired immunodeficiency syndrome (AIDS) and patients who had transplantation years earlier. Treatment with cytarabine (2 mg/kg) should await biopsy determination, but it may retard progression only for several months.

Predictors of Outcome

The prognosis for complete recovery is excellent, and both clinical and MRI resolution are expected

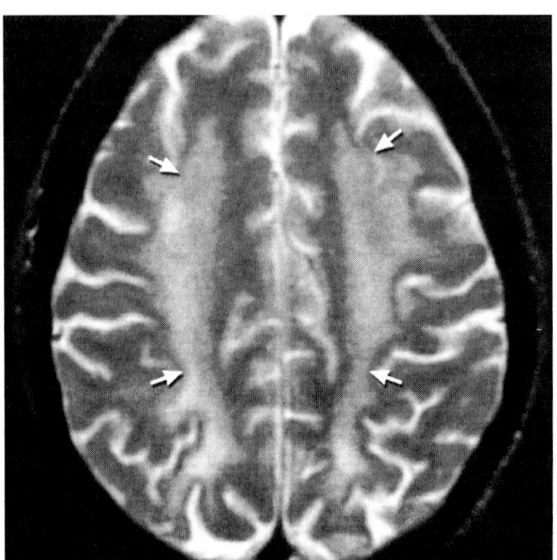

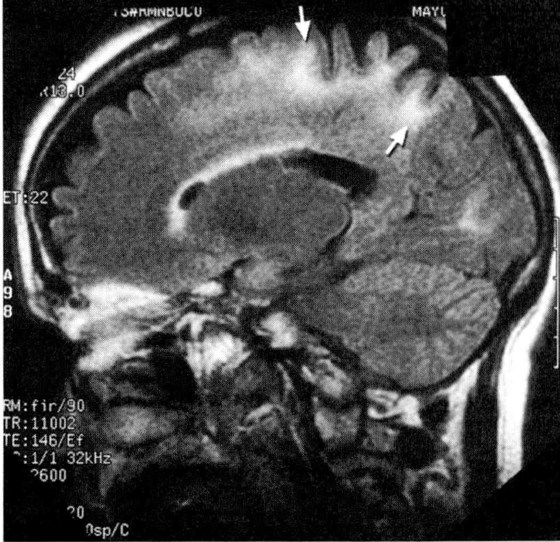

Figure 11.6. Methotrexate leukoencephalopathy on axial T2-weighted and sagittal fluid-attenuated inversion recovery magnetic resonance imaging (similar findings possible with 5-fluorouracil and levamisole).

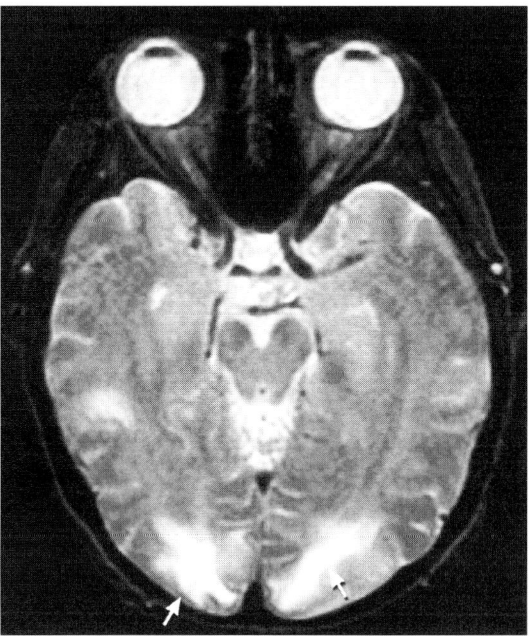

Figure 11.7. Cyclosporine-associated leukoencephalopathy.

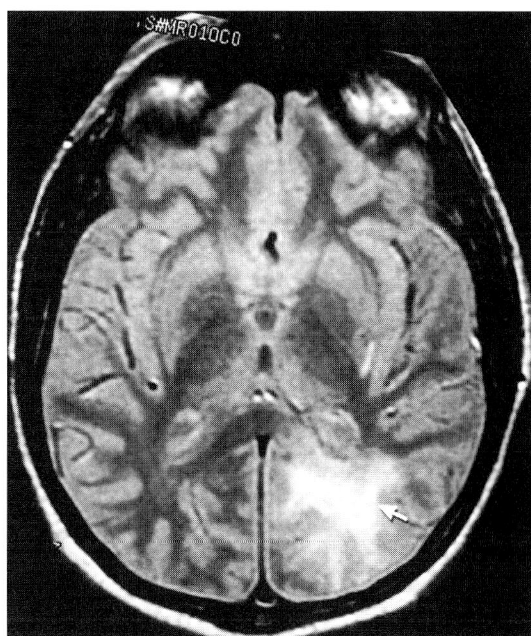

Figure 11.8. Focal posterior leukoencephalopathy due to biopsy-proven progressive multifocal leukoencephalopathy.

after cessation of the immunosuppressive and chemotherapeutic agents. Incomplete recovery has been noted, however, particularly in comatose patients.[50] The median survival with progressive multifocal leukoencephalopathy in HIV infection is 10 weeks, but survival appears prolonged when leukoencephalopathy emerges in patients receiving highly active antiretroviral therapy (HAART), increasing to 46 weeks.[74]

Triage

- Most patients can be treated with supportive care on the ward.
- Status epilepticus or focal partial status epilepticus is very uncommon, but a prolonged series of seizures may justify 24-hour observation with video and electroencephalographic monitoring in an intensive care unit.

References

1. Kornips HM, Verhagen WI, Prick MJ. Acute disseminated encephalomyelitis probably related to a *Mycoplasma pneumoniae* infection. Clin Neurol Neurosurg 1993;95:59.
2. Mills RW, Schoolfield L. Acute transverse myelitis associated with *Mycoplasma pneumoniae* infection: a case report and review of the literature. Pediatr Infect Dis J 1992;11:228.
3. Carrigan DR, Harrington D, Knox KK. Subacute leukoencephalitis caused by CNS infection with human herpesvirus-6 manifesting as acute multiple sclerosis. Neurology 1996;47:145.
4. Atlas SW, Grossman RI, Goldberg HI, et al. MR diagnosis of acute disseminated encephalomyelitis. J Comput Assist Tomogr 1986;10:798.
5. Mader I, Stock KW, Ettlin T, Probst A. Acute disseminated encephalomyelitis: MR and CT features. AJNR Am J Neuroradiol 1996;17:104.
6. Kesselring J, Miller DH, Robb SA, et al. Acute disseminated encephalomyelitis. MRI findings and the distinction from multiple sclerosis. Brain 1990;113:291.
7. Orrell RW. Grand Rounds—Hammersmith Hospitals. Distinguishing acute disseminated encephalomyelitis from multiple sclerosis. BMJ 1996;313:802.
8. Caldemeyer KS, Harris TM, Smith RR, Edwards MK. Gadolinium enhancement in acute disseminated encephalomyelitis. J Comput Assist Tomogr 1991;15:673.
9. Caldemeyer KS, Smith RR, Harris TM, Edwards MK. MRI in acute disseminated encephalomyelitis. Neuroradiology 1994;36:216.
10. Burnham JA, Wright RR, Dreisbach J, Murray RS. The effect of high-dose steroids on MRI gadolinium enhance-

ment in acute demyelinating lesions. Neurology 1991;41:1349.

11. Case records of the Massachusetts General Hospital (Case 1-1999). N Engl J Med 1999;340:127.
12. Markus R, Brew BJ, Turner J, Pell M. Successful outcome with aggressive treatment of acute haemorrhagic leukoencephalitis. J Neurol Neurosurg Psychiatry 1997;63:551.
13. Kanter DS, Horensky D, Sperling RA, et al. Plasmapheresis in fulminant acute disseminated encephalomyelitis. Neurology 1995;45:824.
14. Stricker RB, Miller RG, Kiprov DD. Role of plasmapheresis in acute disseminated (postinfectious) encephalomyelitis. J Clin Apheresis 1992;7:173.
15. Hahn JS, Siegler DJ, Enzmann D. Intravenous gammaglobulin therapy in recurrent acute disseminated encephalomyelitis. Neurology 1996;46:1173.
16. Kleiman M, Brunquell P. Acute disseminated encephalomyelitis: response to intravenous immunoglobulin. J Child Neurol 1995;10:481.
17. Blunt SB, Boulton J, Wise R, et al. Locked-in syndrome in fulminant demyelinating disease (letter to the editor). J Neurol Neurosurg Psychiatry 1994;57:504.
18. Forti A, Ambrosetto G, Amore M, et al. Locked-in syndrome in multiple sclerosis with sparing of the ventral portion of the pons. Ann Neurol 1982;12:393.
19. Johnson MD, Lavin P, Whetsell WO Jr. Fulminant monophasic multiple sclerosis, Marburg's type. J Neurol Neurosurg Psychiatry 1990;53:918.
20. Melin J, Usenius JP, Fogelholm R. Left ventricular failure and pulmonary edema in acute multiple sclerosis. Acta Neurol Scand 1996;93:315.
21. Niebler G, Harris T, Davis T, Roos K. Fulminant multiple sclerosis. AJNR Am J Neuroradiol 1992;13:1547.
22. Paty DW, Oger JJ, Kastrukoff LF, et al. MRI in the diagnosis of MS: a prospective study with comparison of clinical evaluation, evoked potentials, oligoclonal banding, and CT. Neurology 1988;38:180.
23. Powell T, Sussman JG, Davies-Jones GA. MR imaging in acute multiple sclerosis: ringlike appearance in plaques suggesting the presence of paramagnetic free radicals. AJNR Am J Neuroradiol 1992;13:1544.
24. Landtblom A-M, Sjöqvist L, Söderfeldt B, et al. Proton MR spectroscopy and MR imaging in acute and chronic multiple sclerosis—ringlike appearances in acute plaques. Acta Radiol 1996;37:278.
25. Chiappa KH. Evoked Potentials in Clinical Medicine, 3rd ed. Philadelphia: Lippincott-Raven, 1997.
26. Nuwer MR. Evoked Potentials in Multiple Sclerosis. In CS Raine, HF McFarland, WW Tourtellotte (eds), Multiple Sclerosis: Clinical and Pathologenetic Basis. London: Chapman & Hall Medical, 1997;43.
27. Ebers GC, Paty DW. CSF electrophoresis in one thousand patients. Can J Neurol Sci 1980;7:275.
28. Miller DH, Thompson AJ, Morrissey SP, et al. High dose steroids in acute relapses of multiple sclerosis: MRI evidence for a possible mechanism of therapeutic effect. J Neurol Neurosurg Psychiatry 1992;55:450.
29. Rodriguez M, Karnes WE, Bartleson JD, Pineda AA. Plasmapheresis in acute episodes of fulminant CNS inflammatory demyelination. Neurology 1993;43:1100.
30. Rudick RA, Cohen JA, Weinstock-Guttman B, et al. Management of multiple sclerosis. N Engl J Med 1997;337:1604.
31. Paty DW, Ebers GC. Multiple Sclerosis (Contemporary Neurology Series). Philadelphia: FA Davis Company, 1998.
32. Kelley CE, Mathews J, Noskin GA. Acute transverse myelitis in the emergency department: a case report and review of the literature. J Emerg Med 1991;9:417.
33. Berman M, Feldman S, Alter M, et al. Acute transverse myelitis: incidence and etiologic considerations. Neurology 1981;31:966.
34. Barakos JA, Mark AS, Dillon WP, Norman D. MR imaging of acute transverse myelitis and AIDS myelopathy. J Comput Assist Tomogr 1990;14:45.
35. Fukazawa T, Hamada T, Tashiro K, et al. Acute transverse myelopathy in multiple sclerosis. J Neurol Sci 1990;100:217.
36. Fukazawa T, Miyasaka K, Tashiro K, et al. MRI findings of multiple sclerosis with acute transverse myelopathy. J Neurol Sci 1992;110:27.
37. Sanders KA, Khandji AG, Mohr JP. Gadolinium-MRI in acute transverse myelopathy. Neurology 1990;40:1614.
38. Tartaglino LM, Heiman-Patterson T, Friedman DP, Flanders AE. MR imaging in a case of postvaccination myelitis. AJNR Am J Neuroradiol 1995;16:581.
39. Baig SM, Khan MA. Cytomegalovirus-associated transverse myelitis in a non-immunocompromised patient. J Neurol Sci 1995;134:210.
40. Ford B, Tampieri D, Francis G. Long-term follow-up of acute partial transverse myelopathy. Neurology 1992;42:250.
41. Austin SG, Zee CS, Waters C. The role of magnetic resonance imaging in acute transverse myelitis. Can J Neurol Sci 1992;19:508.
42. Arnoldus EP, Van Laar T. A reversible posterior leukoencephalopathy syndrome (letter to the editor). N Engl J Med 1996;334:1745.
43. Donnan GA. Posterior leucoencephalopathy syndrome. Lancet 1996;347:988.
44. Eaton JM. A reversible posterior leukoencephalopathy syndrome (letter to the editor). N Engl J Med 1996; 334:1744.
45. Hinchey J, Chaves C, Appignani B, et al. A reversible posterior leukoencephalopathy syndrome. N Engl J Med 1996;334:494.
46. Williams EJ, Oatridge A, Holdcroft A, et al. Posterior leucoencephalopathy syndrome (letter to the editor). Lancet 1996;347:1556.
47. Cairns H, Oldfield RC, Pennybacker JB, Whitteridge D. Akinetic mutism with an epidermoid cyst of the third ventricle (with a report on associated disturbance of brain potentials). Brain 1941;64:273.
48. Hauben M. Cyclosporine neurotoxicity. Pharmacotherapy 1996;16:576.
49. Wijdicks EFM, Dahlke LJ, Wiesner RH. Oral cyclo-

sporine decreases severity of neurotoxicity in liver transplant recipients. Neurology 1999;52:1708.
50. Figueredo AT, Fawcet SE, Molloy DW, et al. Disabling encephalopathy during 5-fluorouracil and levamisole adjuvant therapy for resected colorectal cancer: a report of two cases. Cancer Invest 1995;13:608.
51. Critchley P, Abbott R, Madden FJ. Multifocal inflammatory leukoencephalopathy developing in a patient receiving 5-fluorouracil and levamisole. Clin Oncol (R Coll Radiol) 1994;6:406.
52. Hook CC, Kimmel DW, Kvols LK, et al. Multifocal inflammatory leukoencephalopathy with 5-fluorouracil and levamisole. Ann Neurol 1992;31:262.
53. Kimmel DW, Wijdicks EFM, Rodriguez M. Multifocal inflammatory leukoencephalopathy associated with levamisole therapy. Neurology 1995;45:374.
54. Worthley SG, McNeil JD. Leukoencephalopathy in a patient taking low dose oral methotrexate therapy for rheumatoid arthritis. J Rheumatol 1995;22:335.
55. Chamberlain MC, Kormanik PA, Barba D. Complications associated with intraventricular chemotherapy in patients with leptomeningeal metastases. J Neurosurg 1997;87:694.
56. Lemann W, Wiley RG, Posner JB. Leukoencephalopathy complicating intraventricular catheters: clinical, radiographic and pathologic study of 10 cases. J Neurooncol 1988;6:67.
57. Tsuboi K, Yoshii Y, Hyodo A, et al. Leukoencephalopathy associated with intra-arterial ACNU in patients with gliomas. J Neurooncol 1995;23:223.
58. Gay CT, Bodensteiner JB, Nitschke R, et al. Reversible treatment-related leukoencephalopathy. J Child Neurol 1989;4:208.
59. Tan TP, Algra PR, Valk J, Wolters EC. Toxic leukoencephalopathy after inhalation of poisoned heroin: MR findings. AJNR Am J Neuroradiol 1994;15:175.
60. Wolters EC, van Wijngaarden GK, Stam FC, et al. Leucoencephalopathy after inhaling "heroin" pyrolysate. Lancet 1982;2:1233.
61. Delanty N, Vaughan C, Frucht S, Stubgen P. Erythropoietin-associated hypertensive posterior leukoencephalopathy. Neurology 1997;49:686.
62. Walker RW, Rosenblum MK. Amphotericin B-associated leukoencephalopathy. Neurology 1992;42:2005.
63. Dahmus MA, Barton JR, Sibai BM. Cerebral imaging in eclampsia: magnetic resonance imaging versus computed tomography. Am J Obstet Gynecol 1992; 167:935.
64. Anders KH, Becker PS, Holden JK, et al. Multifocal necrotizing leukoencephalopathy with pontine predilection in immunosuppressed patients: a clinicopathologic review of 16 cases. Hum Pathol 1993;24:897.
65. Gray F, Chimelli L, Mohr M, et al. Fulminating multiple sclerosis-like leukoencephalopathy revealing human immunodeficiency virus infection. Neurology 1991; 41:105.
66. Poon TP, Tchertkoff V, Win H. Fine needle aspiration biopsy of progressive multifocal leukoencephalopathy in a patient with AIDS. A case report. Acta Cytol 1997;41:1815.
67. Zunt JR, Tu RK, Anderson DM, et al. Progressive multifocal leukoencephalopathy presenting as human immunodeficiency virus type 1 (HIV)-associated dementia. Neurology 1997;49:263.
68. Schaefer PW, Buonanno FS, Gonzalez RG, Schwamm LH. Diffusion-weighted imaging discriminates between cytotoxic and vasogenic edema in a patient with eclampsia. Stroke 1997;28:1082.
69. Wijdicks EFM, Wiesner RH, Dahlke LJ, Krom RA. FK506-induced neurotoxicity in liver transplantation. Ann Neurol 1994;35:498.
70. Wijdicks EFM, Wiesner RH, Krom RA. Neurotoxicity in liver transplant recipients with cyclosporine immunosuppression. Neurology 1995;45:1962.
71. Thyagarajan GK, Cobanoglu A, Johnston W. FK506-induced fulminant leukoencephalopathy after single-lung transplantation. Ann Thorac Surg 1997;64:1461.
72. Jarosz JM, Howlett DC, Cox TC, Bingham JB. Cyclosporine-related reversible posterior leukoencephalopathy: MRI. Neuroradiology 1997;39:711.
73. Lanzino G, Cloft H, Hemstreet MK, et al. Reversible posterior leukoencephalopathy following organ transplantation. Description of two cases. Clin Neurol Neurosurg 1997;99:222.
74. Clifford DB, Yiannoutsos C, Glicksman M, et al. HAART improves prognosis in HIV-associated progressive multifocal leukoencephalopathy. Neurology 1999;52:623.

Chapter 12
Traumatic Brain and Spine Injury

The management of traumatic brain and spine injuries commonly involves patients who have had motorized vehicle accidents, have fallen, or have been shot. The medical complexities in these patients with trauma to the central nervous system may be a predicament for most consulting neurologists. In addition, the life-threatening potential of injuries to vital organs encompasses most of the activity in the emergency department. On closer examination, it appears in some instances that neurologists and neurosurgeons may have only a peripheral role and be consulted only after many hours or days of stabilization of vital organ functions. Quite frankly, the priority to manage chest and abdominal trauma in multitraumatized patients may jeopardize the management of head and spine trauma. Also, as a matter of fact, intoxication often leads to trauma (e.g., bar brawls, intravenous drug use), and its depressing effect on the brain may confound clinical assessment. Some of these patients are found on the street or in the recesses of buildings, often in deplorable clinical condition. In addition, gunshot wounds have increased in frequency, introducing an entirely different scope of problems. This chapter discusses how to determine the severity of the initial injury, accomplish medical management of traumatic brain edema and contusions, and assess the need for acute neurosurgical intervention.

Traumatic Brain Injury

The severity of injury is graded on the basis of the Glasgow coma score (Chapter 1; see Table 1.4 and Figure 1.3) and the presentation computed tomography (CT) scan. Head injury can be classified in several characteristic categories, and each may have different triage options (Table 12.1). Coexisting categories are common in catastrophic trauma.

Clinical Presentation

Traumatic brain injury frequently impairs level of alertness, but the mechanism is diverse. Coma may occur from bihemispheric contusions, mass effect on the opposite hemisphere or thalamus from extracerebral hematoma, penetrating bihemispheric damage, and, rarely, an isolated brain stem lesion.

The Glasgow coma score reliably measures the degree of traumatic coma. Eye opening and motor responses remain the most important leads and often closely correspond with other changes in the brain stem reflexes, such as pupillary and oculocephalic responses. In addition, the Glasgow coma score predicts outcome after traumatic brain injury irrespective of the underlying structural lesion, but assessment is most reliable after cardiopulmonary resuscitation and at least 6 hours after injury.[1] Coma is closely linked to a Glasgow coma sum score of 8 or less (e.g., ability to open eyes only to pain, E_2; incomprehensible sounds, V_2; and arm withdrawal to pain, M_4).

Pupillary light responses and pupil size further differentiate. Unilaterally enlarged pupil is often due to an evolving intracranial mass lesion and may become oval when intracranial pressure is increased.

Table 12.1. Classification of Traumatic Brain Injury

Closed
Parenchymal
Hemorrhagic contusion
Contrecoup contusion
Shear lesion
Malignant brain edema
Diffuse axonal injury
Extracerebral
Epidural
Subdural
Penetrating
Parenchymal
Intracerebral hematoma
Extracerebral
Subdural hematoma
Skull
Fractures
Skull fracture
Vault
Linear or stellate
Depressed
Open or closed
Basilar
With spinal fluid leak
With facial nerve palsy

The fixed pupil of an extracranial hematoma is on the same side, but occasionally a falsely localizing contralateral pupil is seen, an observation not adequately explained. Mydriasis of one pupil after head injury indicates a swollen temporal lobe causing traction of the third nerve or direct compression. However, when a patient with a fixed pupil is seen early after trauma, the most frequent cause is an ipsilateral epidural or large subdural hematoma.

Fixed pupils of midposition size (diameter of 5 to 6 mm) may indicate a mesencephalic stage of herniation and may be the first indication of brain death in the emergency room. Brain death in head injury is a result of massive cerebral edema, multiple hemorrhagic contusions, or a rapidly evolving epidural hematoma causing brain stem compression and downward herniation. It is often observed in subtentorial epidural hematomas, which are not accommodated for in the small compartment of the posterior fossa.

In the midst of multiple trauma to limbs, abdomen, or chest, facial trauma may receive less attention, and neurologists are often the first to point out the injuries when the cranial nerves are examined. Scalp avulsions may cause significant blood loss and shock and should be repaired immediately. It should be emphasized, however, that hypotension in adults is only a direct result of central nervous system trauma in a few instances, such as major external scalp bleeding, spinal shock, and brain death, and in children may occur with a large epidural hematoma. Orbital swelling can be profound and may prevent full examination of fundi and eye movements. If the swelling is associated with ecchymosis of the eyelids (so-called raccoon or panda bear eyes) (Color Plate 21), it may indicate a fracture of the orbital roof or, more commonly, a LeFort II fracture (nasal-orbital-ethmoid midface fracture) or a zygomatic fracture. The orbital roof fracture may extend through the ethmoid or cribriform-ethmoid junction and result in a cerebrospinal fluid (CSF) fistula. Petrous bone fractures may result in facial paralysis from direct injury to the facial nerve, ecchymosis over the mastoid (Battle's sign), and a CSF leak from the external canal. The Battle and raccoon eye signs, however, take several hours to develop, and specificity for basal skull fracture is low. Abrasions of the chin are clues to a possible retroflexion trauma of the spine and should prompt precautionary measures, such as a collar, until a cervical spine radiograph or CT scan has excluded a fracture or dislocation.

Seizures are associated with traumatic brain injury in only up to 10% of patients and are more common in patients with a cortical contusion or traumatic intracerebral hematoma, depressed skull fracture, and dural tear.

Dysautonomia may coexist, but if so, it indicates catastrophic diffuse axonal brain trauma.[2] Patients clench a fist, often pressing the thumb between the index and middle finger ("obscene sign"), grind teeth, and lock the jaw. Other manifestations are profuse sweating (Figure 12.1) and tachycardia.

Many algorithms and trauma scores have been devised and may be helpful in triage; however, it is more important to weigh factors that would justify rapid transportation to a neurotrauma center or neurologic-neurosurgical intensive care unit (Table 12.2).

Interpretation of Diagnostic Tests

Computed Tomography and Magnetic Resonance Imaging

CT scan imaging is imperative in any patient with facial lacerations or hematoma, reduced level of consciousness, a significant impact to the cranium

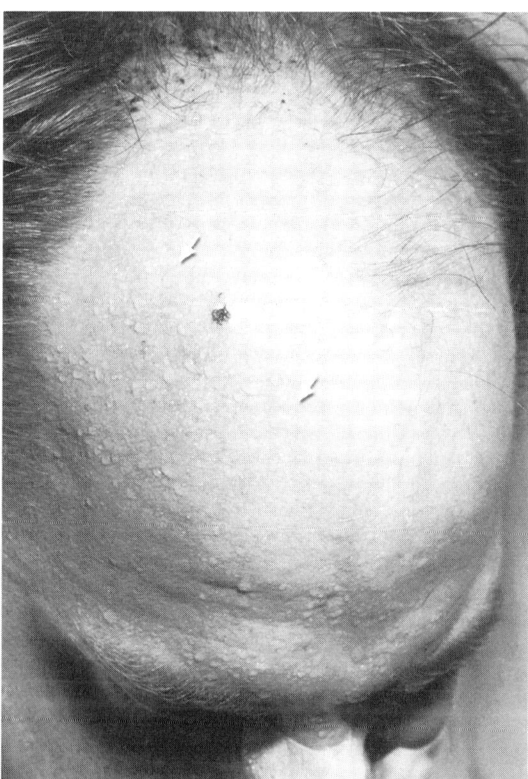

Figure 12.1. Profuse sweating (*arrows*) in a patient with axonal brain injury from dysautonomia.

(particularly a fall or fist fight), any evidence of focal neurologic signs, or pupillary inequality during transport.[3] CT scan of the brain should be part of a complete evaluation in a patient with multitrauma and not be deferred to a later time. Magnetic resonance imaging (MRI) is considered when CT scans do not fully explain the clinical presentation, but it is not readily available and is probably unsafe in mechanically ventilated patients with unstable multiple traumatic lesions to vital organs. Major dissimilarities between CT scan findings after trauma and the patient's state of impaired consciousness should point to confounding insults to the brain, some of which are reversible (Table 12.3).

Several CT scan patterns can be recognized, and they are illustrated in the figures. The severity of head injury in comatose patients can be further classified. Absence of visualization of the basal cisterns, midline shift, and a mass lesion are strong predictors of increased intracranial pressure. Mass effect with absence of a third ventricle and trapping of the temporal horn correlates strongly with increased intracranial pressure.

Table 12.2. Assessment of Severity Indicators of Traumatic Brain Injury

Amnesia for trauma
Fall, fist, car collision
Age >60 yrs
Tachypnea
Hypotension
Scalp or face injury
Penetrating injury
Pupils fixed to light
Abnormal finding on computed tomography scan

Table 12.3. Coma in Traumatic Brain Injury but "Normal" Findings on Computed Tomography Scanning

Drug or alcohol overdose
Postanoxic insult from asphyxia (vomiting, aspiration, foreign body)
Postictal state after seizures or nonconvulsive status epilepticus
Vertebral artery dissection with basilar artery occlusion (rare)

Most parenchymal injuries are a direct effect of a blow to the brain. These contusions are created when brain tissue becomes impacted against the bony protuberances of the base of the skull. They are further subdivided into fracture contusions, contrecoup contusions, and shear lesions.

Fracture contusions, most common in the frontal lobes, are seen in association with a fracture of the anterior fossa (Figure 12.2A). This abnormality may be accompanied by an epidural or subdural hematoma, which may be responsible for the clinical symptoms. In patients with acute subdural hematoma, follow-up CT scans show lacerated brain tissue at the same site, or this becomes apparent during craniotomy and removal of the extradural hematoma (so-called burst lobe) (Figure 12.2B).

Contrecoup contusions (Figure 12.3) are often two or more lesions diametrically opposite to one another. Shear lesions (Figure 12.4) are punctate lesions from disruption of small penetrating arteries due to rotational forces at impact. The localization of shear lesions varies, but often they are identified at the gray-white matter junction. Basal ganglia (predominantly putamen or thalamus) may be involved. Outcome in these patients is poor because of association with other brain contusions.

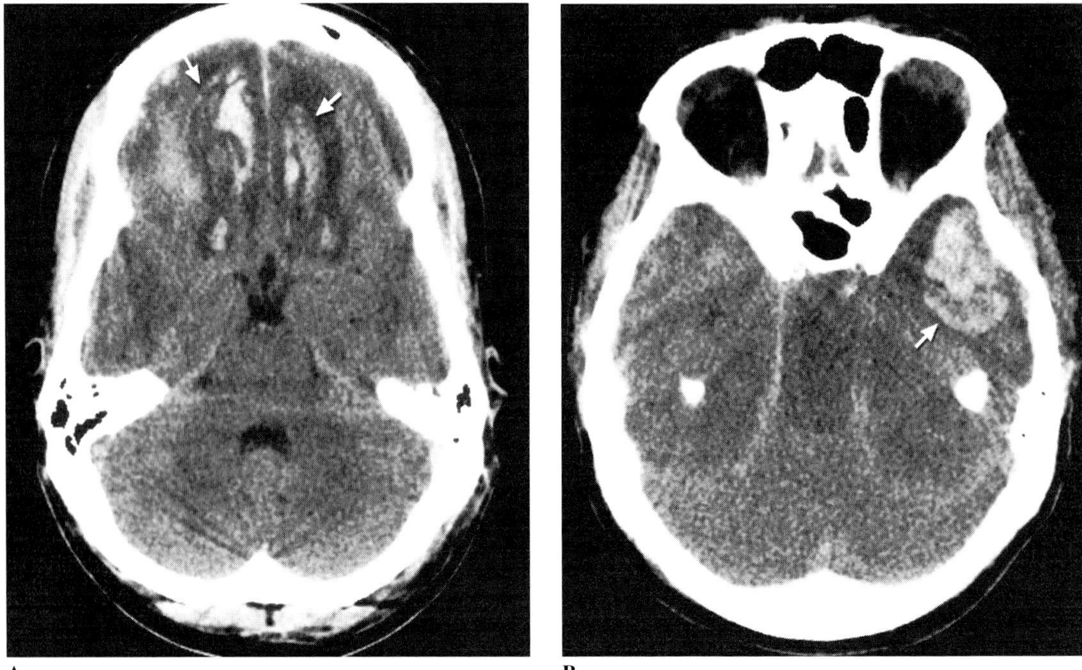

Figure 12.2. A. Frontal lobe contusions (*arrows*). **B.** Temporal lobe burst hematoma (*arrow*).

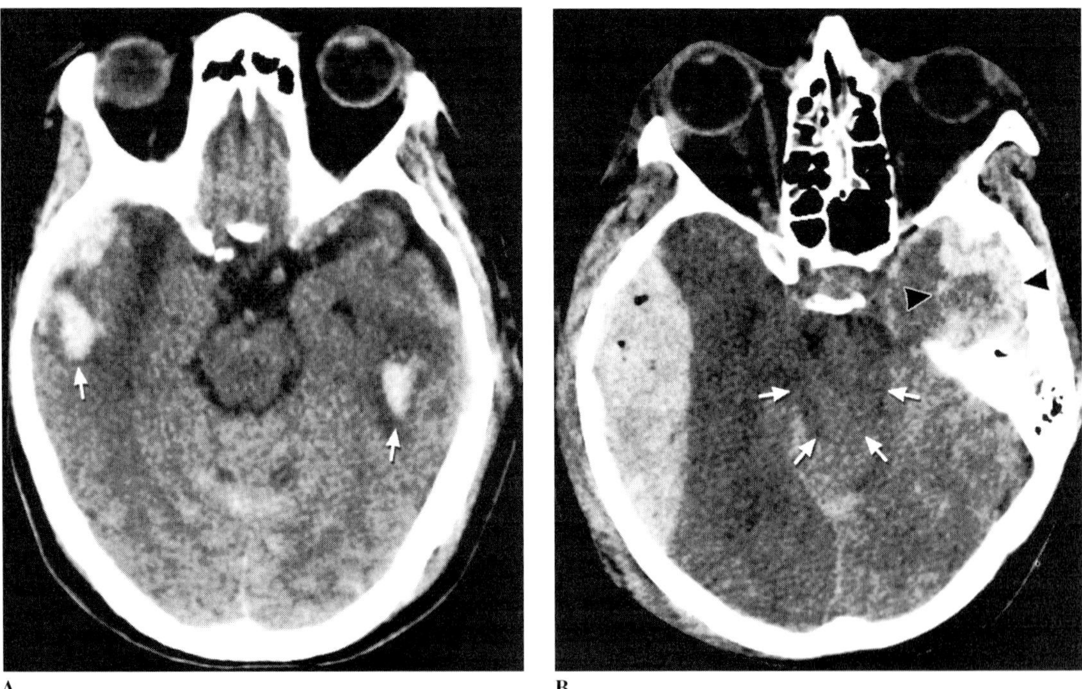

Figure 12.3. A. Contrecoup contusions (*arrows*). **B.** Epidural hematoma with contrecoup temporal lobe contusion (*arrowheads*) and basal cistern effacement (*small arrows*).

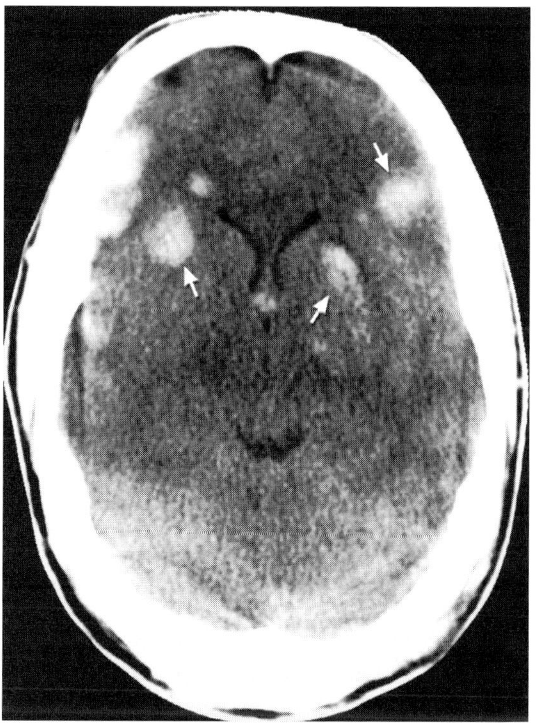

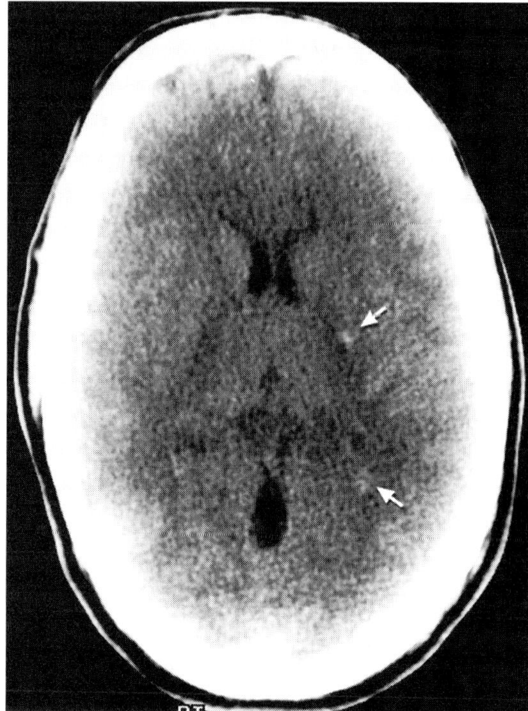

Figure 12.4. Shear lesions (*arrows*), including basal ganglia.

Hemorrhagic contusions are commonly localized in the frontal or temporal lobe and may be bilateral. They may not be evident on initial CT scanning, are unmasked only on repeat studies, and are not always associated with clearly documented clinical deterioration (Figure 12.5). Mass effect from cortical contusions is seldom severe initially but may increase from pericontusional swelling.

Another rather frequent CT scan image is diffuse axonal injury.[4] The pathologic damage is caused by acceleration-deceleration forces,[5] and the overwhelming evidence of axonal destruction may be noted only microscopically at autopsy.[6] CT scan findings can initially be normal, but often subtle changes are present, such as intraventricular blood (small amounts from corpus callosum tearing), punctate shear lesions, or sulci effacement. Later CT scans may show (ex vacuo) enlargement of the ventricles from reduction of the white matter tissue.

Corpus callosum lesions may be demonstrated on MRI but seldom are found by CT scanning. The corpus callosum lesions are in the splenium and posterior body because relative fixation from the posterior falx results in a tensile force rather than release with rotation. Brain stem lesions have been noted, also often with multiple hemispheric lesions. A focal hemorrhage is most commonly seen in the dorsolateral aspect of the brain stem from a blow to the edge of the tentorium or in the interpeduncular cistern. Diffuse cerebral swelling (Figure 12.6) occasionally is seen early after impact and indicates severe axonal damage. Typically, the sulci disappear, but this may be difficult to judge in most young adults. The differentiating features of the white matter and gray matter disappear, and the basal cisterns are obliterated, resulting in a "featureless grayout of the brain." This malignant edema is often fatal and may occur after an asymptomatic interval and "trivial" impact (fall off horse or bicycle).

Gunshot wounds to the brain are complex injuries, with skull fracture, tracks of bone, missile fragments, and often an associated intracerebral hematoma, which determines the initial clinical condition (Figure 12.7 and 12.8). Cerebral contusions may be seen at the entry and exit sites.

A subdural hematoma typically is recognized as a hyperdense lesion with a characteristic crescentic (curving with the skull) collection.[7] Acute subdural

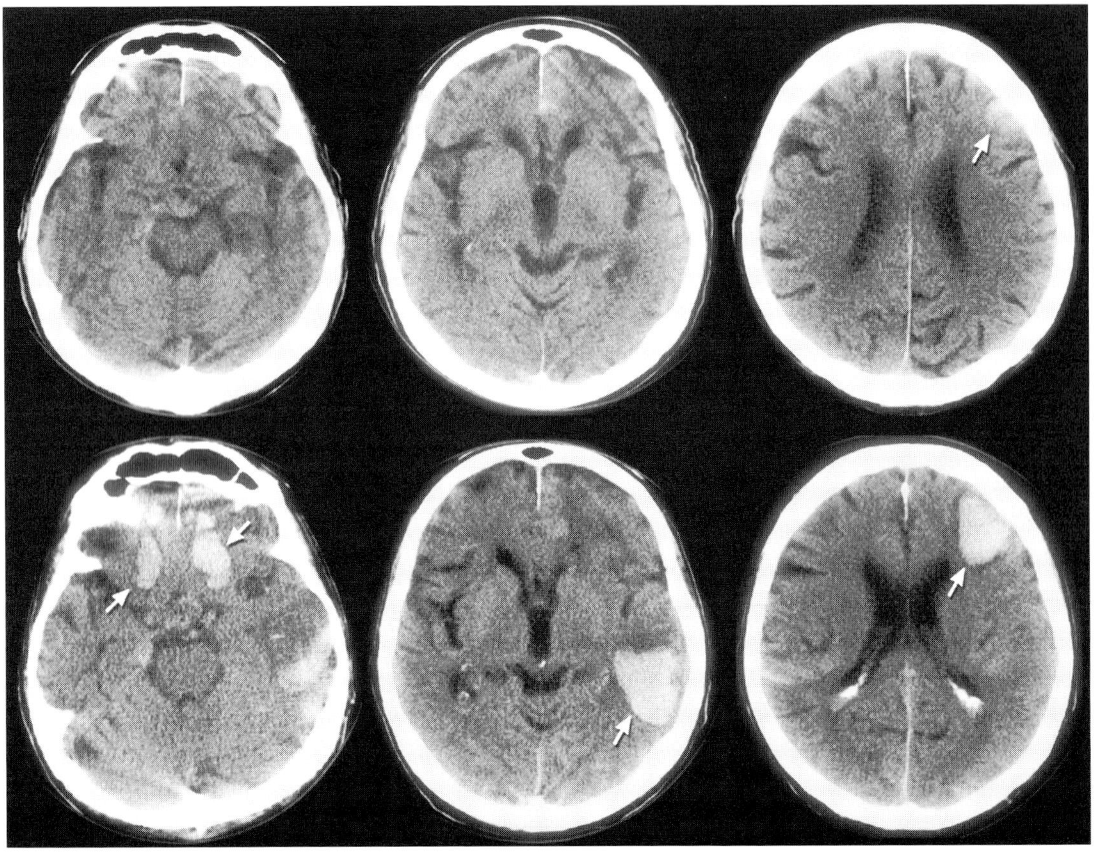

Figure 12.5. Delayed abnormalities on computed tomography scans. *Top row*, Contusion (*arrow*) is barely seen. *Bottom row*, Multiple lobar contusions (*arrows*) develop later.

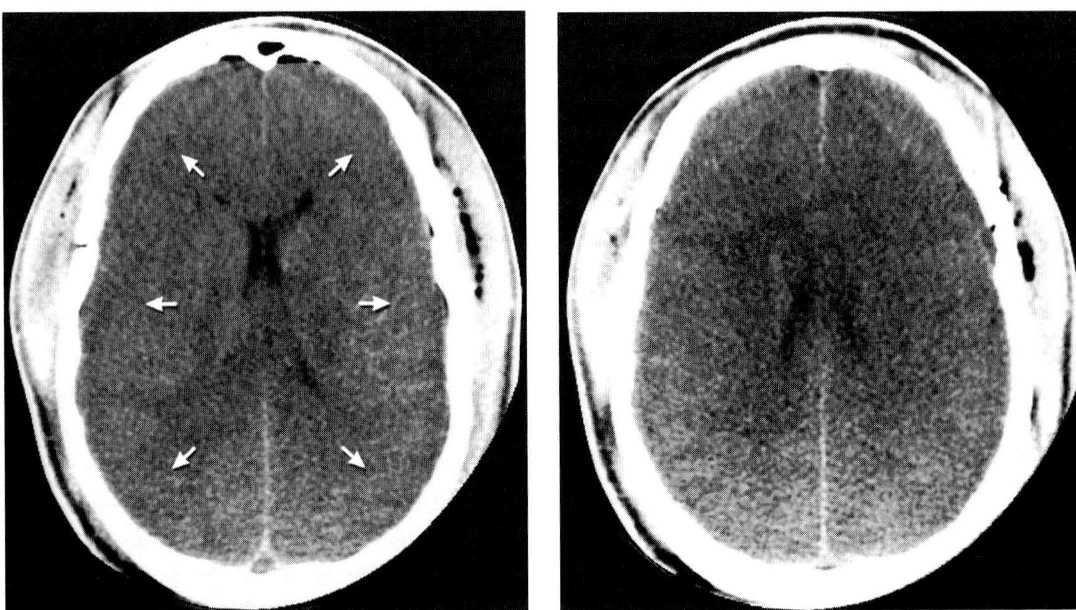

Figure 12.6. Axonal injury to the brain and diffuse swelling (*arrows*), with so-called featureless grayout.

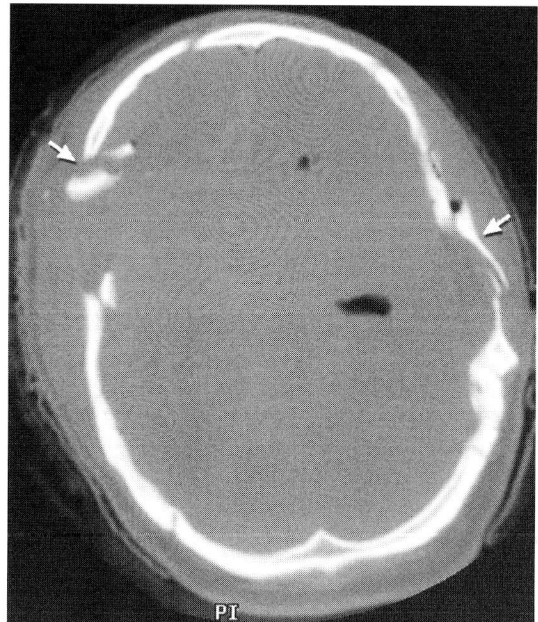

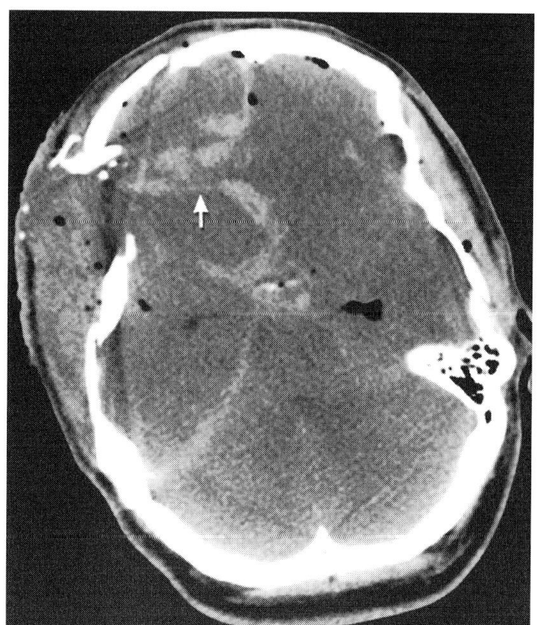

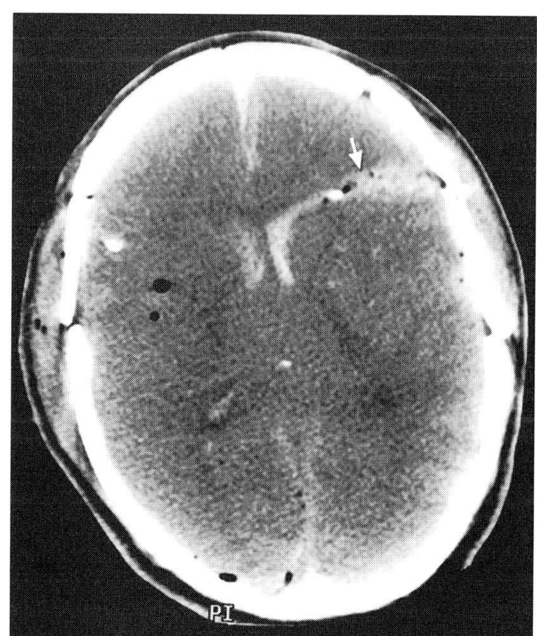

Figure 12.7. Patient example of gunshot-induced fracture with intracranial hematoma. Transventricular injury (track with intraventricular hematoma) with bone destruction (*arrows*) and intracranial air. Entry and exit contusions (*arrows*).

hematomas are hyperdense, but when marked anemia (hemoglobin <10 g/dL) is present, they may approach the density of brain tissue. When hyperdensity is seen within an isodense collection, rebleeding is likely. A fluid-blood interface may distinguish hematomas of different ages (Figure 12.9). Usually, a subdural hematoma isodense to the gray matter is evident 3 weeks after onset. A change to a hypodense collection follows, but estimation of the age of the hematoma on CT images is difficult. In elderly patients, isodense subdural hematomas may be recognized by loss of sulci and small ventricles (so-called hypernormal CT finding for age). Small layers of subdural hematoma may go unde-

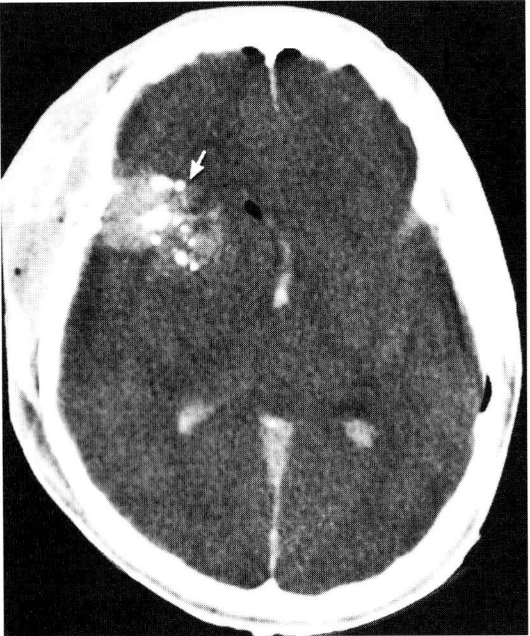
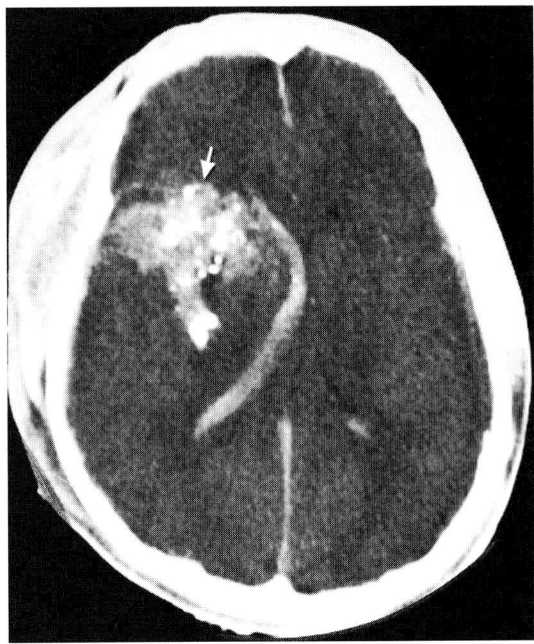

Figure 12.8. Gunshot-induced intracranial hematoma with intraventricular hematoma.

tected on CT scans, because they can hardly be distinguished from bone; MRI visualizes them (see Figure 12.9A). Subdural hematoma can be seen as an interhemispheric collection along the falx, and this collection tends to enlarge.

Epidural hematomas (Figure 12.10) are associated with fracture in more than 95% of cases. The hematoma, which is due to a tear in a meningeal artery, strips the dura away from the inner table of the skull, producing a biconvex, or lens-shaped, configuration. Anterior-posterior extension is usually limited by the skull sutures. Its mass effect is significant in both the supratentorial and the infratentorial spaces and may rapidly lead to brain herniation syndromes. An ominous CT scan feature is a hyperlucent area, which should be recognized on CT images (see Figure 12.10). It indicates active bleeding, because a completed epidural hematoma is uniformly dense. An epidural hematoma in the posterior fossa is caused by a torn dural sinus; it may become large enough to cause full effacement of the brain stem cisterns. Vertex epidural hematomas, which are very rare, are caused by rupture of the superior sagittal sinus. Unlike the rapid evolution of arterial epidural hematomas, involvement of the dural sinus may not become clinically noticeable for several hours.[8]

Traumatic subarachnoid collections in sulci and fissures should not involve any of the suprasellar cisterns. Occasionally some sediment is seen in the ambient cistern (see Figure 6.10 in Chapter 6). Blood from traumatic subarachnoid hemorrhage may have collected in the sylvian fissure alone. The distinction between a ruptured middle cerebral artery aneurysm, with blood deposited in the sylvian fissure, that causes the patient to fall and subarachnoid hemorrhage from trauma alone is impossible if no clear history of a thunderclap headache is volunteered by the patient, and cerebral angiography is always needed to find the answer.

Bone Window Computed Tomography

Bone windows on CT scans are important to show linear fractures in the skull and are equivalent to routine skull radiographs. In many instances, they indicate the site of the blow and are next to the contused area of the brain. In one study, skull fracture was present in 77% of patients with contusion, 87% with an extradural hematoma, 72% with a subdural hematoma, and 66% with an intracerebral hematoma.[9] The degree of depression of skull fracture can be easily visualized. Linear fractures are more commonly associated with epidural or sub-

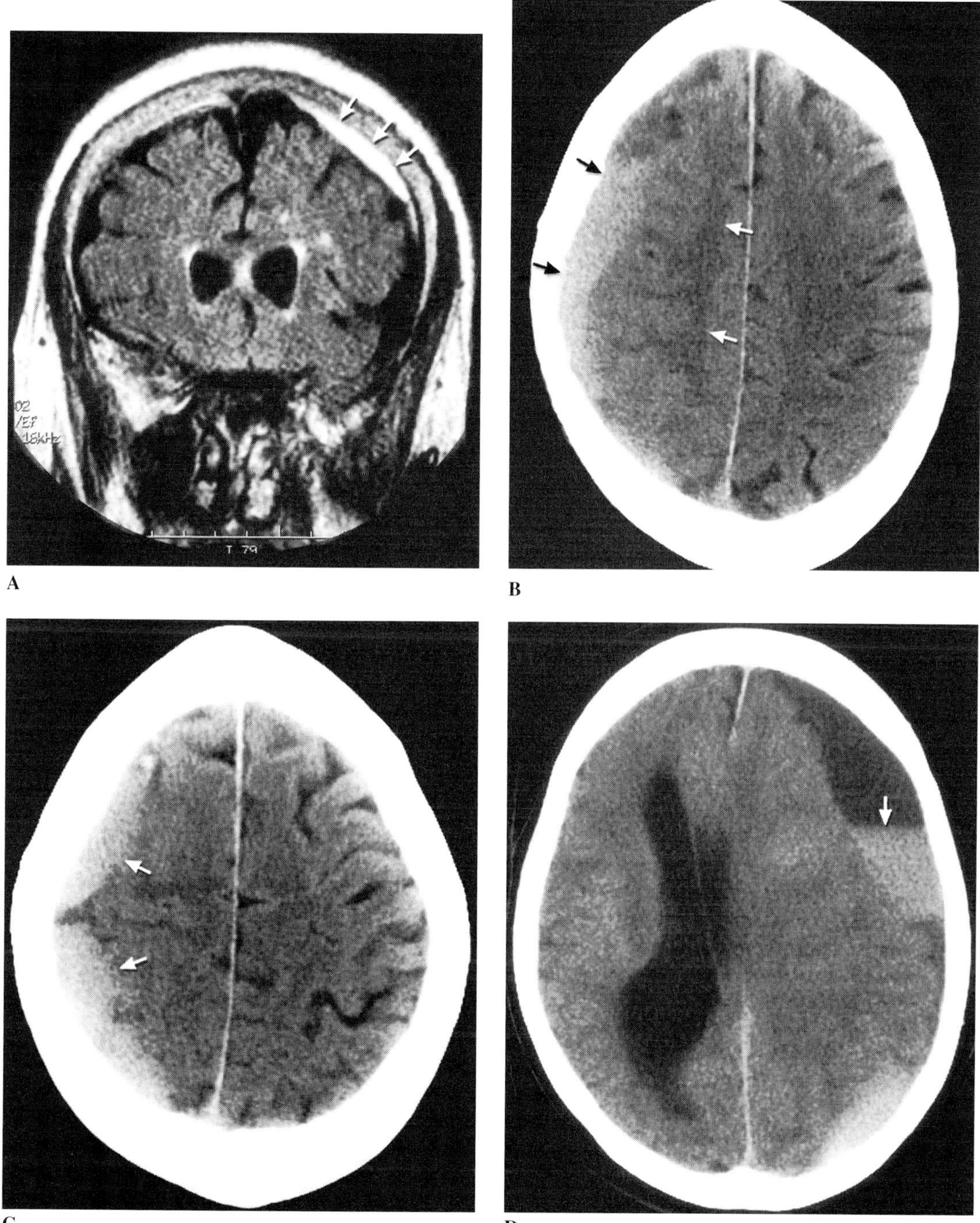

Figure 12.9. Different types of subdural hematomas. **A.** Subdural hematoma (*arrows*) on magnetic resonance imaging (fluid-attenuated inversion recovery) in a patient with transient ischemic attacks on presentation who had normal computed tomography findings but abnormal findings on magnetic resonance imaging. **B–C.** Typical subdural hematoma (*arrows*) with no shift but compression of the white matter (*arrows*). **D.** Rebleeding subdural hematoma with fluid interface (*arrow*) between recent and older collections of blood.

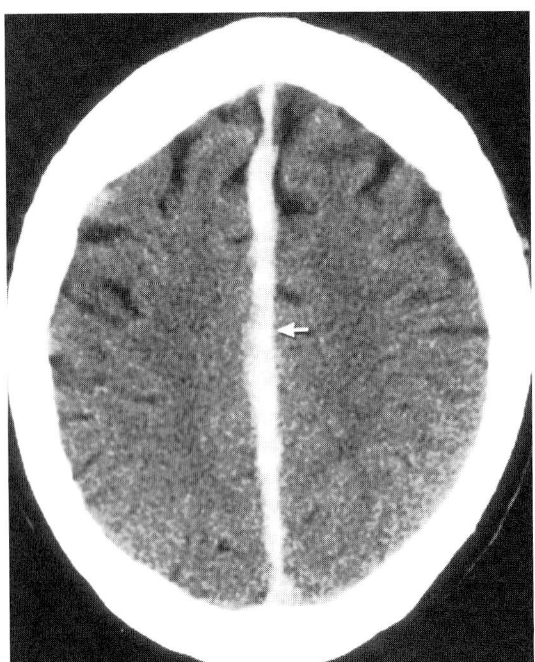

Figure 12.9. *Continued.* **E.** Falx subdural hematoma (*arrow*).

dural hematomas than are depressed skull fractures[9] (Figure 12.11).

Serum

Next to a routine laboratory survey, obtaining a serum (and urinary) toxicologic screen is of value. Blood alcohol level is imperative not only for medicolegal reasons but also for judging its influence on level of consciousness. Increased serum osmolality may also indicate alcohol intoxication (a more detailed discussion is in Chapter 1). Laboratory support of disseminated intravascular coagulation needs to be sought and includes prolonged prothrombin time, thrombocytopenia (<60,000 platelets), increase in fibrin degradation products, red cell fragments in smears, and increased D-dimers. Early appearance of disseminated intravascular coagulation indicates massive destruction of brain tissue.

Miscellaneous

Routine x-ray imaging in a head-injured patient should include the cervical spine with lateral and odontoid views and, when relevant, plain films of the abdomen and pelvis. Diagnostic peritoneal lavage or CT scan of the abdomen is indicated in patients with fluctuating blood pressure after adequate fluid replacement.

First Priority in Management

The main principle of management of traumatic head injury is immediate treatment of increased intracranial pressure, which may involve removal of an extracranial hematoma or contusion with mass effect.[10,11]

Immediate stabilization is summarized in Table 12.4. Rapid triage to CT scanning is essential because it determines the cause of impaired consciousness in most instances. Scalp lacerations should be temporarily repaired in the emergency department unless they are contaminated. It is important to secure the airway, provide fluids with two large-bore catheters, and exclude abdominal trauma with peritoneal lavage if blood pressure remains marginal despite fluid loading with hypertonic saline or dextran.[12,13] Some experts argue for a flat body position to maximize cerebral perfusion pressure.

The focus of management involves not only reduction of intracranial pressure but also maintenance of interrelated cerebral perfusion pressure (Capsule 12.1). It is prudent to hyperventilate the patient (frequency of more than 20 breaths per minute or squeezing the anesthesia bag every 3 seconds) and to give a single loading dose of mannitol (20%), 1 g/kg over 10 minutes, but only if blood pressure has remained stable throughout. Mannitol in multiple doses may have the opposite effect by accumulating within the brain and thus reversing the osmotic gradient between edematous brain and plasma.[15]

A restless patient may require intubation and sedation with propofol (infusion of 0.1 to 0.5 mg/kg per minute)[16] or with morphine (infusion of 1 mg/hour) if the endotracheal tube and mechanical ventilator are not tolerated. Because propofol also reduces increased intracranial pressure, it is a useful drug in agitated patients with early brain swelling.[16] There is no rationale for corticosteroids, barbiturates, or antihypertensive agents, all of which may seriously complicate management and possibly inversely affect outcome

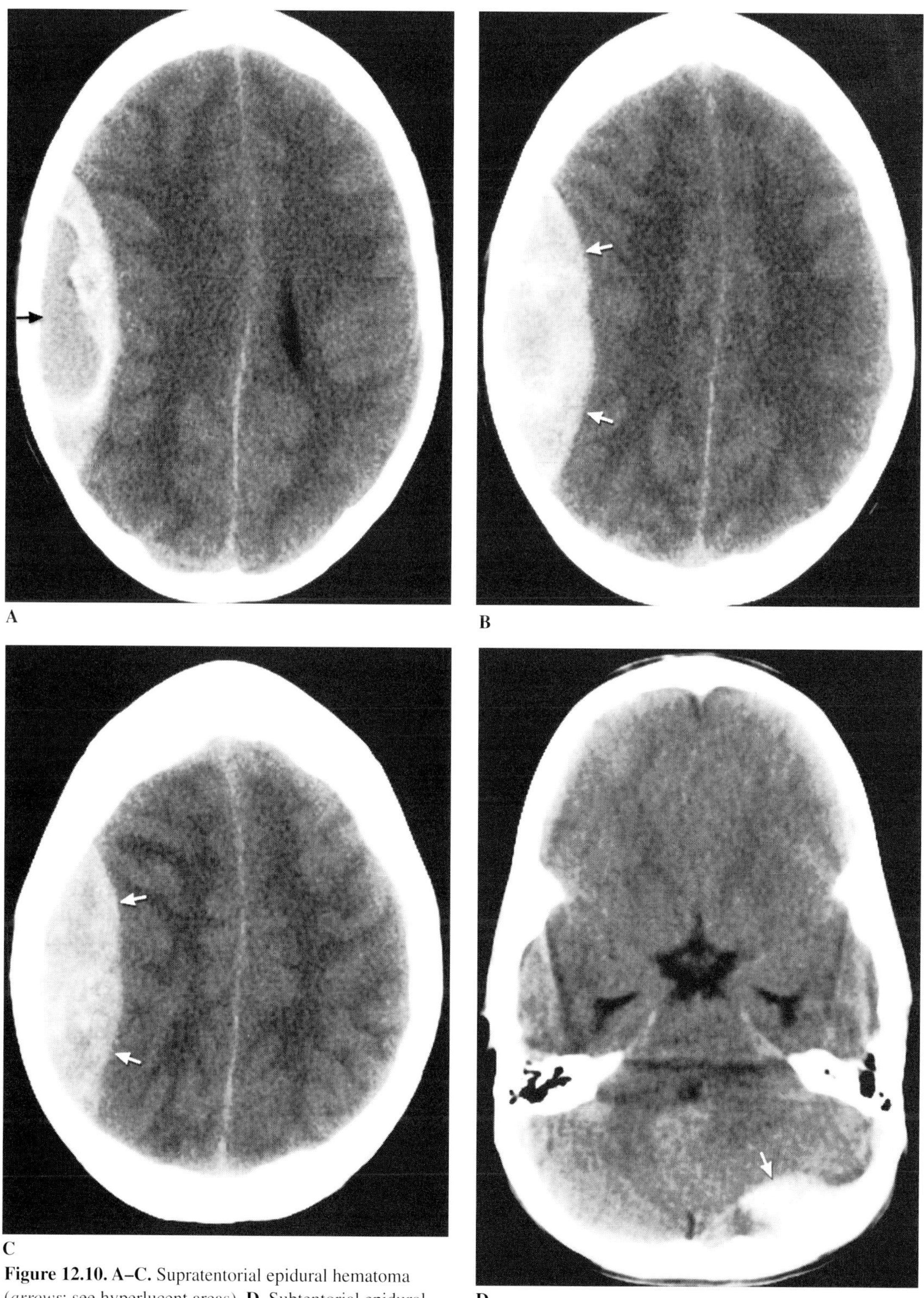

Figure 12.10. A–C. Supratentorial epidural hematoma (*arrows*; see hyperlucent areas). **D.** Subtentorial epidural hematoma.

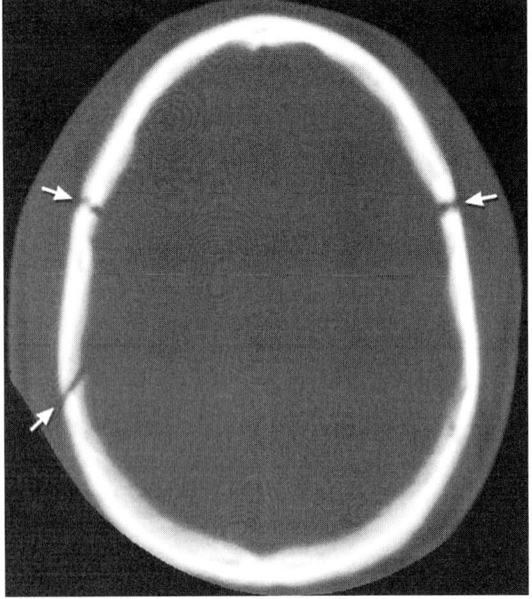

A

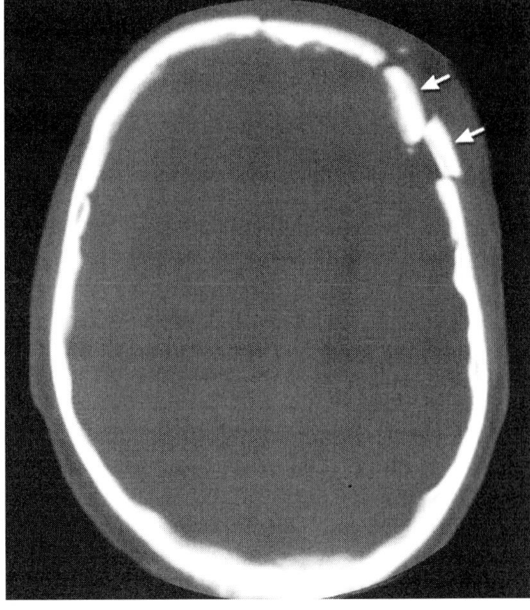

B

C

Figure 12.11. Important skull fractures. Nondepressed (**A**) and depressed (**B**) skull fractures. **C.** Petrous bone fracture.

through adverse effects of hypotension.[17–21] Simple measures also reduce intracranial pressure, such as preventing head rotation to one side (jugular vein compression), suctioning without stimulation of the soft palate or posterior pharyngeal wall, which elicits a gag and cough reflex, suctioning through an endotracheal tube with one passage only. Intravenous administration of lidocaine (1 mg/kg) may blunt these intracranial pressure responses.[22,23] Several drugs may increase intracranial pressure through an increase in cerebral blood flow by vasodilation (Table 12.5).

Hypoxemia should be aggressively managed, and after intubation, positive end-expiratory pressure (PEEP) is needed to improve gas exchange.[24] PEEP may increase intrapleural pressure and superior vena cava pressure and reduce the cerebral venous out-

Capsule 12.1. Management of Cerebral Perfusion in Traumatic Brain Injury: An Alternative Approach

Cerebral blood flow is held constant within the range of mean arterial pressure from 80 to 160 mm Hg. Outside this homeostatic range, cerebral blood flow is linearly coupled with pressure. Below the lower threshold, a decrease in cerebral perfusion pressure (CPP) results in a decrease in blood flow and ischemia. Theoretically, above the upper threshold an increase in CPP results in breakdown of the blood-brain barrier and edema, but recent studies suggest that high perfusion pressures are tolerated for brief periods.

Management of CPP has been advocated, but it assumes intact autoregulation, which may not be present in up to 50% of patients with severe traumatic head injury. Cerebral perfusion is usually aimed at 70 to 80 mm Hg and can be increased by increasing systolic arterial blood pressure (SABP), draining cerebrospinal fluid pressure, and using mannitol (CPP = SABP – ICP [intracranial pressure]).

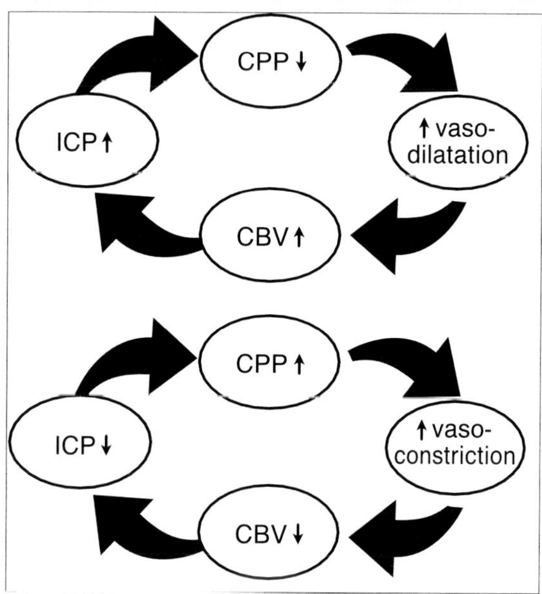

Figure 12.12.

The vasodilatory and vasoconstriction cascades (Figure 12.12) modeled after Rosner and Daughton[14] have led to management of CPP irrespective of ICP. Blood pressure can be increased with α-adrenergic receptor drugs, and normovolemia is maintained with albumin. Early results, albeit observational, suggest good to superior outcome, but this protocol is not generally accepted. (CBV = cerebral blood volume.)

Table 12.4. Immediate Priorities in Head Injury

Secure airway
Remove foreign body
Endotracheal intubation
Immobilize spine
Inspect for scalp laceration and depressed fracture
Peritoneal lavage with hypotension
Secure venous access with two catheters
Use hypertonic saline or dextran (7.4%) in hypotensive patients
Obtain cervical spine x-ray
Chest radiography
Computed tomography scan of the brain
Computed tomography scan of the abdomen (if appropriate)

Table 12.5. Medications To Be Avoided with Increased Intracranial Pressure

Hydralazine
Sodium nitroprusside
Halogenated inhalation anesthetics (halothane, isoflurane)
Ketamine
Calcium channel blockers (nicardipine, nimodipine)

flow. Intracranial pressure may become seriously elevated if PEEP values higher than 10 cm H_2O are needed, but its increase can be countered with mannitol and head elevation. PEEP may increase $PaCO_2$ because of increased physiologic dead space; this effect should be anticipated and managed by increasing the minute volume of the ventilator.

Systemic hypothermia (32°C to 33°C) within 6 hours could be beneficial in severe head injury. Its benefit and potential complications (cardiac arrhythmias, pneumonia, coagulation problems, and increase in prothrombin time) are currently being investigated. However, fever should be aggressively treated with cooling blankets, alcohol rubbing, or, as a last resort, ice gastric lavage. If shivering results, propofol should be sufficient. These measures are certainly needed in patients with a severe sympathetic outburst, who usually have tachycardia, tachypnea, and profuse sweating, with temperature increases up to 40°C.

Surgical management of extracerebral hematomas is urgently indicated. Usually, time can be allowed to evacuate the hematoma in the operating room, but in rapidly deteriorating patients, emergency drilling in the emergency department has been lifesaving.[25] Medical management and observation in extracerebral hematomas are considered only for patients with a maximal Glasgow coma score. Epidural hematomas with a diameter less than 1.5 cm and no midline shift and, as alluded to earlier, no lucent area inside the hematoma suggesting recent bleeding may be managed with observation.[26,27] For subdural hematomas, medical management is considered if the thickness of the hematoma is similar to the thickness of the skull. Large subdural hematomas without any shift caused by atrophy of the brain in elderly patients can be surgically managed in a delayed fashion when the clinical signs are minimal. Burr hole placement after the hematoma has liquefied is preferred above a large craniotomy.

The management of gunshot wounds is similar to that of any other type of penetrating trauma. Reconstructive repair of the bone and dura should begin immediately.[28,29] The wound should be considered contaminated, and broad-spectrum antibiotics (vancomycin with cefotaxime) should be administered early. A major problem is the early development of disseminated intravascular coagulation. Its occurrence is related in general to the volume of tissue damage, and it is frequent in gunshot wounds. Its appearance denotes a poor outcome.

Predictors of Outcome

It is impossible to make an accurate prediction of outcome in the emergency room. Early predictors commonly have been inaccurate, proposed cutoff points in certain scales have been disproven, and successful resuscitation of a patient for systemic injuries may greatly improve the outcome. Prognosis estimates in the 24 hours after injury can be unreliable.[30]

Age remains an important factor in prognosis, with 80% mortality from diffuse axonal injury in patients older than 55 years.[31] Prognosis is worse with the following factors: shock, subdural hematoma,[32] and coma in the elderly; early diffuse edema and increased intracranial pressure;[33] and failure to decrease intracranial pressure with conventional methods. In a recent study of MRI in 80 severely injured patients, corpus callosum lesions and dorsolateral brain stem lesions predicted an unfavorable outcome, including vegetative state.[34]

Poor outcome in patients with gunshot wounds is expected in patients with a low Glasgow coma score at admission, abnormal pupils, CT scan demonstration of ventricular involvement, crossing of midsagittal or midventricular horizontal planes, intraparenchymal hemorrhage, and a high volume of contused or damaged brain.[29]

Triage

- Evacuation of any epidural or subdural hematoma if the patient has a decrease in consciousness, hemiparesis, or speech deficit.
- Evacuation of hemorrhagic contusion if mass effect occurs.
- Placement of intracranial monitor and monitoring of intracranial pressure in neurologic-neurosurgical intensive care unit.

Spinal Cord Injury

Spinal cord injury may be from traffic accidents in more than 50% of patients arriving at emergency departments. The demographic profile consists of men in their thirties seen most often during weekends in the summer months. Complete cord lesions have decreased in prevalence, a decrease tentatively explained by improved care in the field, increased

Capsule 12.2. Surgical Management of Spinal Cord Injury

Surgical management of spine injury in a patient with spinal cord injury is pursued to prevent further injury in incomplete lesions, to ensure stability, and to prevent deformity. Unstable cervical lesions should be expected if anterior or posterior elements are destroyed, sagittal diameter of the spinal canal is less than 13 mm, or sagittal displacement is more than 3.5 mm or 20%. A stable lesion allows for earlier mobilization and transfers. Operative stabilization has not been shown to improve recovery in complete or incomplete lesions, although a recent survey calls for a trial based on suggestive data review.[37]

Deformity requires instrumentation and posterior fusion in many instances.[38]

use of seat belts, and, possibly, surgical care of unstable spine trauma. It is prudent to assume that spinal cord injury may have occurred in patients who have had multiple trauma, motor vehicle or sports accidents, or a documented spine fracture.[35,36]

This section is not intended to comprehensively discuss the entire gamut of spinal traumatic lesions and surgical management, which can only be properly addressed by experienced spine surgeons or neurosurgeons with special qualifications in the management of spine trauma. Recently, guidelines for surgical management were outlined (Capsule 12.2). The field has evolved into a subspecialty in which the role of a neurologist or emergency physician is important but limited to accurate clinical description of the damage, appropriate stabilization, recognition of unstable spine fractures or dislocations, and, when necessary, early specific medical management.

Clinical Presentation

Traumatic spinal cord injury involves the cervical cord in approximately 50% of cases, the thoracic segment in 35%, and the lumbar segment or conus in the others. Subtle signs of cervical spine injury are physical signs of an injury above the clavicle, neck pain, and tilting of the head to one side.

Tetraplegia or paraplegia is evident from the insult, but most clinical challenges involve the management of its commonly associated dysautonomia and urogenital manifestations.

In the spinal shock phase, a generalized state of hypoexcitability occurs. The marked reduction of sympathetic outflow results in peripheral vasodilatation, decreased cardiac output, bradycardia (from cardiac chronotropic activity), and venous pooling, all factors reducing blood pressure. Blood pressure typically is less than 100 mm Hg and depends on position and volume; reduction in the sitting or upright position may result in syncope. The lower extremities may show a bluish discoloration from vasodilatation and venous pooling. Passive engorgement of the penis (priapism) occurs as a consequence of sympathetic loss and always indicates an extensive spinal cord lesion. Typically, pain does not produce an increase in heart rate or blood pressure.

Temperature may be unregulated. Shivering cannot occur below the lesion because of loss of sympathetic tone, and lack of increase in metabolism may result in hypothermia. Paradoxically, core hypothermia may be present in patients with otherwise warm extremities. The bladder is completely paralyzed, causing urinary retention and overflow. Detrusor muscle contraction only later results in spontaneous or external stimuli-induced voiding.

It is important to determine the sensory level by use of the cutaneous innervation of the dermatomes. Pinprick sensation should be evaluated serially (Appendix 12.1). It is important to memorize and document clinical markers (nipple, T4; navel, T10; midway from arm to chest, C4-T2 border). It may be difficult to determine whether the level is cervical or thoracic, because the C4 and T2 levels abut each other, but examination of motor function and reflexes of the arm further helps localization.

Reflexes such as the anal wink (puckering of anus with stimulus to the perianal region) and the bulbocavernosus reflex (traction on a Foley catheter or digital pressure on the clitoris or penis while anal sphincter contraction is monitored with a gloved finger in the rectum) should be examined. Neurologic examination should be carefully documented by use of the American Spinal Injury Association neurologic classification of spinal cord injury (Appendices 12.1 and 12.2). The American Spinal Injury Association improvement scale can be used to monitor progress as well.

Interpretation of Diagnostic Tests

Neuroimaging of the spine and spinal cord has a high priority. The extent of imaging is determined by neurologic findings at presentation. Careful clinical delineation of level of involvement and accurate elucidation of possible forces during trauma may further tailor orientation and selection of the studies.

Neuroradiologists should have access to clinical information that may further determine certain MRI sequences. The priority in the emergency department is to diagnose unstable cervical or thoracic spine fractures or spine compression.

Spine Plain Films

Screening cervical spine radiographs for alert patients with no neck tenderness and no neurologic abnormalities have a very low yield.[39] Combined lateral, anteroposterior, and odontoid views have a high diagnostic yield and should recognize more than 90% of the lesions, although a false-negative rate of 26% was found in a study of 70 patients. The lateral cervical spine radiograph and odontoid views (Figure 12.13) should be viewed systematically.[40,41] A common pitfall is focusing on a single fracture or misalignment while overlooking other abnormalities. The essentials of cervical spine plain film viewing are shown in Table 12.6. Evaluation is very difficult. Only the trained eye of an experienced physician can identify fractures, but even then a CT scan is often needed for confirmation. The threshold for ordering a CT scan of the cervical spine must be very low, particularly when plain films of the cervical spine give dubious information or are of marginal quality.

First, the cervical vertebral bodies should be identified, and particular attention should be paid to the lower cervical spine. Hand traction should be used to pull both arms and shoulders of the patient down. Inadequate films should prompt CT scanning of the spine. When a lateral spine film is evaluated, four lordotic curves and alignments are assessed to look for displacement (see Figure 12.13A).

Common findings are compression of the vertebral bodies (vertebral body often several millimeters less anteriorly than posteriorly), displacement in the lateral view (more than 3 mm between adjacent vertebral bodies), and displacement of the odontoid bone (odontoid tip should be aligned with the tip of the clivus).

Indications of instability are displacement of a vertebral body, widening of the interspinous or interlaminar distance, widening of the facet joints or spinal canal, disruption of the posterior spinal line, and anterolisthesis or retrolisthesis with flexion or extension. The odontoid bone typically lies within 13 mm of the posterior cortex of the anterior C1 arch.

Hyperflexion injuries of the cervical spine can be seen in various degrees from mild widening of the posterior intervertebral space to subluxation of the vertebra, and the inferior articular facet may become lodged on the superior facet of the vertebra below (so-called perched facet). A cord lesion is common or easily induced with further manipulation.

Unilateral facet distortion can be recognized by an alteration in the laminar space, namely, the distance between the spinolaminar line and the posterior margin of the articular mass.

Hyperextension injuries produce fairly characteristic features, such as a hyperextension teardrop fracture (avulsion of the site of attachment of the anterior longitudinal ligament), hangman's fracture with bilateral fracture through the pars interarticularis of C2, Jefferson's fracture (fracture of the ring of C1), and odontoid fractures (tip is type I, base is type II, and extension into the body of C2 is type III). Figure 12.14 illustrates the most common unstable cervical fractures.

Computed Tomography and Magnetic Resonance Imaging

CT scans added to a plain cervical spine film are unsurpassed in diagnostic value for demonstration of fractures. Myelography combined with CT can more clearly demonstrate the cord and nerve roots and determine whether they are compressed by the misalignment or fracture. In most instances, specific areas are scanned with axial slices 1.5 to 3 mm thick for the cervical spine and 3 to 5 mm thick for the thoracic and lumbar spines. CT scan reconstructions are very useful in imaging loose bone fragments and facet dislocation.

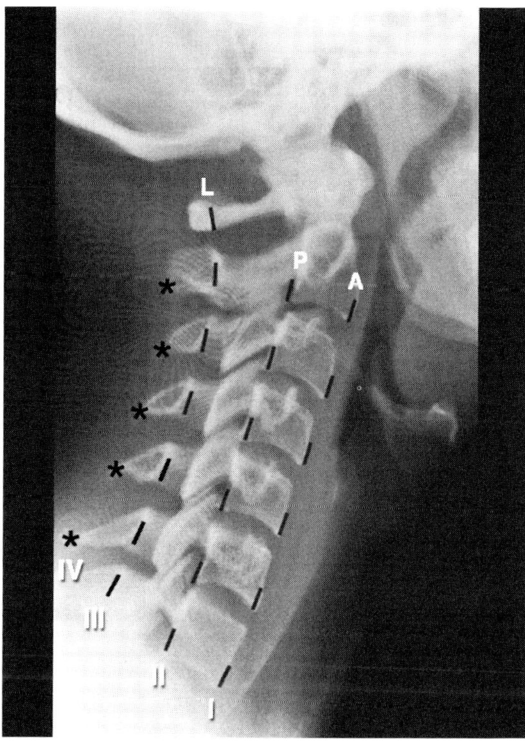

A

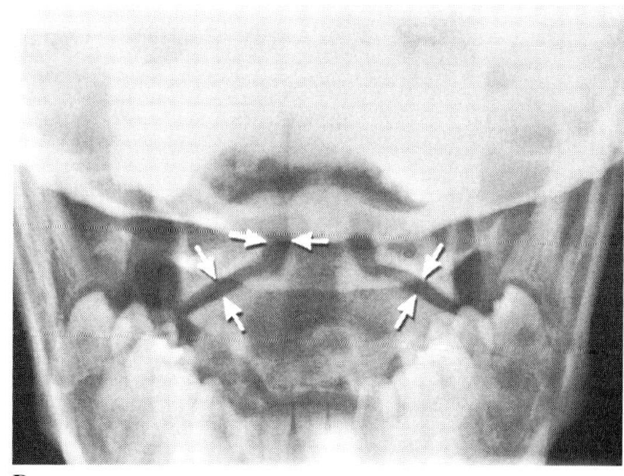

B

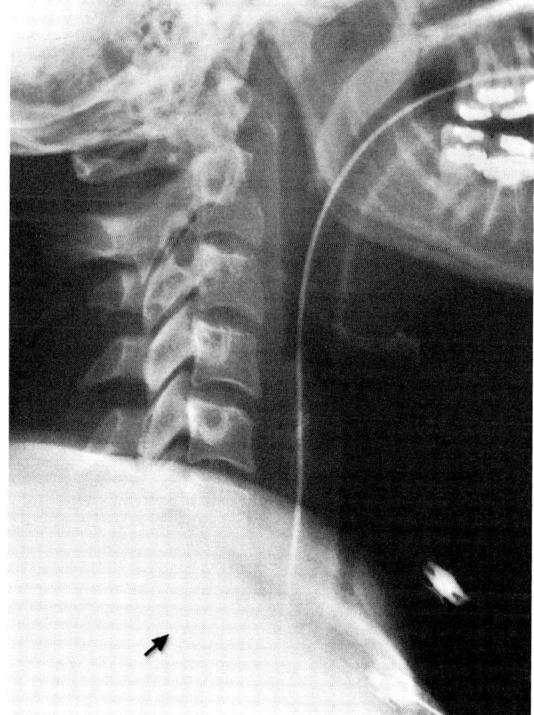

C

Figure 12.13. Plain spine radiographs with examination techniques to uncover fractures and dislocations. **A.** Normal alignment lines: I = normal alignment along the anterior (A) vertebral margins; II = posterior (P) vertebral margin alignment line; III = spinal laminar (L) line ; IV = relation of the dorsal spinous processes. **B.** Indicators of normal odontoid interspace (*arrows*). **C.** Incomplete cervical spine examination (C7 is missing) (*arrow*).

The intrathecal administration of contrast medium (myelography, CT scanning) is usually reserved for patients who cannot undergo MRI (pacemaker, aneurysm clips, cochlear implants, bullet fragments, or morbid obesity). It has become the second-choice imaging modality in spine injury because it is time-consuming and requires patient movement.

MRI in spine injury should first obtain sagittal T1-weighted images, with axial images through abnormal areas.[42] A T1-weighted image is important to rule out major abnormalities and can be followed by T2 or gradient echo sequences (short time to acquire and sensitive for early hemorrhages in the spine). On T1-weighted images (short TR, 300 to 1,000 msec; TE, 10 to 30 msec), subacute hemorrhage is bright and CSF is dark. On T2-weighted images (long TR, 1,500 to 3,000 msec; TE, 60 to 120 msec), CSF is bright, cord edema is bright, and acute hemorrhage is dark.[43] An example of cord trauma and swelling is shown in Figure 12.15.

Table 12.6. Essentials of Disciplined Cervical Spine Viewing

Count the number of cervical vertebral bodies; seven cervical spine bodies and the superior endplate of T1 should be visible
Trace the contour of every body to detect fractures
Evaluate the alignment lines (see Figure 12.13A)
1. Anterior spinal line along the anterior longitudinal ligament
2. Posterior spinal line along the posterior longitudinal ligament
3. Spinolaminar line along the base of the spinous processes
4. Line of the spinous processes
Assess soft tissue
Assess facet lines
Assess the craniocervical junction
Assess the space between the dens axis and lateral masses of C1

First Priority in Management

Immediate cervical spine immobilization and endotracheal intubation are needed.

Hypotension from unopposed parasympathetic tone is common, particularly with change in position or in the first minutes after connection to the mechanical ventilator. Volume resuscitation or an α-adrenergic receptor agent, such as phenylephrine, is needed. In occasional patients, autonomic dysregulation is manifested as marked hypertensive surges, which should be treated with labetalol. Administration of methylprednisolone has resulted in better recovery 1 year after injury (Third National Acute Spinal Cord Injury study).[44] Maintenance therapy depends on first initiation of therapy (Table 12.7).

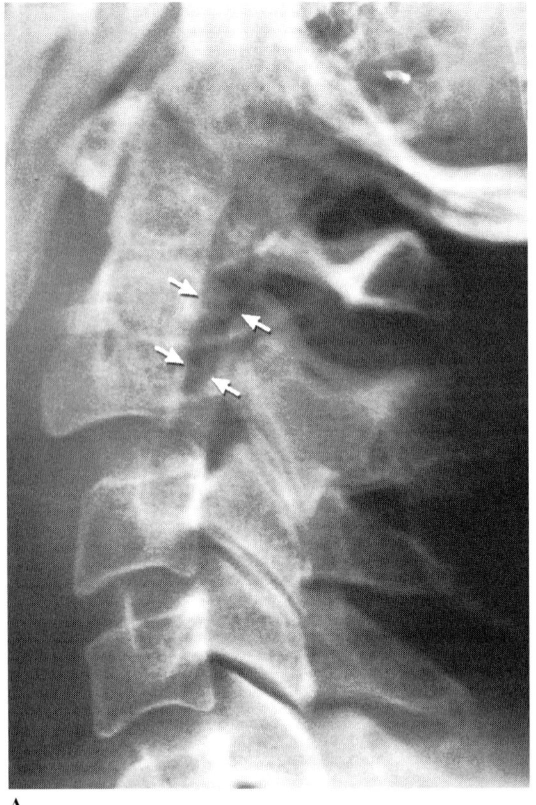

A

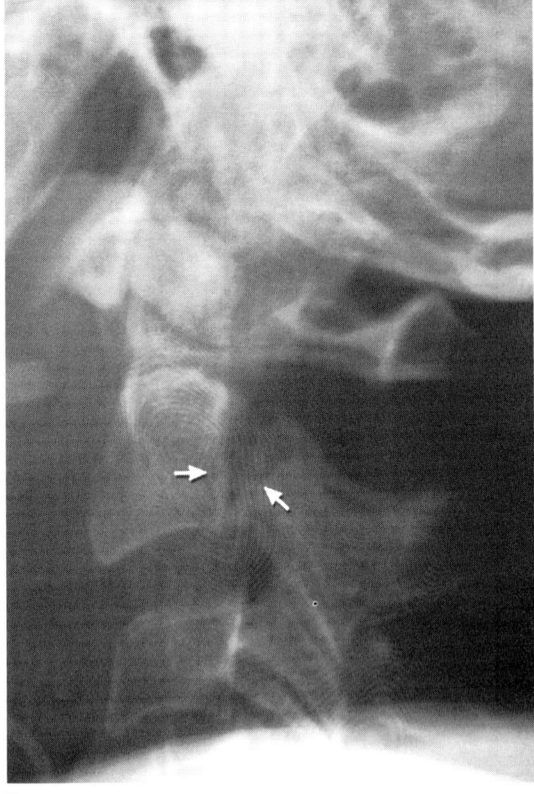

B

Figure 12.14. A–B. Two examples of hangman fracture (C2 bilateral fracture through pars articularis); common with windshield injuries.

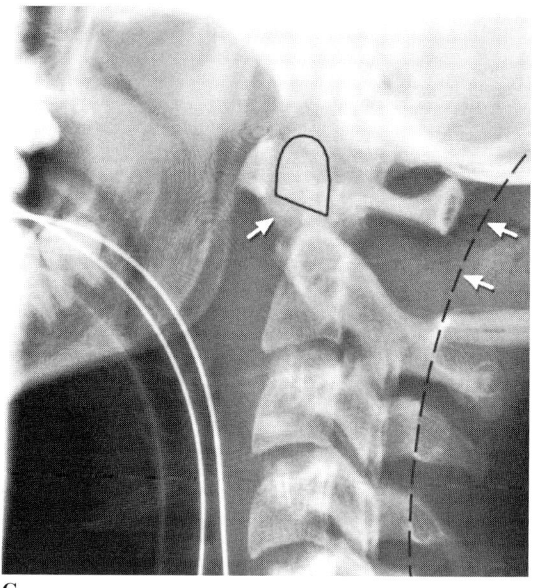

C

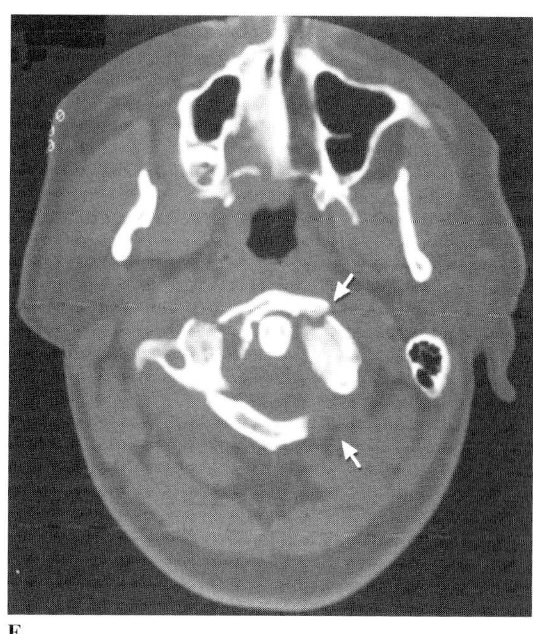

E

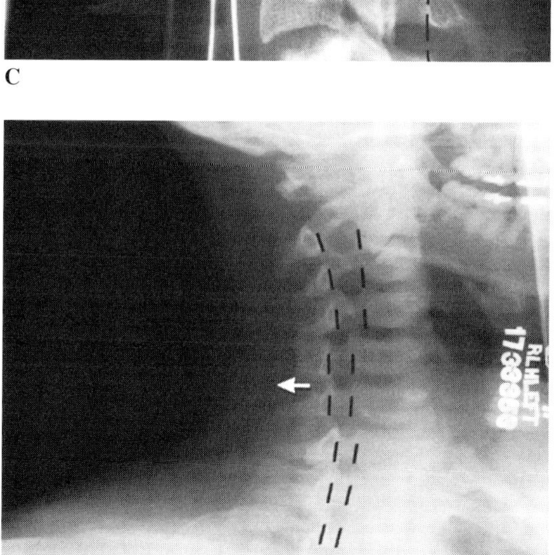

D

Figure 12.4. *Continued.* **C.** Odontoid fracture. The spinal laminar line is disrupted. Dens is outlined *(arrow)*. **D.** Locked facet dislocation *(arrows)* (hyperflexion injury). **E.** Jefferson C1 fracture *(arrows)*.

Catheter placement, gastric ulcer prophylaxis (ranitidine or sucralfate), correction of core hypothermia, and deep venous thrombosis prophylaxis (subcutaneous heparin) are important before triage.

Predictors of Outcome

The degree of cord injury at presentation determines initial outcome. Patients with complete cervical transection and apnea usually do not recover. Patients are tetraplegic, depend on a mechanical ventilator, and can only operate devices for communication and locomotion (speech may be possible through a special tracheostomy). Patients with injuries above the C3 level are uncommonly weaned. One study claimed weaning in 28% with C2 injury, 51% with C3 injuries, and an average of 80% in lower level lesions.[45]

Complete cord lesion very rarely changes to an incomplete lesion and vice versa. Patients with incomplete lesions but no motor function and only sensory function have a 10% to 30% chance to regain some motor function in more than half the

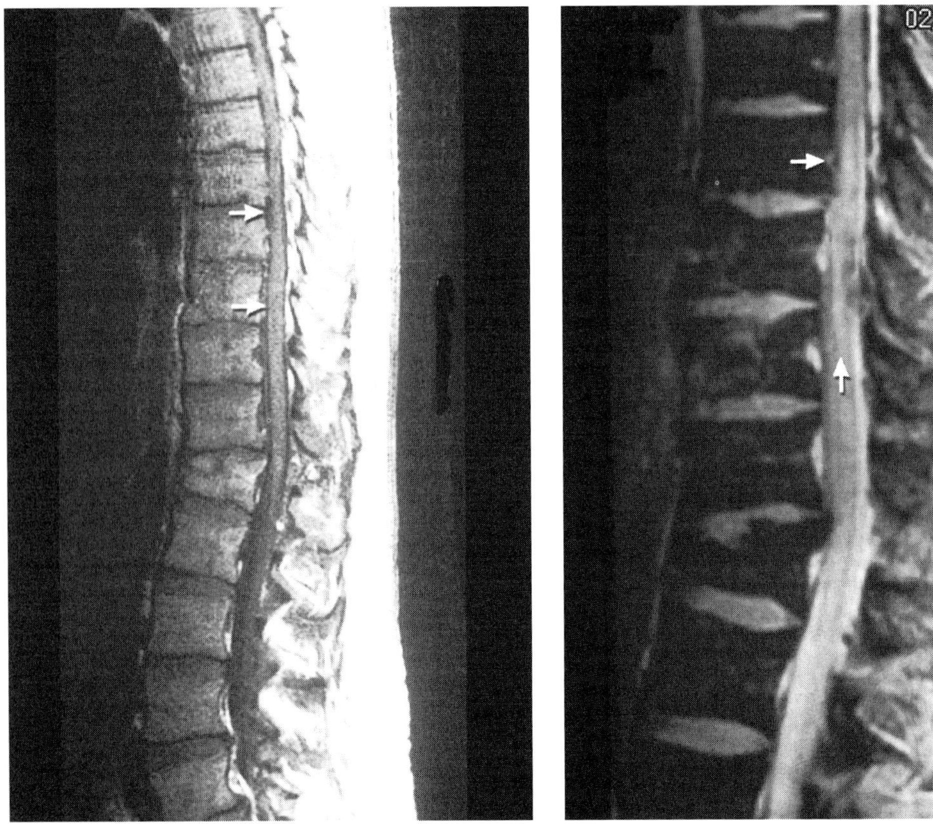

Figure 12.15. Magnetic resonance images of traumatic cord swelling (*arrows*).

Table 12.7. Emergency Room Management of Traumatic Spine Injury

Intubation and mechanical ventilation with lesion at C3 or lower
Intubate if aspiration and diaphragm failure
Volume loading with albumin or Ringer's lactated solution
Epinephrine drip
Body warming with blanket; warming intravenous fluids
Subcutaneous heparin, 5,000 U
Codeine for pain
Sucralfate to prevent gastrointestinal bleeding
Interval 0–3 hrs, methylprednisolone, 30 mg/kg
Infusion of methylprednisolone, 5.4 mg/kg/hr for 24 hrs
Interval 3–8 hrs, methylprednisolone, 30 mg/kg
Infusion of methylprednisolone, 5.4 mg/kg/hr for 48 hrs

common extremity muscles below the level defined as a Medical Research Council muscle grade of 3 or greater. Patients with incomplete lesions but returned motor function have a 50% chance of improvement to half of the common muscles defined as a Medical Research Council muscle grade of 3 or more.[46]

MRI abnormalities with intramedullary hematoma or contusion involving more than one segment predict a worse outcome. Central low signal intensity on T2 images may represent central cord contusion, with poor prospects. Central high signal intensity without areas of low signal intensity with normal T1 may represent cord edema or ischemia but no infarction. Mixtures of patterns are possible and make the use of MRI for prognosis indeterminate.

Triage

- Neurologic-neurosurgical intensive care unit for management of dysautonomia; bladder, skin, and bowel care; and planning for stabilizing spinal surgery.
- Spinal rehabilitation center if surgery is not indicated and dysautonomia is absent.

References

1. Marion DW, Carlier PM. Problems with initial Glasgow Coma Scale assessment caused by prehospital treatment of patients with head injuries: results of a national survey. J Trauma 1994;36:89.
2. Baguley IJ, Nicholls JL, Felmingham KL, et al. Dysautonomia after traumatic brain injury: a forgotten syndrome? J Neurol Neurosurg Psychiatry 1999;67:39.
3. Thornbury JR, Masters SJ, Campbell JA. Imaging recommendations for head trauma: a new comprehensive strategy. AJR Am J Roentgenol 1987;149:781.
4. Adams JH, Graham DI, Murray LS, Scott G. Diffuse axonal injury due to nonmissile head injury in humans: an analysis of 45 cases. Ann Neurol 1982;12:557.
5. Gennarelli TA, Thibault LE, Adams JH, et al. Diffuse axonal injury and traumatic coma in the primate. Ann Neurol 1982;12:564.
6. Blumbergs PC, Jones NR, North JB. Diffuse axonal injury in head trauma. J Neurol Neurosurg Psychiatry 1989;52:838.
7. Piek J, Chesnut RM, Marshall LF, et al. Extracranial complications of severe head injury. J Neurosurg 1992;77:901.
8. Di Rocco A, Ellis SJ, Landes C. Delayed epidural hematoma. Neuroradiology 1991;33:253.
9. MacPherson M, MacPherson P, Jennett B. CT evidence of intracranial contusion and haematoma in relation to the presence, site and type of skull fracture. Clin Radiol 1990;42:321.
10. Gibson RM, Stephenson GC. Aggressive management of severe closed head trauma: time for reappraisal. Lancet 1989;2:369.
11. Miller JD, Dearden NM, Piper IR, Chan KH. Control of intracranial pressure in patients with severe head injury. J Neurotrauma 1992;9(Suppl 1):S317.
12. Bickell WH, Wall MJ Jr, Pepe PE, et al. Immediate versus delayed fluid resuscitation for hypotensive patients with penetrating torso injuries. N Engl J Med 1994;331:1105.
13. Mattox KL, Maningas PA, Moore EE, et al. Prehospital hypertonic saline/dextran infusion for post-traumatic hypotension. The U.S.A. Multicenter Trial. Ann Surg 1991;213:482.
14. Rosner MJ, Daughton S. Cerebral perfusion pressure management in head injury. J Trauma 1990;30:933.
15. Kaufmann AM, Cardoso ER. Aggravation of vasogenic cerebral edema by multiple-dose mannitol. J Neurosurg 1992;77:584.
16. Kelly DF, Goodale DB, Williams J, et al. Propofol in the treatment of moderate and severe head injury: a randomized, prospective double-blinded pilot trial. J Neurosurg 1999;90:1042.
17. Bouma GJ, Muizelaar JP, Bandoh K, Marmarou A. Blood pressure and intracranial pressure-volume dynamics in severe head injury: relationship with cerebral blood flow. Neurosurgery 1992;77:15.
18. Braakman R, Schouten HJ, Blaauw-van Dishoeck M, Minderhoud JM. Megadose steroids in severe head injury. Results of a prospective double-blind clinical trial. J Neurosurg 1983;58:326.
19. Cottrell JE, Patel K, Turndorf H, Ransohoff J. Intracranial pressure changes induced by sodium nitroprusside in patients with intracranial mass lesions. J Neurosurg 1978;48:329.
20. Rea GL, Rockswold GL. Barbiturate therapy in uncontrolled intracranial hypertension. Neurosurgery 1983;12:401.
21. Ward JD, Becker DP, Miller JD, et al. Failure of prophylactic barbiturate coma in the treatment of severe head injury. J Neurosurg 1985;62:383.
22. Yano M, Nishiyama H, Yokota H, et al. Effect of lidocaine on ICP response to endotracheal suctioning. Anesthesiology 1986;64:651.
23. Evans DE, Kobrine AI. Reduction of experimental intracranial hypertension by lidocaine. Neurosurgery 1987;20:542.
24. Chesnut RM, Marshall LF, Klauber MR, et al. The role of secondary brain injury in determining outcome from severe head injury. J Trauma 1993;34:216.
25. Mahoney BD, Rockswold GL, Ruiz E, Clinton JE. Emergency twist drill trephination. Neurosurgery 1981;8:551.
26. Hamilton M, Wallace C. Nonoperative management of acute epidural hematoma diagnosed by CT: the neuroradiologist's role. AJNR Am J Neuroradiol 1992;13:853.
27. Sagher O, Ribas GC, Jane JA. Nonoperative management of acute epidural hematoma diagnosed by CT: the neuroradiologist's role. AJNR Am J Neuroradiol 1992;13:860.
28. Helling TS, McNabney WK, Whittaker CK, et al. The role of early surgical intervention in civilian gunshot wounds to the head. J Trauma 1992;32:398.
29. Shaffrey ME, Polin RS, Phillips CD, et al. Classification of civilian craniocerebral gunshot wounds: a multivariate analysis predictive of mortality. J Neurotrauma 1992;9(Suppl 1):S279.
30. Lang EW, Pitts LH, Damron SL, Rutledge R. Outcome after severe head injury: an analysis of prediction based upon comparison of neural network versus logistic regression analysis. Neurol Res 1997;19:274.
31. Choi SC, Narayan RK, Anderson RL, Ward JD. Enhanced specificity of prognosis in severe head injury. J Neurosurg 1988;69:381.
32. Wilberger JE Jr, Harris M, Diamond DL. Acute subdural hematoma: morbidity and mortality related to timing of operative intervention. J Trauma 1990;30:733.
33. Signorini DF, Andrews PJ, Jones PA, et al. Adding insult to injury: the prognostic value of early secondary insults for survival after traumatic brain injury. J Neurol Neurosurg Psychiatry 1999;66:26.
34. Kampfl A, Schmutzhard E, Franz G, et al. Prediction of recovery from post-traumatic vegetative state with cerebral magnetic-resonance imaging. Lancet 1998;351:1763.
35. Hills MW, Deane SA. Head injury and facial injury: is there an increased risk of cervical spine injury? J Trauma 1993;34:549.

36. Michael DB, Guyot DR, Darmody WR. Coincidence of head and cervical spine injury. J Neurotrauma 1989; 6:177.
37. Fehlings MG, Tator CH. An evidence-based review of decompressive surgery in acute spinal cord injury: rationale, indications, and timing based on experimental and clinical studies. J Neurosurg 1999;91:1.
38. Donovan WH. Operative and nonoperative management of spinal cord injury. A review. Paraplegia 1994;32:375.
39. Bachulis BL, Long WB, Hynes GD, Johnson MC. Clinical indications for cervical spine radiographs in the traumatized patient. Am J Surg 1987;153:473.
40. Kreipke DL, Gillespie KR, McCarthy MC, et al. Reliability of indications for cervical spine films in trauma patients. J Trauma 1989;29:1438.
41. Mirvis SE, Diaconis JN, Chirico PA, et al. Protocol-driven radiologic evaluation of suspected cervical spine injury: efficacy study. Radiology 1989;170:831.
42. Kalfas I, Wilberger J, Goldberg A, Prostko ER. Magnetic resonance imaging in acute spinal cord trauma. Neurosurgery 1988;23:295.
43. Wittenberg RH, Boetel U, Beyer HK. Magnetic resonance imaging and computer tomography of acute spinal cord trauma. Clin Orthop 1990;260:176.
44. Bracken MB, Shepard MJ, Holford TR, et al. Administration of methylprednisolone for 24 or 48 hours or tirilazad mesylate for 48 hours in the treatment of acute spinal cord injury. Results of the Third National Acute Spinal Cord Injury Randomized Controlled Trial. JAMA 1997;277:1597.
45. Wicks AB, Menter RR. Long-term outlook in quadriplegic patients with initial ventilator dependency. Chest 1986;90:406.
46. Ditunno JF Jr, Formal CS. Spinal Cord Injury. In JM Gilchrist (ed), Prognosis in Neurology. Boston: Butterworth-Heinemann, 1998;287.

Appendix 12.1

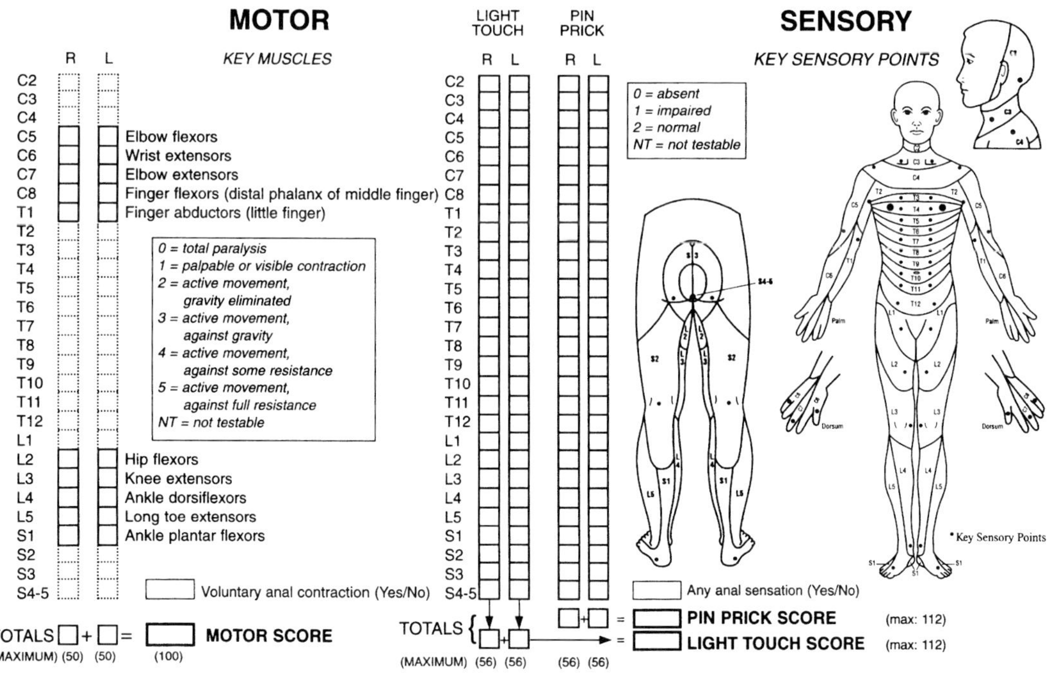

STANDARD NEUROLOGICAL CLASSIFICATION OF SPINAL CORD INJURY

MOTOR

KEY MUSCLES

	R	L	
C2			
C3			
C4			
C5			Elbow flexors
C6			Wrist extensors
C7			Elbow extensors
C8			Finger flexors (distal phalanx of middle finger)
T1			Finger abductors (little finger)
T2			
T3			
T4			
T5			
T6			
T7			
T8			
T9			
T10			
T11			
T12			
L1			
L2			Hip flexors
L3			Knee extensors
L4			Ankle dorsiflexors
L5			Long toe extensors
S1			Ankle plantar flexors
S2			
S3			
S4-5			Voluntary anal contraction (Yes/No)

0 = total paralysis
1 = palpable or visible contraction
2 = active movement, gravity eliminated
3 = active movement, against gravity
4 = active movement, against some resistance
5 = active movement, against full resistance
NT = not testable

TOTALS ☐ + ☐ = ☐ **MOTOR SCORE**
(MAXIMUM) (50) (50) (100)

SENSORY

KEY SENSORY POINTS

	LIGHT TOUCH R	LIGHT TOUCH L	PIN PRICK R	PIN PRICK L
C2				
C3				
C4				
C5				
C6				
C7				
C8				
T1				
T2				
T3				
T4				
T5				
T6				
T7				
T8				
T9				
T10				
T11				
T12				
L1				
L2				
L3				
L4				
L5				
S1				
S2				
S3				
S4-5				

0 = absent
1 = impaired
2 = normal
NT = not testable

Any anal sensation (Yes/No)

TOTALS ☐ + ☐ = **PIN PRICK SCORE** (max: 112)
☐ + ☐ = **LIGHT TOUCH SCORE** (max: 112)
(MAXIMUM) (56) (56) (56) (56)

• Key Sensory Points

NEUROLOGICAL LEVEL *The most caudal segment with normal function*	R	L	**COMPLETE OR INCOMPLETE?** *Incomplete = Any sensory or motor function in S4-S5*	**ZONE OF PARTIAL PRESERVATION** *Partially innervated segments*	R	L
SENSORY			**ASIA IMPAIRMENT SCALE**	SENSORY		
MOTOR				MOTOR		

Version 4p
GHC 1996

Appendix 12.2

Functional Independence Measure (FIM)

L E V E L S	7 Complete Independence (Timely, Safely) 6 Modified Independence (Device)	No Helper
	Modified Dependence 5 Supervision 4 Minimal Assist (Subject = 75%+) 3 Moderate Assist (Subject = 50%+) **Complete Dependence** 2 Maximal Assist (Subject = 25%+) 1 Total Assist (Subject = 0%+)	Helper

	ADMIT	DISCH
Self Care		
A. Eating	☐	☐
B. Grooming	☐	☐
C. Bathing	☐	☐
D. Dressing-Upper Body	☐	☐
E. Dressing-Lower Body	☐	☐
F. Toileting	☐	☐
Sphincter Control		
G. Bladder Management	☐	☐
H. Bowel Management	☐	☐
Mobility		
Transfer:		
I. Bed, Chair, Wheelchair	☐	☐
J. Toilet	☐	☐
K. Tub, Shower	☐	☐
Locomotion		
L. Walk/Wheelchair	W☐ C☐ ☐	W☐ C☐ ☐
M. Stairs	☐	☐
Communication		
N. Comprehension	A☐ V☐ ☐	A☐ V☐ ☐
O. Expression	V☐ N☐ ☐	V☐ N☐ ☐
Social Cognition		
P. Social Interaction	☐	☐
Q. Problem Solving	☐	☐
R. Memory	☐	☐
Total FIM	☐	☐

NOTE: Leave no blanks; enter 1 if patient not testable due to risk.

ASIA IMPAIRMENT SCALE

☐ A = **Complete:** No motor or sensory function is preserved in the sacral segments S4-S5.

☐ B = **Incomplete:** Sensory but not motor function is preserved below the neurological level and includes the sacral segments S4-S5.

☐ C = **Incomplete:** Motor function is preserved below the neurological level, and more than half of key muscles below the neurological level have a muscle grade less than 3.

☐ D = **Incomplete:** Motor function is preserved below the neurological level, and at least half of key muscles below the neurological level have a muscle grade of 3 or more.

☐ E = **Normal:** motor and sensory function is normal

CLINICAL SYNDROMES

☐ Central Cord
☐ Brown-Sequard
☐ Anterior Cord
☐ Conus Medullaris
☐ Cauda Equina

Index

Page numbers followed by *t*, *f*, and *c* denote tables, figures, and capsules, respectively.